Kentucky's
First Asylum

Kentucky's First Asylum

A Saga of the People and Practices

Alma Wynelle Deese

iUniverse, Inc.
Bloomington

Kentucky's First Asylum
A Saga of the People and Practices

iUniverse books may be ordered through booksellers or by contacting:

iUniverse
1663 Liberty Drive
Bloomington, IN 47403
www.iuniverse.com
1-800-Authors (1-800-288-4677)

Because of the dynamic nature of the Internet, any web addresses or links contained in this book may have changed since publication and may no longer be valid. The views expressed in this work are solely those of the author and do not necessarily reflect the views of the publisher, and the publisher hereby disclaims any responsibility for them.

ISBN: 978-1-4620-7303-0 (sc)
ISBN: 978-1-4620-7305-4 (hc)
ISBN: 978-1-4620-7304-7 (e)

Printed in the United States of America

iUniverse rev. date: 01/16/2012

Asylums were established to care for the unfortunates of society.

It was later that they acquired a negative image: why?

Contents

Preface

—◆·•◆·•◆—

My journey into writing this book started back in the 1970s, when the new superintendent of Eastern State Hospital told some employees to empty out a storage room full of old documents. Rather than throwing them away, I allowed them to store the old documents in my office; some of them dated back to the 1800s. After reading through them, I realized that these documents reflected the early history of Eastern State, the first asylum in Kentucky and the second state-supported asylum in the United States. That history was unknown to me at the time, but I did extensive research and continued to add to that history throughout my remaining years of employment in that facility. The history of Eastern State Hospital had been ignored for many years, which motivated writing this book.

I tried to get others interested in that history by giving lectures and writing presentations. Those presentations became part of the orientation for students working at Eastern State Hospital. To improve my writing and presentation skills, I joined the History Division of the American Psychological Association and the International Historical Association of the Behavioral Sciences. While these groups were very supportive of my goal of writing a book about Eastern State's history, publishing companies were not interested in another book on an early mental institution.

Their argument was that there were already many histories of mental institutions, and Eastern State did not deviate from the general trends found in American mental hospitals. True! While the Kentucky Lunatic Asylum was one of the first, it did follow the general psychiatric trends of the times. Since there appeared to be nothing unique about the topic, I agreed with their conclusion. There were many other good books on the history of psychiatric care.

Some psychiatric histories are related to a specific institution, such as Norman Dain's *Disordered Minds: First Century of Eastern State Hospital in Williamsburg, Virginia.* Another book is the most excellent *Empty Beds: A History of Vermont State Hospital,* by Marsha Kincheloe and Herbert Hunt. That book has wonderful old pictures and a concisely written history from the hospital's beginning in 1891 up through its closing in 1988. These histories correspond to today's current community mental system policy of deinstitutionalization. Vermont State Hospital is now closed and has been converted into a nursing home.

There are also many histories of private asylums; Dr. Francis Braceland wrote *The Institute of Living: The Hartford Retreat from 1822 to 1972,* and Alex Beam's *Gracefully Insane: The Rise and Fall of America's Premier Mental Hospital* showed the unusual individuals who worked and lived there. Both books examined the long, proud tradition of workers who cared for the wealthy mentally ill.

There are more general books related to the early asylums and society's influence upon those facilities: David Rothman's *Conscience and Convenience: The asylum and Its Alternative in Progressive America,* Andrew Scull's *Madhouses, Mad-Doctors, and Madmen: The Social History of Psychiatry in the Victorian Era,* and Janet Oppenheim's *Shattered Nerves* all add perspectives in understanding social influences upon American asylums.

There are other books about specific people in asylums, such as Charles Schlaifer and Lucy Freeman's *Heart's Work: Civil War Heroine and Champion of the Mentally Ill, Dorothea Lynde Dix,* and Barbara Sapinsley's *The Private War of Mrs. Packard,* about a nineteenth-century woman who was committed to an institution by her husband; later, laws were passed to protect wives from husbands who could commit them to mental institutions without legitimate cause. Finally, Mark E. Neely and R. Gerald McMurtry wrote *The Insanity File: The Case of Mary Todd*

Lincoln, giving a family perspective of dealing with the institutionalization of the president's widow.

While this list of asylum-related books is not in any way complete, it does show the proliferation of such books and the range of interests that can be related just to asylums. So at the time of my retirement in 1996, I concluded that there was no need for another book on asylums.

Prior to my retirement, we held a birthday celebration for Eastern State Hospital in 1994; a colleague and I created ninety-nine posters from copies of old historical documents about the hospital. I donated all the original documents to the Lexington Archives and Records Department, hoping to save them for future generations. I took copies of those early documents with me when I moved to Florida, although I had given up on the idea of writing this book.

Three things changed my opinion about writing a book after retirement. First, I attended a workshop given by the Florida Psychological Association on writing a book. The presenter, a psychologist in private practice, had written several books and convinced me that the general public was the best audience for my book. I had never before considered writing for the general public.

Second, I wrote several books for the general public using old postcards. My collection started when I found some Eastern State Hospital postcards from 1905—before there were any pictures of the hospital. My collection grew over the years to include cards from asylums throughout the United States. After writing several books with old postcards, I learned a lot about publishing.

I am still trying to find a publisher interested in a book on asylums in the United States before 1900. The lack of interest is an example of the stigma shown toward the old asylums. It is sad, because many of the early postcards were in beautiful color, and they displayed a long-forgotten pride in such facilities.

The third reason for writing this book came when I reread copies of Eastern State Hospital's history. There was a close relationship between Lexington citizens and the first asylum. Colonel John R. Allen, attorney general in Lexington in the early 1900s, was the son of Dr. John R. Allen, superintendent of the Kentucky Lunatic Asylum from 1844 to 1855. Although Colonel Allen was born in Iowa in 1857, he returned to Lexington to attend the Kentucky University Law School and stayed the rest of his life. Other prominent families include the Duncans, Chipleys, and Hunts.

While the association between local families and the Kentucky Lunatic Asylum continued for years, such connections often go unexplored in psychiatric histories. Current mental health programs claim to work toward a "new idea" of local community involvement, but these Lexington families were a part of Kentucky's first asylum. That story has not been told and needs to be.

The first chapter jumps to 1906 as a pivotal year of changes: four employees in the first asylum were charged in the murder of a patient. That issue and two other major changes in that year set the stage for the past and present history of that facility. The major changes followed social and political attitudes. Colonel Allen's involvement with the incident of 1906 shows the situation in the asylum at that time while reflecting upon his father, Dr. John R. Allen, who had been the first superintendent at the asylum. Allen's law partner, Henry T. Duncan III, was the son of Henry T. Duncan II, a previous mayor of Lexington and newspaper owner, while both were well connected with earlier members of the asylum's board and leaders in the Transylvania Medical School and Law Department. This first chapter ends with this question: How did the asylum become so eroded, when it had previously been a source of pride by the local people and politicians?

Chapter 2 reverts back to the beginning to show how the already established Transylvania Medical School and Law Department helped to establish a Fayette Public Hospital in 1817. That hospital was later opened as the first Kentucky asylum. John W. Hunt was the original chairman of the Board of Commissioners of the asylum from 1824 until 1844 and was on the Board of Trustees at Transylvania. Several of his sons attended the Transylvania Medical and Law Schools. One son served on the asylum board in the 1870s, and a grandson was employed at the asylum in the 1880s. The families involved with these three early institutions have had little historical attention, yet their influence was significant.

The Transylvania Medical School, which existed from 1817 into the 1860s, was closely related to the early asylum; two of its graduates were the first two superintendents of the asylum, and both were professors there. It had the best medically qualified leaders in medical education at that time period; the professors were pioneers in medicine.

Chapters 3 through 8 follows the history from 1824 to 1969 when the Transylvania Law Department provided many legally trained members to the Board of Commissioners to administratively managed the early Asylum. The Law Department of Transylvania merged into the Kentucky University of Law, from which Colonel Allen graduated. Later, that law school became part of the current University of Kentucky. Some of the best legal minds of the time served on the Board of Commissioners at the Kentucky asylum; Colonel Allen was well respected as a lawyer and attorney general. This book documents the changing processes of caring for the mentally ill through the 1960s. That first Asylum has had many name changes; currently it is called Eastern State Hospital.

All characters in this book were actual people living in Lexington, Kentucky. Characters such as the sheriff or deputy, whose specific names were not known, were drawn from a collective knowledge that such historical individuals did exist during that time. They were added to help with the cohesiveness of the historical story.

Actual patient names were used in this book when they were identified by other sources such as the local newspaper, or other public sources such as Collins's *History of Kentucky,* or family histories such as the Henry Clay Sr. papers. Otherwise, no names were used.

While the dialogue between individuals was developed by the author, it was dependent upon available data; no dialogue was created unless there was sufficient historical data. Other times, when just the facts were available, the author used her experience as an employee of the current Eastern State Hospital to interpret the scene. For example, the author's examinations of old pictures or maps helped to describe the asylum, but actually walking those same hallways or being where those wards were have helped even more.

Many things were left out of the book just because the research was not there. Sources are identified at the end of each chapter.

This second edition was developed after extensive research produced additional data relating to the original book, *The Early Gatekeepers: A Saga of Three American Institutions,* published in 2005. That book showed how the early community was part of the development of the Kentucky Lunatic Asylum, but it missed the psychiatric history market.

The second edition of this book includes two more chapters. Chapter 9 shows how Eastern State Hospital decreased in patient population while having more professionally trained staff than in its whole past history. The typical "snake pit" attendant described in 1950 was changed by the 1990s, as employees were more professionally trained with fewer patients. This equal (1:1) patient-to-employee ratio allowed better treatment programs as more patients were discharged. American mental health care shifted toward closing or downsizing many similar institutions as employees faced threats of termination or job losses. These conflicts are reflected in chapter 9. The history of that facility was celebrated on May 2, 1994.

While the facility is still called Eastern State Hospital, it has been changed into a privately administered facility and the employees are no longer state employees; as private employees, they have no state job protection. A new facility at a different location is expected to be completed in the future and funded by the state of Kentucky. The old location will be taken over by a local junior college.

In 2009, Dr. Oliver Sacks and Christopher Payne wrote a book about the current closure of the old mental institutions. They reviewed the histories and destruction of twenty-five state mental hospitals. A few of the hospitals have been converted successfully into residential, commercial, or academic communities, while others reopened as prisons. Few Americans realize that these institutions were once examples of civic pride and places of refuge for therapy and healing.

Other old state hospital buildings were left for decay, demonization, and ghost hunters as old state mental hospitals continued to close throughout the United States. The total effects are alarming. Currently, more Americans are receiving mental health treatment in prisons and jails than in hospitals or treatment centers. Fifty years ago, there were six hundred thousand state hospital beds; today the number has dwindled to forty thousand. The jail is the only institution that can never say no to the mentally ill. American psychiatric care is facing a new crisis as the old asylums and state hospitals are being closed and the mentally ill are being abandoned to the streets. While current medications only work on a percentage of patients, hospitals still are needed for long-term care. Any long-term care was ignored in the rush toward deinstitutionalization, as Isaac and Armant (1990) have described.

Today, there are other horrifying examples, such as Kleier (2005), who wrote about her mentally ill daughter killing her sister. As the mentally ill continue to be isolated and disenfranchised from the rules of society, the rate of violence grows, and forced treatment becomes the norm through the courts and jails because the asylums are gone; psychiatric history is repeating itself. Jails and prisons were the warehouses of the insane before the state hospitals and asylums were built, and now, we have come full circle as the jails once again become the major source of American mental health care.

The lone voice of Dr. Sacks (2009) points to activities and social opportunities that were present in the early asylums; now, they are forgotten or not financially feasible in today's world of budget tightening. Often the pharmacological approach to treatment ignores the human and social needs of the mentally ill. Although there have been some clubhouses established for the mentally ill with dedicated employees and volunteers, they depend upon private funds that decrease with economic downturns.

There are no simple solutions. However, ignorance of the history of psychiatric care leads to quick but inadequate solutions. While no one wants to return to the asylums, an honest critique of those early processes can improve the current understanding of that care.

Chapter 10 reviews a unique article that was based on the effect of the process of court-imposed commitment upon two sons of Henry Clay Sr., who were patients at the Kentucky Lunatic Asylum. This review is unique because the court commitment process of that time is mostly unknown. This history of the early legal process at the Kentucky's first asylum is just part of a whole maze of asylum histories that need to be told.

Sources for the Preface

Additional contributors: Dan Britton (St. Petersburg, Florida) and Dr. Debby Cassill (associate professor, USF, St. Petersburg).

Dees, J. *Snake Pit Attendant.* New York: Exposition Press, 1950. This book describes the poorly trained and often disrespectful employees working in the state hospitals at that time.

Isaac, R. and V. Armant. *Madness in the Streets.* New York: The Free Press, 1990.

Kleier, M. O. *Possessed Mentalities.* Lincoln, Nebraska: iUniverse, 2005.

Sacks, O. and C. Payne. *Asylums: Inside the Closed Work of State Mental Hospitals.* Cambridge, Massachusetts: MIT Press, 2009.

Sacks, O. "Lost Virtues of the asylum." *New York Review* LVI, no. 14 (2009), 50.

Acknowledgments

While this history was long in achieving publication, a second edition would appear to complicate the acknowledgments, but such is not true. Many people encouraged me to write this book after I retired as an employee of Eastern State Hospital; they all continued to support this project during the second revision process, except for three, who have passed away.

Jane Atwell of the Psychology Department spent many long hours typing data for me. She died before I retired from Eastern State Hospital. I eventually got my own computer and did my own typing, but Jane's help was rarely recognized during her lifetime. She was one of the first people to show an interest in the history of Eastern State Hospital and enjoyed saving it.

Harold Barker was with Records and Archives of the Lexington Fayette Urban County government before retiring; he was always willing to share his information with me. After I moved to Florida, he sent me copies of articles I needed. He introduced me to the Duncan family while he was collecting information related to the past mayors of Lexington. He also introduced me to many other researchers who proved to be helpful in developing this history. He served as a historical consultant for my book *Lexington, Kentucky: Past and Present*, published by Schiffer Publishing Co. in 2009.

Psychologist Dr. Anne Shurling encouraged me in my interest in the history of psychiatric care. She often provided psychology students to whom I could present the history, starting with her community psychology class at Transylvania College. Her interest in Eastern State Hospital's history supported me at a time when it was not so popular within the psychology profession. She continued to be a dear friend until her death.

Peggy Brown was always looking for postcards of Lexington or other asylums for me. Her interest in the history of Eastern State Hospital (due to both her nursing training and her knowledge of some of the patients) was helpful over the years. She could always find the most unusual postcards. She continues to be a dear friend.

Jean Newman, a fellow employee at Eastern State Hospital, has always encouraged me to write this history. We often shared historical discoveries where we worked. She helped me during the 1994 Birthday Celebration of Eastern State Hospital; we produced ninety-nine posters displaying the history of that facility. Even in retirement, she kept reminding me that I had always wanted to write this history and would not let me forget that. She collaborated with me on chapter 9 and continues to be a source of support.

Last but certainly not least, my late husband, Judge J. W. Deese, was supportive both financially and emotionally of my interest in the history of Eastern State Hospital, the history of psychiatric care, and the history of Lexington. He was always an intelligent sounding board for many of my ideas. He died on March 3, 2008, leaving a void after forty-two years of marriage.

These supportive friends in Kentucky and Florida have kept me going with this project.

Chapter One

———◆◆◆◆———

1906

D r. Redwine, Superintendent of the Kentucky Lunatic Asylum, ordered Colonel John Rowan Allen to come to his office in Lexington immediately. At least, Colonel Allen felt it was an order, since the message had been sent directly to him by Dr. Redwine's office. The message had none of the usual politeness that Colonel Allen always expected. The arrogance of those who ran the Kentucky institution had become a sore spot to the Colonel, and today it was especially tiresome to him.

Colonel Allen had heard that Governor Beckham had organized all the charitable organizations, including the asylum in Lexington, under one Board of Control. This new Board of Control was supposed to reduce bickering among the charitable institutions. Instead, the board eliminated the experienced Board of Commissioners, who had been administratively governing the asylum for over eighty-two years. The local citizens and Colonel Allen watched helplessly as the experienced Board of Commissioners was eliminated; to many, it was just another political scheme.

While the politicians had always used Kentucky University and the asylum to provide local jobs for their own supporters, the university and law school were able to limit political appointees by establishing educational requirements. The asylum had no such limitations, and politically appointed employees often manipulated the asylum. Internal

1

loyalty of employees was dependent upon the controlling political party rather than the needs of the patients.

Colonel Allen had visited the Kentucky Lunatic Asylum back in the 1890s, when they held weekly dances. They were pleasant occasions, and citizens were expected to dance with the unfortunates. They had to work for the privilege of attending the dances. During his last dance in 1891, Colonel Allen observed the superintendent and Board of Commissioners bickering among themselves. Colonel Allen preferred to stay out of the local bickering. He had avoided being around any of the local Asylum employees and citizens who talked about the battles between political parties and administrators while he observed how the asylum suffered.

The message from Dr. Redwine was that a patient at the asylum had been killed, and the newly created Board of Control wanted Colonel Allen to prosecute several employees for that death. Colonel Allen considered himself to be neutral and wished to stay that way. He especially disliked this new Board of Control telling him what to do.

In this year of 1906, Colonel Allen was forty-nine years old, had been practicing law in Lexington for twenty-eight years, and was currently the attorney general. As he was leaving his office, Colonel Allen observed with pride two tall buildings on Short Street that dominated the Lexington downtown skyline. Between those two tall buildings was the Northern Bank Building, which housed the prestigious law firm of Colonel Allen and Henry Timberlake Duncan III. Colonel Allen's office occupied the same building where his grandfather and uncle had practiced law. After these reflections, he got into his buggy to go see Dr. Redwine.

Leaving Short Street, Colonel Allen turned left onto Limestone Street. He continued north on Limestone Street and turned left onto Fourth Street. He observed many old, beautiful homes for several blocks and noticed how the area was changing as he got closer to the stockyards on Fourth Street.

The stockyards had developed on the east side of the railroad and across from the asylum. The area was losing its appeal because the smell was drawing complaints from many of the neighbors. The changes were disturbing to Colonel Allen as he continued on with his journey.

Colonel Allen approached the asylum's two-story entrance gate and knew that he had to ask the guard on duty for permission to enter. Permission was granted since the guard knew that he was expected. He followed the road leading to the original building of Kentucky's first asylum. He knew that this older building was used when his father had been superintendent. On the left was the newest building, called the Administration Building, built around 1894; Colonel Allen stopped his carriage in front of it. He tied his carriage to a post and entered onto the front porch.

Colonel Allen opened the front door and walked inside to a foyer. A young man got up from a desk and approached him.

"Colonel Allen, I presume?" the man asked, shaking his hand.

"Yes, sir; to whom am I speaking?"

"I am Mr. Hiram McElroy, Dr. Redwine's personal secretary. Dr. Redwine requested that I greet you; I will now check to see if he is available."

"Thank you, sir," Colonel Allen said; he noticed the wide hallway and a beautiful oak stairway on the left, curving up and around toward the right side onto another landing.

He noticed how clean the building appeared. On the left side of the hall was a sign boldly displaying Dr. Redwine's name.

McElroy returned from that direction with a very dignified man following him.

He approached Colonel Allen and said, "I'm Dr. Redwine; I sent the message for you. Would you come into my office, here on the left?"

"Yes," Colonel Allen said. "I have not been inside this building before. It is nice and clean." He followed Dr. Redwine into his office.

"We are happy with it," Dr. Redwine said, "but the whole facility is still inadequate. I understand that your father was employed here before the newer buildings were added?" Dr. Redwine sat in his chair while offering Colonel Allen another chair.

"Yes, he was in the oldest building, but that was before my birth, and now, even as a longtime citizen of Lexington, I have not kept up with the current changes in this facility." Colonel Allen sat comfortably in his chair.

"I will be happy to show you around after we have our discussion. But what we must discuss at this time is more important."

"Yes, I understand." Colonel Allen asked, "I heard you had a death here?"

"Yes, we did; Mr. Fred Ketterer recently passed away." Dr. Redwine lowered his voice, indicating a sadness and reverence, and added, "Any death is bad but this one raised questions for the Ketterer family."

"Is that really unusual? I thought it was common for lunatics to die outside and even inside of institutions from poor health."

"Yes, it is not unusual, except that there are new members on our Board of Control. They wish to prove that the patient died from neglect by four of our employees. They have a witness who says that R. R. Champion, an employee, admitted to hurting Mr. Ketterer."

"What did this Mr. Ketterer die from, sir?"

"We do not know. His body was badly beaten, so the Board of Control wants you to charge the four employees on duty with Mr. Ketterer's death."

"They want me to file charges against all four employees?"

"Yes, and prove their guilt," added Dr. Redwine.

"Dr. Redwine!" Colonel Allen showed his irritation by standing up. "I have trouble believing that any employee would do that. I know there have been many disputes among the employees, board members, superintendents, and even governors over wages, hiring, and anything else you can imagine, but employees killing a patient? I have trouble accepting that." He remained standing.

"Colonel Allen, I am doing what I have been told to do by the Board of Control. I'm not saying I believe that the employees did this. Please, sit down and hear me out."

Colonel Allen returned to his seat. "Oh yes, sir, I'm sorry for my lack of manners. Please continue."

"The incident must be reviewed by the legal system because the Ketterer family is suing this institution. The Board of Control believes that the only way a state institution can keep from being legally liable is to bring charges against the employees who were involved," Dr. Redwine finished, reclining back into his chair.

"Well, I will certainly need to interview all four employees and others to determine if criminal charges are appropriate," Colonel Allen said.

"Yes, please. We are trying to have a progressive institution here," Dr. Redwine stated emphatically. "Employees must be held accountable for what happens."

"I have trouble believing that employees are at fault, as most employees are duty bound and care about their charges," Colonel Allen responded quickly, "but I will reserve my opinion."

"In the past, no one, including employees, was held accountable." Dr. Redwine tried to maintain control of his voice as he continued. "Now, the Board of Control wants someone made accountable, and the employees are the ones providing the care!"

"But, sir," Colonel Allen stated firmly, "my investigation must prove that the employees involved had the intention of killing this patient. It is up to you, as administrator, to control the board and politics of this facility. The politicians could also prove to be the ones responsible, by putting their own interests ahead of the needs of the patients of this institution."

"Oh, yes, I will agree with you, but that is not the issue at this time." Relaxing, Dr. Redwine stood up to gather some files and returned to his desk. "I will offer you my services, their files, and any office you wish." He handed Colonel Allen the employee files. "But the Board of Control insists that you bring criminal charges against these employees."

Colonel Allen tried to control his anger as he said, "Sir, this Board of Control does not tell me what to do! I will determine if such charges are necessary when I conduct my own investigation. I hope that is understood." Colonel Allen started looking through the employee records.

"Yes, we understand each other," answered Dr. Redwine.

"Sir, one question for you," Colonel Allen said as he looked over the four suspected employee files. "The employees whom you and the board have specified, how many of these four did you hire?"

"Three," he replied. "The fourth, Mr. Champion, was appointed in 1896 by Dr. W. F. Scott. He is reported to have done the beatings."

"If I remember correctly, Dr. Scott was appointed by his brother-in-law, Governor William O. Bradley; he was a Republican, wasn't he?"

"Yes, there was a lot of trouble with Dr. Scott, here."

"But now," Colonel Allen concluded, "the Democrats are in control. Since Mr. Champion was appointed by a Republican, isn't he a political scapegoat for the current board?" Having difficulty controlling his anger, Colonel Allen rose again from his chair.

"Now, Colonel Allen, you cannot make such a conclusion, regardless of politics. There has been a wrongful death here that no one can explain. Please be seated again."

"Yes, you are right," Colonel Allen said as he returned to his chair. "I just don't like being put in the middle of a political war, as I now fear I have been."

"I would hope to avoid that also," Dr. Redwine added as he discussed the details of Fred Ketterer's death. Following Ketterer's death, his body was shipped to relatives, who noticed excessive bruises and broken bones and called for further investigation.

Dr. Redwine told Colonel Allen that the family did not notify him, as the superintendent, which was the regular procedure, but rather notified the new Board of Control. The board saw this death as evidence of mismanagement within the asylum.

Dr. Redwine showed his dismay; he looked tired and weary. "This new board does not listen to me, Colonel Allen, and you are the only one who can help."

"Well, I need time to review the cases. I will start the interviewing tomorrow. I must excuse myself for the rest of the afternoon."

Dr. Redwine agreed and noticed that Colonel Allen had lost interest in the Administration Building as he was leaving. Hoping to encourage him, Dr. Redwine said, "I would be glad to show you around this new building."

"Thank you, but I would prefer to see it later," Colonel Allen said as he left; he was feeling disgusted with the whole process and trying to hide his own internal uneasiness. "I just need some time to review some facts on my own." He rose from his chair for the last time.

"Well, then, can I expect you early tomorrow morning, sir?" Dr. Redwine asked as he escorted Colonel Allen out of his office.

` "Yes, you can. Thank you for your kindness," Colonel Allen said as he walked out. He needed time to review the disputes that had been part of that institution for the last few years. He needed time to think, as he hurriedly left the building. Forgetting his usual manners, Colonel Allen ignored Dr. Redwine's secretary and rushed to his buggy.

Returning to his office, Colonel Allen preferred to think about Lexington's history. The city was part of the Old Buffalo Trail, which steered the early settlers from the northeastern to the southwestern part of Kentucky. The Buffalo Trail started from the northernmost settlement, Limestone (later renamed Maysville), and continued through Lexington as Mulberry Street, which was officially changed to Limestone Street in 1902.

As a child, John R. Allen Jr. had grown up with stories about the Kentucky Lunatic Asylum from his father, who was the superintendent. While Colonel Allen had not grown up in Lexington, his mother's family did, and he often visited there after returning to Kentucky to study law. He achieved the military title of "colonel" in the Kentucky State Guard. He retired at the age of twenty-eight from his regiment and started practicing law.

Both his father's and mother's families were from Green County, Kentucky, but his mother's family moved to Lexington in the early 1800s as her father, Richard A. Buckner Sr., practiced law and became a judge. Colonel Allen's father had studied at the Transylvania Law Department and returned to Green County. By 1835, he left Green County after being a Kentucky senator and returned to Lexington to study medicine at the Transylvania Medical School. He had rejected the common practice of "bleeding" the lunatics and had expected to provide better care methods when he became superintendent of the Kentucky asylum. Dr. Allen experienced both successes and failures as superintendent, but he felt the defeat most because he left Kentucky in 1855 with his family, moved to Keokuk, Iowa, and returned to politics until the Civil War. Dr. Allen and his family moved to Memphis as John R. Allen Jr. grew into adulthood, and Dr. Allen provided medical care for Civil War soldiers.

After Colonel Allen arrived back at his office on Short Street, he saw his partner, Henry Timberlake Duncan III. Colonel Allen had married his partner's sister twenty-one years earlier, while Duncan was still single at the age of thirty-eight. They still had a great deal in common with their families, law, and the history of Lexington. He asked Henry to come into his office as his mind kept returning to the mess at the asylum.

As both settled down into office chairs, Colonel Allen asked, "Do you remember the last time there was a dispute between the superintendent of the asylum, Board of Commissioners, and governor?"

"Well, the last one, I think, was this year when the governor did away with the previous Board of Commissioners," Henry stated. The governor claimed that the previous commissioners were incompetent, and therefore, he was justified in appointing his own friends to a new Board of Control. This new board would control all Kentucky asylums from Frankfort, from where they make all decisions, not where the asylums are located.

"But I hear the previous commissioners were all well-respected Lexington citizens," Colonel Allen said.

"Oh, there were negative rumors spread against the local Board of Commissioners to allow a new Board of Control for the governor's own supporters," added Henry. "That is Kentucky state government as usual." He shrugged his shoulders in disgust.

"That was early this year?" asked Colonel Allen.

"Yes, but years earlier, Governor William O. Bradley, a Republican, replaced the hospital superintendent with Dr. W. F. Scott. That was a real mess."

"Yes, I remember hearing about that," added Colonel Allen.

"I understand that Dr. Scott fired all the employees, including the experienced ones, and put his supporters into those jobs. This was around 1896–1897," concluded Henry in his usual casual way.

"How can someone be so uncaring about the needs of the patients? That facility needs caring employees, not political supporters," Colonel Allen said.

"If you are the governor of Kentucky, you can do as you wish," Henry said as he smiled.

The Board of Commissioners had threatened to resign if the governor did not remove Dr. Scott. The governor took his time, so the National

Guard had to be called in to maintain peace among the employees until the dispute was settled. Several patients were left unsupervised, and some of them died.

"Why don't lawyers question what happens in a state asylum?" asked Colonel Allen.

"They never have, but if they did, the politicians would attempt to corrupt the lawyers more than ever." Henry laughed, trying to add humor to cheer the too serious Colonel Allen. "The asylums have always been a major source of political jobs; it is so sad."

"One of the employees appointed by Dr. Scott, R. R. Champion, will be charged with murder if the Board of Control has its way," Colonel Allen added.

"Oh, no, so the politicians have a scapegoat!" said Henry.

"I hope not, but it's my job to investigate it. I had hoped not to be involved with all this, since this asylum is so different when my father was there. But it seems that I must be involved," concluded Colonel Allen.

"You need to do your duty at this time, as our families did during their time. It is now your job as attorney general to investigate. Actually, it is about time the law got involved with state-supported asylum care," Henry added.

"My father viewed our asylum as a caring and benevolent place for the unfortunates of society rather than what it is now: just a job for incompetent political stooges." Colonel Allen, disgusted, stood up and reached for his hat.

"Yes," added Henry, "when my father was editor of our local newspaper, he often reported negative impressions of that asylum. That did nothing. I especially like his last article, called, 'Another muddle at the asylum.'" Henry stood up from his chair, waiting to see what his partner would do.

"I'm afraid your father's article is still accurate, but I heard that all this turmoil started after Dr. William S. Chipley left in 1870."

"Yes, Father often stated that Dr. Chipley was fired because of his politics during the Civil War. Since Dr. Chipley, various political parties have used the institution to provide jobs for their supporters with no thought about what is best for the institution or the unfortunate patients," Henry said.

"Oh, I have heard of so many rumors," added Colonel Allen.

"Worse, the buildings deteriorate while they use the money for their own projects and point their fingers at each other," Henry stated. "Oh, don't get me started. I don't like what I have heard."

"Did you know that I knew Dr. Chipley? He was a close friend of my father. I never remember him being fired, but he was a really nice, brilliant, respected man," added Colonel Allen.

"Yes, he was well known in Lexington, but he was fired by the prevailing political parties who were pro-Southern during the Civil War. My father can sure tell you about all that, since he served on the Northern side," stated Henry.

"Obviously you still keep up with the local politics?" said Colonel Allen.

"I have to; my family would get ahead of me if I didn't keep up with it." Henry laughed, again trying to lighten up the conversation.

"Well, do you think the current politicians would go so far as to charge someone with murder, just to gain their own purposes?" asked Colonel Allen.

"Yes, anything is possible."

"I don't like this."

"So you are in the middle," observed his partner.

"No, I refuse to be in the middle. Talking with you has helped me see things more fully, but I must do my job." Colonel Allen looked at his watch and realized the time of day.

Henry suggested that Colonel Allen talk to some of the early community leaders, such as Charlton Hunt Morgan, who was fired as a steward in the 1880s. Also, he should talk to his father; as the local newspaper editor and later mayor, Henry Timberlake Duncan II had fought the misuse of public funds.

Henry noticed the time and realized that they should be going.

"Yes, I hope to see your father tonight," Colonel Allen said. "I will do a full investigation and present the results to the grand jury. While I don't like what I see, as attorney for the commonwealth I must do my job to the fullest. Oh, I guess you know that Miss Lilly is having one of her parties tonight. Elizabeth wanted me to remind you."

"Yes, your wife called and reminded me this morning. Miss Lilly says my Uncle John Brand, her brother, is in town. This is her reason for having a party.".

"Well, Miss Lilly never needs a reason to have a party, but she is expecting us tonight at Ingleside. She expects all family members to be at her parties. Are you bringing a date?" asked Colonel Allen.

"If I had a date, I would not expose the poor girl to our family. No, I will come alone," Henry added as he smiled. "You know I love her parties, but not with a girlfriend."

"I will pick up Elizabeth, and we will meet you later at Ingleside." Colonel Allen left the building.

Henry returned to his office. He recognized the agitation that Colonel Allen had about the asylum but realized that there were many local citizens who were also upset over the same issues. The asylum had been such a local source of pride, and now, it had fallen into much disrepair and political hassle.

That night, Colonel and Elizabeth Allen approached Ingleside's entrance on the south end of town, where South Broadway turned into Harrodsburg Road. A half-story three-bay arched gatehouse faced South Broadway. Once entering past the gatehouse, a large fifteen-room mansion was set among three hundred acres. The Allens were frequent visitors there. Miss Lilly was Elizabeth Allen's aunt.

Miss Lilly Duncan and her sister, Mary Duncan Gibson, lived at Ingleside. Ingleside was built in 1852, and Mrs. Gibson's late husband, Hart, purchased the mansion for his wife and son, Henry. When Mary became a widow, she was in danger of losing Ingleside until Lilly paid off the remaining loans and moved in with her. Since then, Miss Lilly and Mrs. Gibson made the mansion into a showplace of Lexington. Ingleside was often called the Castle.

While Mrs. Gibson was more reclusive, Miss Lilly enjoyed entertaining many friends at their mansion. That night, Miss Lilly was in her usual prime as she welcomed all her guests.

"Oh, dears, how good to see you, do come in," said Miss Lilly, smiling. "Do meet my guests in the other room."

"Miss Lilly, we are always happy to come," Colonel Allen said.

She looked at Elizabeth and said, "Your father is in the dining room, you might like to see him first; he is grumpy tonight. See if you can improve him a little."

"Yes, I will," Elizabeth said as she walked toward her father, Henry Duncan II. They met in the hall and hugged, as they usually did. Henry Duncan II, at the age of seventy, still yearned for his late wife, Lilly Brand, who had been dead for over twenty-five years. Yet his daughter, Elizabeth, was so much like her mother.

"Elizabeth, I hope you are well; where is that husband of yours? I want to talk to him. I hear that he will be investigating the killing at the asylum."

"Now, Dad, no politics tonight," Elizabeth said, knowing she was wasting her breath. "How are you?"

"How do you think a seventy-year-old man is? As well as can be; I'm old but I'm glad my little girl is fine."

Colonel Allen entered the room and shook hands with his father-in-law. "Sir, it is so good to see you; I had heard that you would be here."

"I hear you are investigating the asylum. You know that is a very political situation, don't you?"

"Yes, sir, I'm aware of that. Do you have any suggestions?"

"Well, make sure you don't get caught in the middle, especially with the corrupt bosses here in Lexington."

"Sir, I am doing my best, but I don't expect to be in the middle."

"You know that the asylum has been their source of jobs for years, and if you disturb their plans, they will make your life miserable," stated his father-in-law.

"Sir, I have no choice; I must investigate as I see fit and let the grand jury decide if the patient was murdered by any employees."

"Yes, I know you will do as you have always done. Just let me know if I can help." Duncan felt the same pride in his son-in-law that he had experienced with his own children.

"Colonel," Miss Lilly said as she tapped him on the shoulder, "I want you to meet my brother, John H. Brand."

Colonel Allen shook hands with the visitor. "I'm so glad to finally meet you. I have always heard so much about you from the family."

"I haven't visited my Kentucky relatives in years," Brand said, "but you have always been out of town when I did visit."

"Well, I'm so glad to finally meet you." Colonel Allen put his arm around Elizabeth.

Miss Lilly continued talking to Elizabeth, saying, "He is also the brother of your mother and my sister, Lilly Brand, God rest her soul. You both were always away when he visited Kentucky; my brother is staying here at Ingleside before returning to New York."

"Yes, sir," Colonel Allen continued, "I know you lived in Louisville for several years before moving to New York. We are pleased to have you visiting now."

"I wanted to visit my roots in Lexington. As you know, my father, George W. Brand, was raised in Lexington, and my grandfather, John Brand, lived in Lexington all his life. I was named after him."

The first John Brand was on the board of Kentucky's first asylum when John Hunt was the chairman. The Brand family owned a house on Walnut and Fourth Streets until it was sold in the early 1900s.

Many different guests were moving around in the living room; Colonel Allen noticed Joseph W. Rhodes, sheriff of Fayette County for the last two terms. He excused himself from Uncle John and went over to him.

"Sir, I'm so glad to see you enjoying Miss Lilly's party."

"Yes, I am." Both men had known each other for years. Sheriff Rhodes was one year older than Colonel Allen, and they had worked together on several cases when Colonel Allen needed a sheriff.

"Are you working on another case?" Colonel Allen asked.

"Actually no, and I'm considering not running for sheriff this third term. This is more of a job for a young man."

"Your son is still a deputy sheriff?"

"Yes, but he is still young," added Rhodes. "Politics in Lexington has gotten pretty tight for me, now."

"Yes, I can understand what you are saying," said Colonel Allen; he had heard that the current political cronyism of Lexington was taking over the sheriff's office.

Lexington had many older soldiers who knew how to handle guns. For years, they served as assistants to the sheriff or even as the sheriff. They were always part of the history of the town. They helped with the early settlement of Lexington and maintained peace. They served the early wilderness town well but those jobs were becoming more politically controlled by the early 1900s.

Miss Lilly came into the living room to introduce another guest, James Lane Allen, a popular novelist. He had often been a visitor with Miss Lilly, so the family knew him.

Miss Lilly announced that dinner was ready to be served, and everyone moved to the dining room. The dining room was elaborately decorated with fresh flowers from the grounds of Ingleside. Miss Lilly seated each guest at the table, and the hired help brought in the food. Everyone was delighted, especially Miss Lilly.

Uncle John Brand was impressed with the food and started the conversation. He asked Colonel Allen if he and James Allen were related.

"No, sir," replied Colonel Allen. "There are many Allens in Lexington. Although there were four Allens from Lexington in the War of 1812, none were from my family. My grandfather was from Green County, Kentucky, and he died during the next war."

"Well, I'm impressed with your history."

Colonel Allen continued, "There was a Sterling Allen, brother to my father, living in the next county, but there is no one there now. I know of no other connections, do you, Mr. Allen?"

"I don't know about any others," James Allen said. "My father was working here in Lexington when I was born. I graduated from Kentucky University in 1871. I did find out that my father was appointed as manager at the Eastern Kentucky Lunatic Asylum in 1853, the same time when your father was superintendent."

"Oh, that is a surprise," Colonel Allen added as he was passing food to his wife.

"Yes, but my father did not stay long. I really don't know why; I would guess that he did not take to being a manager," Mr. Allen stated while eating the delicious food.

"He may not have liked the lunatics; some were very difficult, as I recall my father saying so," Colonel Allen said.

"Well, the facilities were not very good," added Uncle John Brand. "My grandfather often took me as a child to visit, and I remember the screams and cries of many people there. It scared me. I never wanted to go back, but my grandfather enjoyed knowing the patients and helping them."

"Yes," added Miss Lilly, "I remember visiting there. The buildings and sanitation were poor. It was a horrible experience for me. I think it is a horrible subject to talk about now." She attempted to change the subject by passing more food around the table.

"But that was the best available at the time," stated Colonel Allen. "I know my father was always seeking the newest and best ways to do things there. He and Dr. Chipley really tried." He commented about the food as others added to the compliments.

Miss Lilly beamed in response to the compliments and stated, "Yes, I guess you are right, but to children, it was scary. All the loud noise from people crying; it was bad."

"I remember hearing some of the early sheriffs talking about the days before Kentucky's first asylum," stated Sheriff Rhodes. "They were so proud of that asylum, since it was a big improvement over what they had seen previously."

"Do you mean before the asylum was even opened?" asked Colonel Allen. "That had to be before 1824."

"Yes, the old sheriffs often talked about people who were paid to care for the lunatics on their farms; this was before the asylum was opened," added Sheriff Rhodes. He had finished his food and was sitting back in his chair.

"You mean the State of Kentucky paid farmers to care for the lunatics?" asked Colonel Allen.

"Yes, there were few requirements, and many saw it as an opportunity to get cheap labor," added Sheriff Rhodes. "They called it the 'boarding-out' system, but it had no organization to it, just people who were willing to take a lunatic on their farm."

"I did not know that," stated a surprised Colonel Allen.

"Oh, yes, the lunatics lived in horrible conditions, and no one could do anything about it," stated Sheriff Rhodes. "It was perfectly legal not to provide for a lunatic under the boarding-out system, and the keeper got paid."

"I understand," Miss Lilly said, trying to interrupt, "Colonel Allen will be investigating the asylum. Isn't this the first time it has really been investigated by the law?"

"Actually, Miss Lilly," responded Colonel Allen, "many lawyers have been associated with that asylum in the past, mostly in administrative roles. My law professor, M. C. Johnson, was on the board for many years. The second chairman of the board, Richard Pindell, was legally trained and served in my position as commonwealth attorney in the early 1830s."

"Also, your uncle, Judge Buckner, was considered one of the best legal authorities around, and he was on the board for many years," stated the colonel's father-in-law.

"Of course," Colonel Allen said. "Also, F. K. Hunt, son of John Wesley Hunt, who was the first chairman of the board at the asylum, was a lawyer, and he served on the board for many years. However, after that, politicians were always changing the leaders, and no one stayed long in those positions. The constant political changes created chaos."

"So, there have been many good lawyers who have served," Duncan added.

"Yes, but Miss Lilly is also correct," continued Colonel Allen, "this is the first real investigation into criminal charges against employees. That is a very different role from all the previously trained lawyers who served that asylum. The employees are being held legally responsible for those under their care; it's a new and different concept."

"But instead, they should be investigating the political powers that have contaminated it for years," Duncan said. "Each politician wants his people in the paying jobs, disregarding any institutional goals or needs."

"Maybe so, but that is not the task given to me. I will do as I am required by the law," claimed Colonel Allen. "Hopefully, the whole system will improve when problems are exposed to the public."

"I assume you do not expect to get rid of the political cronyism that you find?" Duncan asked.

Smiling back, Colonel Allen stated, "The public will need to do that when they hear about the investigation. You did not get rid of the political cronyism in Lexington when you were mayor."

The colonel's father-in-law smiled back and said, "I sure tried my best. I left the asylum alone while the city was open range for my investigations. My paper, the *Lexington Daily Press,* was constantly investigating corruption. As mayor, I instituted methods of fund disbursements and efficient government, hoping to eliminate any future corruption, but I was not very successful."

"Unfortunately," added his son, Henry, "your swearing-in ceremony as mayor on January 1, 1900, was overshadowed by the increasingly disturbing news from the capital in Frankfort."

"Oh, yes, the newly elected Democratic governor, William Goebel, was shot the day before and died three days later," Henry continued. "Instead of a new era of progress, Goebel's assassination launched a new wave of anger and bitterness."

"But wasn't that just in Frankfort?" asked Colonel Allen.

"No, our politics are controlled from Frankfort, even though Lexington is a hundred miles away. My term as mayor of Lexington was affected," Duncan continued.

"You also had the Big Six, who wanted you to do things their way in Lexington. They included Representative Klair, Judge Bullock, Louis DesCognets (a contractor), Lieutenant Governor Beckham, Ernest Ellis (another contractor), and Thomas Combs, now the current mayor," Henry stated. "All ruled by the two mangy rats, Klair and Combs. They still have their way here."

"If you feel that way, why not run for mayor yourself?" asked Sheriff Rhodes. "You are the only one who can win against them."

"I might," said Henry. "I will wait until they mess themselves up, and I plan to be there to show it to the public. Thomas Combs uses state money to buy contractors and jobs. These next few years will reveal their corruption."

The conversation continued way into the night, until the guests had to leave. Miss Lilly had had another of her great parties. She was known for her political as well as social parties. Everyone enjoyed the party.

*   *   *

Colonel Allen arrived early at Kentucky's first asylum, now called the Eastern Kentucky Lunatic Asylum (EKLA), one of three asylums in the state. He was hoping to look around, putting together what he had heard from his father and what had changed in the last years. The original building had two additions on each side, and a back part had been added after his father came in 1844. Colonel Allen could see the back of that building. He looked around at all the others and observed that the grounds were well cultivated with many trees and plants.

Another much larger building nearer to Newtown Pike was added during Dr. Chipley's time as superintendent. A "Negro" building nearer to the railroad tracks was added after the Civil War. More recently, three other major buildings were added: an Administration Building, the Dr. B. W. Dudley Infirmary, and the superintendent's home. An earlier superintendent's house, built prior to the Civil War, had faced Newtown Pike nearer the cemetery but the newer superintendent's home was closer to the front of the facility.

Colonel Allen observed the pump house on the right of the original building, next to a spring of water. This was their original water supply. He remembered being told that the water had once been a source of health problems for those living in the asylum. There was now a different source of water: city water was brought into the institution. A small fence protected individuals from the sink hole that had originally been a proud source of "unfailing water." There was a strange quietness surrounding the now unwanted water.

A train track bordered the facility on the northeast side, while the asylum grounds continued on to Fourth Street. The entrance had always been off of Fourth Street, but a new iron fence had been added to the old two-story gatehouse.

Colonel Allen proceeded northwestward to the back of the institution, where small buildings were scattered along the farming area. The farm consisted of around 230 acres, with crops and cattle providing the main source of food. Patients provided the labor for the chores. Colonel Allen stood and took in the whole feel of the institution, as he observed people moving around.

Colonel Allen was not nostalgic, since this facility never meant anything to him, but it had been meaningful to his father. He had heard other stories about how the Transylvania Medical School professors had worked here, searching for cures in medicine and teaching the philosophy of phrenology.

Colonel Allen recognized that phrenology was now criticized as a boneheaded medicine that was not based on science. Yet he also understood that it was the first organized science about human behavior in his father's day. While it soon proved to be inadequate for helping lunatics, his father often read journals that covered the philosophy of his time.

Dr. Allen had accepted the challenge of this facility, even though it held so many frustrations and failures for him. But he still believed in the possibilities of a retreat for those who needed it. Yet his son was unable to comprehend what this institution meant to the early city or his father, when all he could see was the political exploitation.

Colonel Allen returned to the Administration Building to meet Dr. Redwine and to start his investigations. The first employee, Mr. J. M. Claggett, was present and waiting.

"Mr. Claggett, please sit down," Colonel Allen said as they went into the office. Dr. Redwine followed both men into the office. Colonel Allen noticed that Dr. Redwine was not leaving, so he said, "Sir, I would like to do my own interviewing; may we be left alone?"

He thought it was important to have independent interviews without the presence of another person, especially Dr. Redwine.

Dr. Redwine responded, "I would like to be part of the investigation and know what my employees are saying."

"Sir, I feel that this interview should be independent, without the presence of any supervisor. I must insist that you leave or I will refuse to conduct this investigation," Colonel Allen stated firmly.

"We will discuss this later," Dr. Redwine said as he left the room.

Colonel Allen was relieved. He did not believe that any employee would talk freely if his supervisor was present.

"Mr. Claggett, let us continue. What wards do you work on?"

"On Ward 15," Claggett said. "I also help with Wards 13 and 14."

"I understand this death occurred on Ward 15, which is considered the worst men's ward of the institution?"

"It's bad," Claggett said.

"You were on the day shift when this happened on June 22?"

"Yes, this Champion, he's bragging about hitting the lunatic here in the eye. He'd asked for a mop to clean the blood."

"That lunatic was Mr. Ketterer?"

"Yes, that were his name, I've not had much learning, so I don't remember much," added Claggett.

"Did you ask Mr. Champion how it happened?"

"No, I just saw him rough him up before. Those lunatics always mean too. This Mr. Champion just pushed the lunatic to the floor, tied him, and put him in a chair."

"What would the other employees do?" asked Colonel Allen.

"Huh? They just left the lunatic alone."

"What would happen when employees left Mr. Ketterer alone?" asked Colonel Allen.

"He would fall, hurt himself. That Mr. Champion did more. He would tie him to the chair. We can't help it if the lunatic hurt himself. Sometime, the lunatic would stay in a chair, but not if he were not tied there. Then, the stupid lunatic would get hurt."

"If Mr. Champion fought the lunatic to tie him down, would he still get loose?" asked the colonel, wondering why other employees would not help.

"No, but the lunatic would fall anyway; he was always falling. I see that Champion man looked to fighting that lunatic. I had watched this many times. The lunatic is hopeless and nothing can be done for him. That Champion man wasted time on that hopeless lunatic."

"So what you are saying, is that Mr. Champion was cruel to Mr. Ketterer and murdered him?"

"He was mean to him. I did not see him kill him. He was found dead many hours later."

"So you did not see Mr. Champion kill Mr. Ketterer?" Colonel Allen moved closer with his chair.

"No, I had just saw Mr. Champion being mean to the lunatic." Claggett sat back in his chair, smiling and revealing several broken teeth.

"Mr. Claggett, may I ask you some personal questions?"

"Okay, sure, I have nothing to hide," he said as the smile faded.

"How long have you worked at this institution?"

"One year. Dr. Redwine hired me, and I was sure glad to have a job."

"Have you had any previous experience in this work?"

"No, I did not go far in school and needs money."

"Does the job pay well enough?"

"The pay is okay if you look at everything you get with it."

"So what are the benefits?"

"I get a room, meals, clean bed, and spending money. I want to buy a farm, but I not got the money to get it. It is okay for now. I ain't got no family to help so I's got make my own way. I's hope to get something better, but this here is okay for now. I can save money here."

"Did you support the current governor?" Colonel Allen was getting more skeptical about the dedication that he had hoped to find among employees.

"Y—yes." He looked around to see who could hear and whispered, "I vote the way the party wants me. It has been good to me and to my dead father."

"Oh, I just had a guess," Colonel Allen stated casually, but then he remembered his legal responsibilities. He reminded himself that he was not there to judge the employees but to find the truth about Ketterer's death and present it to the grand jury and let them judge.

"Are you the only person to witness Mr. Champion's brutality?"

"I guess no one else was around; we have more lunatics than we have room for them."

"Do you know if there were no other employees around?"

"I don't reckon so. The officers are spread all over but they only visit once in a while. They are in charge. We keepers stay on a ward during our whole shift while the officers have many wards, and they check on what we do."

"So you were the only one to work with Mr. Champion on this Ward 15. He is an officer and you are a keeper?" Colonel Allen was writing the facts down. "How many patients are on this ward?" He was making sure the facts were correct.

"I heard of fifty on this ward, and many of them is mean. They is always fighting. They're many lunatics. Dr. Redwine is working to do something about it."

"Where were the other two employees, Mr. Pharris and Mr. Adams? They are also considered in this murder, right?"

"They just work on the same ward at night," Claggett said as he shrugged his shoulders. "Thems found the lunatic dead while working. There is always someone dying. I don't know why all the fuss over this one."

"Do you know anything about how the others treated Mr. Ketterer?"

"No, but Dr. Redwine hired and trained them. They do not make them lunatics do anything. I just see Mr. Champion, spending too much time with the mean ones."

"What do you mean?" Colonel Allen could not distinguish if employees were spending time with a patient to teach him better control or to punish him. Colonel Allen wondered if an uneducated employee, such as this one, could know the difference.

Claggett continued with his observation, "This here Mr. Champion tried to teach them lunatics to feed themselves when they are really hopeless."

"Is that being cruel?"

"Yes, when they are so hopeless."

"Have you observed other employees being so cruel?"

"No, I hardly see others since I am off the ward sleeping when the other keepers are working."

"Thank you, Mr. Claggett. Will you be willing to testify at the grand jury of what you just told me?"

"Yes, I'm sure this Mr. Champion hurt this lunatic. He expects too much from such filthy lunatics."

"I will see that you are called as a witness," stated Colonel Allen. "By the way, I guess you understand that you are still a suspect, since you are one of the four employees on that ward when Mr. Ketterer died. Do you understand this?"

"Yes, but if this here Mr. Champion is found wrong, then we, the others, can go free?"

"Maybe not; if you did nothing to stop it, you can also be found guilty."

"I can't do anything. This Mr. Champion is a senior officer and I am under him. I can't do anything."

Colonel Allen jumped up and shook hands with Mr. Claggett, saying, "Sir, thank you; I will be getting in touch with you." He sighed with relief and stated to himself, "How depressing!"

After Claggett left the office, Colonel Allen started to review his notes. Dr. Redwine came into the office, obviously upset, and said, "Sir, I must protest you interviewing my employees without my presence. I need to know the problems of this institution. I insist on being part of your interviews, or I will call the Board of Control about this."

Colonel Allen sat down in his chair and caught his breath after hearing Dr. Redwine; he replied, "Sir, you can call anyone you wish. I will not have another person interfere with the interviews. If you insist, I will refuse to participate in this case."

"Well, uh," Dr. Redwine sputtered as he turned around, "I will notify the governor of this disagreement."

"Sir, you do that; I will wait until I am allowed to do the interviews as I feel best. I must find the truth, and that can only be done alone. I will wait for a decision to be made." The colonel left the Administration Building and tipped his hat.

Colonel Allen got into his carriage, believing that the whole process was over for him. He knew the state's attorney general would support him, but he fully expected the governor to side with Dr. Redwine. He went back to his office. He was disappointed that the legal process was not allowed to run its full course. He could now concentrate on his law practice.

Two days later, Mr. Percy Haley stormed into Colonel Allen's law office. Haley insisted upon seeing Colonel Allen, telling his secretary he was a representative from the governor and needed to see the colonel. His tall and slim body was pacing back and forth in the waiting room as the secretary notified Colonel Allen of his presence. His expensive clothes and jewelry set him apart from ordinary clients, but his manner was very offensive. He was someone who was used to getting his way.

"Does he have an appointment?" Colonel Allen asked his secretary.

"No, sir, he does not, but he insists that he see you."

Colonel Allen went into the waiting room and said, "Sir, you wanted to see me? You insist, when I have other clients to see?"

"Yes, Colonel Allen, I am Percy Haley, president of the newly created Board of Control, representing all the charitable institutions in the state of Kentucky. I have a state office in Frankfort, so I have statewide responsibilities."

"I'm not sure that information is important to me," Colonel Allen said.

"Sir, I say that, just to notify you that I am not always in Lexington. I made a special trip to see you. The previous Board of Commissioners had their offices at the asylum. Now, it is harder for me to see you, since my office is located in Frankfort."

"I presume you are here about the investigations at the Eastern Kentucky Insane Asylum; do you know my position? I see no reason to talk unless you agree with my position on the issue." Colonel Allen started to walk back to his office.

Stopping him, Haley stated, "Wait, Colonel. The governor and I agree with you. Please, can we talk in your office?"

"Well, I guess so." Colonel Allen led Haley into his office. However, he did not offer him a chair.

Haley sat down anyway without waiting for an offer; he continued, "We are asking that you continue with the investigations as previously started and only report the results to me. I am responsible for the whole state of Kentucky, and I need to depend upon you for this investigation."

"Sir, I don't have to report to anyone except to the grand jury, which represents the citizens of Lexington. The question is, will I be allowed to conduct the investigations independently, excluding any other parties, including Dr. Redwine? I am also busy and do not wish to waste any more time." The Colonel gestured for Haley to leave. He knew Haley was one of Kentucky's political bosses. He had no patience for political bosses and was finding it difficult being polite to this one.

"That's what I'm here to tell you; yes. You drive a hard bargain. Dr. Redwine was completely out of line. The governor is just waiting for the investigation to be finished before he fires Dr. Redwine."

"So Dr. Redwine will be gone too, after being here over six years. How can that asylum achieve any stability with those constant changes?" Colonel Allen returned to his chair.

"Dr. Redwine does not know that, and I must ask that you keep it confidential."

"Sir, I have no wish to be involved in your political games. I'm just concerned about that institution."

"The governor is trying to clean up the mess by organizing a statewide Board of Control and clearing up the current problems."

"Certainly you cannot expect this investigation to achieve all that," Colonel Allen said.

"No, but it will be a start. All Kentucky institutions will be treated the same, with uniform business practices and administrative management by full-time employees in Frankfort. This will improve all of the facilities."

"It will take away the strong local community connection; will that really benefit the institution? Since early on, Lexington was closely involved with this institution, but all that will be lost." Colonel Allen forcefully stated his opinions. He realized his opinions were growing stronger as he debated with this powerful representative of the state government. He realized that ordinary citizens never have that opportunity.

"Well, the institution will be for the better; local people tend to take advantage of any employment opportunities."

"I don't see it that way, sir," stated Colonel Allen. "Local people also care more and can be more closely involved. I see the politicians taking all the paying jobs for their own friends."

"Well, I'm not here to debate the merits of the governor's programs. We need your help to continue a full investigation, and I will give you my full support. I hope to make the employees responsible for what happens at the asylum. So we need a complete, independent investigation, which only you can objectively and legally provide," responded Haley.

"That means I report to no one," Colonel Allen stated, "just to the grand jury, who will determine who is responsible for that death following my investigation."

"Okay, okay, I will not ask you to report to me, but if you have any more problems, let me know. I will give you any resources you need. Do we understand each other?"

"Yes, but what do I say to Dr. Redwine?" asked Colonel Allen.

"I will notify Dr. Redwine that you are not to be interfered with in any way, including total privacy for your interviews. Is that adequate?"

"Yes, sir," Colonel Allen replied as he sighed with disbelief. "However, I will only report my results to the grand jury."

"Yes, yes, Colonel Allen, I heard you and agree to your terms. I had hoped that you would keep me informed of your results, but I will not require it. I expect you to do your best job."

"I will do my job fairly, that I believe in," stated Colonel Allen.

"And sir, I believe that the governor is interested in creating a progressive Board of Control. My job is to achieve that goal, in any way. We must have some external review of these internal problems."

Then, Haley stood up and politely left. Colonel Allen did not make his usual friendly gesture of inviting out-of-town visitors to his home for supper. Instead, he hoped to never see Haley again.

Such a negative attitude toward someone was unusual for Colonel Allen, who was always a gentleman toward everyone. However, his tolerance for political power was decreasing.

When Colonel Allen continued with his investigations two days later, Dr. Redwine was politely cooperative. Fred Pharris and Daniel Adams, the night shift keepers on Ward 15, had not seen Champion treat Ketterer brutally but confirmed that Ketterer was violent and difficult to keep clean. Both keepers admitted that they had often allowed Ketterer to stay in filth rather than to attempt to clean him.

They admitted that they were supposed to tie Ketterer in a chair to keep him from wandering on the ward, but the night he died, they had forgotten.

Neither employee had any idea of how the patient had died, since they were in the opposite ends of the ward. They were both new employees and concerned over the dirty conditions on the ward. Neither said anything negative about Dr. Redwine's administration, believing that the superintendent was doing his best to improve conditions.

Colonel Allen had difficulty accepting the fact that only four employees were in charge of fifty severely disturbed patients for all hours of each day; how deplorable the conditions on that ward must be.

Colonel Allen left the Administration Building to walk around the grounds, again, trying to understand the place. He just could not understand why these job positions were so sought after by political parties when the conditions that he had heard about were deplorable. None of the employees that he interviewed were motivated beyond the financial gains of the job. Was this the same facility that his father had invested so much personal energy into? Had the facility changed so much? Were there really good employees who cared like his father, or was it just a job? He needed answers for his own personal satisfaction.

While walking around the grounds along Newtown Pike, he noticed an employee in his late twenties helping several patients work in the greenhouse. He observed them for a while. The patients were obviously enjoying their work.

Colonel Allen approached the one in charge and asked, "Do you work here?"

"Yes, sir, I'm James H. Reed, the steward. I have been here since 1900. And who are you, sir?"

"I'm Colonel Allen, investigating the death of Mr. Ketterer. I'm sure you have read about it in the newspaper, if you did not already know about it?"

"Oh, yes. How sad. I never saw Mr. Ketterer because he was confined to Ward 15. I had heard that he was a difficult one."

"Yes, he was. Sir, your being the steward, may I ask, what do you do here?"

"Well, my job is supervising the farm and greenhouse and buying the supplies for the whole institution. I especially enjoy supervising the farm and greenhouse, because the patients really like working here."

"You appear to enjoy it here too," observed Colonel Allen.

"Oh, yes, there are lunatics here who, if they lived in town, would be cast aside, neglected, and eventually die from a lack of care. Here, they are useful and find satisfaction in work."

"Oh, you are really a bright spot here," said Colonel Allen. "I had wanted to know the good parts of this asylum."

"Well, sir," continued Reed, "here, lunatics are active, they enjoy having responsibilities equal to what they are able to do, and I enjoy seeing them gain confidence in themselves from the work. Many see this farm and greenhouse as their only bright spot. They live for their time here and their help within the asylum."

"Is this the only good part of this facility?"

"Well, I hope not; there are others. I'm a businessman and farmer, but helping these lunatics to become productive is really my bright spot."

"Who appointed you to the position?"

"Dr. Redwine! He chose me because of my farming and business background. My family was part of this facility for years."

"Oh, who were they?"

"My grandmother, Catherine Hunt Reed, was the granddaughter of John Wesley Hunt. He was the first chairman of the Board of Commissioners here. There is a lot of history here for me."

"Oh, I remember hearing about John W. Hunt; he hired my father as superintendent in 1844. See, I also have some history here but have avoided this place because of the current negative politics here."

"Yes, I know of the negative politics, but I also know that there are lunatics here who have caring keepers."

"Now, you are the steward. Weren't there other stewards that were fired?" asked Colonel Allen. He was remembering some of the past conflicts that he had heard about.

"Yes, Captain Charlton H. Morgan, a grandson of John W. Hunt, who was the steward from around 1880 to 1883, was fired. Captain Morgan and my father, J. Henry Reed, were both Confederate veterans. Captain Morgan and the superintendent did not agree on how to purchase items for the institution. They were also of different political parties, and the Civil War was another source of division. I am most fortunate that Dr. Redwine lets me conduct my business as I see best to do it."

"So you are not having problems with the current administration?"

"I have no problems with Dr. Redwine. Before him, the steward answered to the Board of Commissioners, and conflicts often developed between stewards and the superintendent."

"Of course, you know of the political interventions reported here?" asked Colonel Allen.

"Yes, I do but I run a tight accounting system, which I learned at Transylvania College, and no one can claim any misuse of state funds or abuse of monies. I also know farming."

"What do you enjoy most about your job?"

"I employ as many lunatics as possible," Reed said.

"Do you pay them?"

"No, the state does not allow that, but we give them special attention, and they often are given pies for their work. I enjoy seeing their faces light up. But their best reward is feeling useful and part of the work at this facility. Outside, they would not have that."

"How nice; is your salary adequate?"

"Yes, it is, especially with the benefits, but I could make more money elsewhere. I just enjoy working here."

"Sir, can I talk with you later? I need to go now; I have someone waiting on me."

"Yes, I am here most of the time. I have an apartment on the grounds, but my family's home is located on a farm south of Lexington. I go home on weekends."

Colonel Allen shook hands with Reed and proceeded back to the Administration Building. Dr. Redwine was waiting for him.

"Where have you been?" the superintendent asked. "I have people waiting for you to interview." Dr. Redwine demonstrated an obvious agitation with Colonel Allen. He disliked undependable employees, and Colonel Allen seemed beyond his control.

"Yes, I am sorry, Dr. Redwine, but I was talking to one of your outstanding employees, Mr. James H. Reed. He spoke highly of you."

Dr. Redwine simmered down; his hostility melted, and he smiled. "Yes, he is outstanding. I do have some real good employees here."

"How did you hire him, since most politicians hire whom they wish here?"

"Well," Dr. Redwine explained, "Mr. Reed did have the right political connections. And he was recommended by Governor Beckham. As you know, Governor Beckham is the grandson of Charles Wickliff, who lived in Lexington. The Wickliff and Hunt families have always been close, and Mr. Reed is related to the Hunt family."

"However, James Reed is also competent and caring," added Colonel Allen as he found his chair.

"Yes, he is. While I take recommendations from the governor, I can choose not to hire someone, which was not always true in the past. I have made some significant changes here, hopefully for the better. Mr. Reed is such an example."

"So you inherited many problems with the institution?"

"Oh, yes," Dr. Redwine said as he started to relax; however, he avoided sitting down, since he was in a hurry. "I am trying to get good employees. I had hoped to only hire good people, but the facility was so depleted of good employees, I have to take what I can. Unfortunately, this death has magnified our problems to the public, and I'm busy handling the press and reporters. I have no time for unnecessary things."

"Such as me?" said Colonel Allen, relaxing against the wall.

"Maybe, but you are different; you are concerned with getting to the bottom of a problem, instead of just stirring things up."

"Thank you; so what problems did you inherit?"

"All the on-ward employees left the institution in 1899, except for Mr. Champion and two others. They refused to leave, even knowing that they may not get paid."

"How could they do that?" asked Colonel Allen.

"They stayed without pay until finally they were paid. Many patients were left untended, with no one to care for them. Some patients can care for themselves, but most on Ward 15 are helpless. I have had to hire anyone that I could. Some employees are good, like Mr. Reed, while others will have to do until we get someone better."

"What are the requirements for these jobs?" asked Colonel Allen.

"There are none. Some state asylums require training before being employed; those workers are called attendants. Most of ours are just keepers, because they are not trained and must be trained on the job. Many do not care to learn and only stay a short period of time, and then we must start training all over again."

"So many employees leave after they are hired and go elsewhere?"

"Yes; in 1896, Dr. W. F. Scott fired all employees and replaced them with all his friends. Scott was fired by the governor in 1897, and his friends left to protest him being fired. The next two years, Dr. E. M. Wiley took any employees he could get."

"So you came after Dr. Wiley?"

"Yes, I did with the expectations of improving things, but it has been slow."

"So why did Dr. Wiley leave?" asked Colonel Allen.

"He was too disgusted, could not get enough employees for basic care, and just left. Previous employees saw how unstable their jobs were and took other opportunities when they had them."

"So what do you enjoy most about your job?"

"Being part of a team with caring employees is inspiring. There is enjoyment in the process of helping the unfortunates. We have some very good employees, as I said," stated Dr. Redwine.

"What is the worst part of the job?" asked Colonel Allen.

"The hopelessness and lack of caring, as often shown by state officials, is very discouraging. Because this asylum is overcrowded, it is difficult to see any progress. I can barely maintain just basic care. It is sad; so much more could be done. Any improvements get lost in the overwhelming numbers of patients."

Recognizing Dr. Redwine's despair, similar to what his father had experienced, Colonel Allen stated, "Hopefully, this investigation will help clarify things for you to do your job. Where do I interview Mr. Champion?"

"He is on Ward 15. He had come earlier to my office but I did not know where you were. He had to get back to his patients there."

"I'm sorry for not letting you know when I would be back," added Colonel Allen. "I just got interested in Mr. Reed's job."

Dr. Redwine said, "I'm sorry for our misunderstanding also. Now, let's see, if I take you on Ward 15, you could see the ward and get a chance to talk to him. I will leave you with him. All wards are locked, and he can help you get off the ward and back outside after you are finished."

"That is better; I'd like to see the ward." He was expecting to see a very unpleasant ward.

"Then you can come back to my office and I will show you the Administration Building. We are very proud of its beautiful ballroom."

"Oh, yes, let's do that!"

"I must warn you, experiences on the ward may not be pleasant," added Dr. Redwine.

"Well, we will see," Colonel Allen responded as they walked out of Dr. Redwine's office and toward the hallway leading to the locked wards. Instead of going to those wards, they went down a stairway into what looked like a basement. It was dark and musty. The floor consisted of bricks laid on dirt, and the ceiling was low.

"Colonel Allen, this leads to the kitchen, which was in the back of the female wards," Dr. Redwine said, pointing. "The kitchen is connected by this basement under the male and female wards. Trays of food are transported through this basement to the locked wards by dumbwaiters. The dumbwaiters provide a quicker way to get the warm food to the wards, much better than before."

"So you have warm food on each ward?" asked Colonel Allen.

"Oh, yes, we sure do. Now, we will go back under the original building, away from the other basement, under the male wards." Dr. Redwine pointed down another long basement hall.

"Is this a brick floor?" asked Colonel Allen while looking around.

"Yes, the bricks were laid by one of our lunatics. There are three male wards on each floor of this three-story building. The keepers live on their wards in adjoining rooms."

Colonel Allen was amazed at the size of the building as he observed others walking around. "Are they lunatics?" he asked.

"Oh yes," stated Dr. Redwine. "Those lunatics have earned yard privileges. I guess you saw the recent article about the death of our oldest patient, Sarah E. Norton. She was eighty-eight years old, admitted in 1845 at the age of twenty-seven; she had been here sixty-one years. She lived much longer by being here."

"Someone like her would have died younger through neglect if she had not gotten the proper care here, right?" asked Colonel Allen.

"Oh, yes. She was severely demented, but very sweet; everyone loved her. All the keepers favored her, and she enjoyed the special attention that she got here. We will all miss her smiling face. She was very childlike but able to follow directions."

"I see; the institution provided her with love and care that would not have been found in the community. Did she have family?"

"No, the family rejected her years ago," responded Dr. Redwine.

"Are there many like that here?" asked Colonel Allen.

"Yes, unfortunately there are many. Often families do not care for their lunatics, so we have many patients without families."

"I am really beginning to see the real purpose of any asylum," stated Colonel Allen.

"Yes, it is home for many who have no home or family," added Dr. Redwine. "Well, we are here at the stairway, leading to the top ward, 15. The first ward on this floor is 13, the next is 14, and 15 is on the top floor. We try to keep the worst cases on top floors, away from others."

They climbed the iron stairs. "Are these new?" asked Colonel Allen.

"Yes, these stairs recently replaced wooden ones. They are much safer in case of a fire." Dr. Redwine took out a large key and unlocked the door. It made a loud sound.

The ward was surprisingly quiet. The lunatics heard the key in the door and rushed to the door's entrance. They pushed to be greeted and made any noise to seek attention. The smell was not bad, and everything was neatly arranged.

Dr. Redwine gently patted each one and put his arm around some to prevent them from touching Colonel Allen. He called several by name, and they responded to the special attention.

"See, they tend to get excited when someone comes. They rarely have visitors. I see Mr. Champion over by the desk." They walked toward the back of the large ward. An ordinary-looking man in a white uniform came forward.

Colonel Allen noticed a big room with rows of what looked like wooden boxes the size of beds. The ward was surprisingly clean. Several lunatics followed him as he patted them.

"I'm R. R. Champion, sir; you are Colonel John R. Allen?"

"Yes, I am," Colonel Allen said, looking around at the surrounding lunatics, who were curious about the stranger. Some were feeling his clothes, and others were looking at his hat.

Dr. Redwine turned to Colonel Allen and said, "Sir, I will leave you here. If you need anything else, do not hesitate to let me know."

"Yes, Dr. Redwine, and thank you. I am glad that we understand each other better now," concluded Colonel Allen, while the lunatics continued to surround him.

"I still want to show you our beautiful ballroom after you finish here," Dr. Redwine said as he shook hands and left. Dr. Redwine was careful not to overlook any of the surrounding lunatics following him back to the door. It took him a while to reach the door, as each patient wanted to be patted on the head. He was careful not to neglect anyone.

"Colonel Allen, let's go over to my desk where we can talk," Champion said as he gently led him over to the side. "I might get interrupted, but if so, you can stay seated here."

Colonel Allen had expected some resentment from Champion over the interview, but the discussion turned out to be very pleasant. He asked, "You have fifty patients on this ward, is that correct?"

"Yes. Dr. Redwine had hoped to reduce that number, but there are too many new ones coming in. We have no empty beds unless someone dies. The beds are lined up against each other."

"Sir, I understand you hit Mr. Ketterer, causing blood on his head. Is that correct?"

"Oh yes, he was fighting with me, and I restrained him, causing an injury to his head. I did not mean to do that but it happened. He was difficult to restrain and was injured in the scuffle."

"Did you mean to hurt him?"

"Oh, I certainly did not! That day, he came at me and I had to restrain him. I tried to keep him tied in a chair, but he would often pull out. He always had bruises on his body from fighting me or others."

"How long have you worked here, sir?"

"I was appointed by Dr. W. F. Scott. Now, I know Dr. Scott made some serious mistakes, but he helped me by hiring me."

"What do you mean?"

"I took care of my father during his last years. He was injured in the Civil War, and my mother said he was never right after that. By the 1880s, he became much worse, and I took care of him. He was a fighter then, and I was the only one who could restrain him. Restraining him always calmed him down."

"So you had some personal experience before coming to work here?" asked Colonel Allen.

"Yes; after my father died, I had no purpose and just gave up on myself. Dr. Scott hired me, knowing that I had cared for my father for many years, and it really helped me."

"So you enjoy taking care of these people?" Colonel Allen asked while observing a confidence that he had not seen in the other keepers.

"Did you give your best to Mr. Ketterer?" Colonel Allen continued.

"Yes, I did. What happened was unfortunate, but it would have been much worse without my caring for him. He was difficult, and I know of no other methods that would have helped him. Medical science just cannot help people like him; he needed more than what is known here, but I did my best."

"Did you kill him?"

"No, sir; I accidentally caused an injury to his head, but he had many injuries, some from other lunatics who fought him if he was not restrained in his chair. There was no way to control him unless we locked him up in seclusion. I did not want that; locking him up would have been cruel. He was often better after being tied in the chair."

"You know that charges may be brought against you?"

"Yes, all I can do is to explain what happened."

"Do you have any witnesses?"

"Not of the actual event, since he was found dead. There are other officers and keepers who will testify for me."

"How about Mr. Claggett; is he a friend?"

"No, he is part of the new keepers who are always criticizing the experienced ones. I really do not think Mr. Claggett is very helpful; he is too critical of the patients."

"He does not always agree with you," stated Colonel Allen.

"He hasn't been here long enough to understand that there is a difference between idealism and the reality of this asylum. This ward is unpleasant at times. But some of the lunatics can learn; I try to teach them and reward their efforts. New employees expect instant results rather than a slow process of encouraging them to learn. They must be motivated to learn. I do the best I can."

All of a sudden, a lunatic ran over to him, choking. Champion grabbed him, bent him over, and hit him on his back. The lunatic spit out a piece of cookie and stopped choking. Champion turned him around, spoke kindly to him, and patted him. Then another lunatic ran over and started hitting the first one. Champion separated them, talked firmly to both while hugging each one separately. They went away in separate directions.

The noise on the ward returned to its usual quiet level as Champion redirected others who were upset over the incident. Throughout this whole incident, Champion showed concern to all who needed special attention. He returned to Colonel Allen.

"I'm sorry, Johnny is always grabbing food and then chokes on it. He is easily choked but always trusts me to help him. If he was on the outside, he would have died. Then the other one, Richard, was mad because Johnny took his cookie."

"Well," added Colonel Allen, "they trust you."

"Yes, they are like children, they just need someone to intervene for them. They depend on me to solve their problems. The other lunatics get upset over such incidents and need reassurance."

Colonel Allen was amazed by the incident; he stood up and stated, "I guess I have all the information I need. Feel free to call me if you have any questions."

"I guess I need to be worried, but I don't see that I did anything wrong. There was no other way. Do I need to worry?"

"Well, it may not be pleasant. My investigation will be turned over to the grand jury, and they will decide what to do."

"Do you think I might lose my job?"

"I don't know, but I can't see how this ward could function without you. You are an asset to the whole asylum."

"Thank you, sir, but Dr. Scott proved that all of us keepers are replaceable. However, caring keepers are really difficult to find, and politicians rarely understand that. These patients," he pointed to several on the ward, "don't trust just anyone. It took time for me to gain their trust, and any change would upset them."

"Thank you, sir. Could you show me out?"

"Yes, I have the key; we will walk down to the stairs, but I need to give out water before I go." Champion handed out water to everyone on the ward and assured them that he would be back soon.

Several lunatics followed both men to the door. Champion unlocked the door and waved to those remaining inside while they walked off the ward. Colonel Allen followed him down the stairs to the bottom of the stairway. Champion opened the door for Colonel Allen.

Pointing to another door across the grassy way on the left, Champion stated, "This is the back side of the Administration Building; you can go through that door. The stairway leading up will put you in the back of the hallway, to Dr. Redwine's office."

"Thank you, I think I can find my way," Colonel Allen said. There were screened porches and two octagonal buildings off the back of a three-story building. Many lunatics were screaming from the screen porches.

"If you are interested, those wards on the right are female wards," Champion said. "They were built in the late 1880s, as you might know, but the male wards are in this original building."

"Yes, Dr. Redwine told me. What are these buildings in front of us?"

"That is the kitchen below with a keeper's dining room on the next floor and sewing room on the top floor. Further back is the vegetable room and storage for our fuel, which is coal. The smoke stack is at the end, and the coal is burned in that back room."

"This is a big place," Colonel Allen remarked.

Champion continued, "I understand there used to be a fence back here where patients could gain fresh air, but that is no more. Now, they just stay on stuffy wards. I just wish the politicians could understand our need for better facilities."

"Yes, it would certainly help you to do your job; again thank you for your time," Colonel Allen said as he left. He stood and stared at the other large buildings.

As he listened to the screams from the other wards, he realized that Champion's ward had been much quieter, although it is a much more difficult ward. Colonel Allen wondered why the wards were so different.

He couldn't help but speculate about the small octagonal-shaped additions on the back of the buildings, as he walked by. *I wonder what those octagonal rooms provide.* The old buildings and their history was fascinating despite other sounds of screams.

He went into the designated door and spotted McElroy, Dr. Redwine's secretary

"Sir, is Dr. Redwine available?"

"No, he was called over to the Infirmary; a patient has become seriously ill, and Dr. Redwine has been checking on him regularly."

Colonel Allen knew about the Dr. B. W. Dudley Infirmary, which had been built about six years ago. It was named for Dr. Benjamin Winslow Dudley. He was a very influential physician in the early years of the asylum and the previous Transylvania Medical School. Recognizing the name, he said, "My father knew Dr. Dudley and had a great deal of respect for him. The Infirmary is used for medical cases?"

"Yes, the physically sick are isolated from the other patients, especially when there is an epidemic. It is a very nice infirmary with the most up-to-date equipment," added McElroy. "However, it is getting crowded."

Dr. Redwine had returned from the Infirmary and came upon McElroy and Colonel Allen talking. "Well, I'm pleased that I am free before you left, Colonel Allen; now I can show you the ballroom."

"Yes, I would like that." They continued walking toward the front of the Administration Building door. "But tell me more about the Infirmary; what do you hope to accomplish with a separate place?" asked Colonel Allen.

"Well, we isolate the more serious cases with physical problems, and it is helpful with epidemics. As you know, there have been several epidemics at this asylum, and it is most important to isolate them, keeping them away from the others."

They stopped at the front of the Administration Building, and Dr. Redwine turned for them to go up the beautiful oak stairway. Colonel Allen followed.

"Do the lunatics get well from the Infirmary or just die there?" asked Colonel Allen as they reached the first landing.

"I hope they can get well, but unfortunately, most die there. I'm hoping to implement homeopathic methods following some of the teachings of Dr. Hering and the earlier writings of Dr. Hahnemann, the German physician."

"That is interesting," replied Colonel Allen.

"All the remedies in homeopathic medicine are made from natural ingredients."

"Yes, I've heard of recent developments in homeopathy," added Colonel Allen. He observed the large rooms on the second landing as they continued walking.

Dr. Redwine continued, "Homeopathy was used during three recent devastating cholera epidemics, and they had fewer deaths than those treated in allopathic hospitals." Dr. Redwine's eyes lighted up as he enthusiastically explained his plans for the Infirmary. "Oh, yes, these are apartments for the medical staff," he said, pointing to the surrounding rooms. "We will go up to the top floor."

They took another set of stairs from the second landing to the third floor. At the top of the third floor, they walked into a large room. It had walnut paneling with a beautiful chandelier in the center of the room. There were full-length windows, and the space was large enough to allow over five hundred people to attend. A bandstand was at the rear of the room. They walked around. It was breathtaking.

"This is beautiful!" exclaimed Colonel Allen.

"Yes, it is. The windows can be opened up to provide full circulation of air," added Dr. Redwine. "As you might know, weekly balls were always a part of this asylum."

"Yes, I attended one a few years ago when they were in Megowan Hall; it was more in the back of the original building and much smaller," added Colonel Allen.

"The asylum was left money by a patient, James S. Megowan, to provide funds for recreation. Some of that money paid for the early Megowan Hall. It also paid for finishing this ballroom. As you know, the state will not pay for any recreation since it is considered a waste on lunatics, but the ballroom is used weekly."

"I would think it would help them," added Colonel Allen.

"Yes, it does. The early Board of Commissioners invested the money and it has continued to grow to provide this asylum with recreation funds that the State of Kentucky would not pay."

"Do the citizens of Lexington still attend the balls?"

"Yes, some still do. They understand the value of weekly balls for the lunatics, who must work for the privilege to attend. However, the local support is much less than in the past; I hope that will improve. The weekly balls are very important to the lunatics," added Dr. Redwine.

"Yes, I can remember that it did mean a lot to the lunatics. Each time I attended, they were well dressed and very appropriate." Colonel Allen did not wish to reveal his reasons for not attending more often.

"We work with them to be appropriate and remove them from the ball if they display unacceptable behaviors. Most work hard for the privilege to attend the ball," Dr. Redwine said.

As they were walking around, Colonel Allen noticed a woman cleaning the dressing rooms. "Is she a lunatic?" he asked.

"Yes, that is Rosie; she has lived here since 1889 and was a housekeeper in previous jobs. Her mania causes her to lose jobs, and then she has no place to live. She is a good worker when she is not having a manic attack."

"So she lives here?"

"Yes; if she becomes manic, she is allowed time off from her job and her place to live is still available for her. When she improves, she enjoys keeping this area clean and is amply rewarded."

Both men started toward the back exit. Colonel Allen observed a long metal slide leading from a back window, down to the ground outside. It looked steep and dangerous. "What is this?" he asked.

Dr. Redwine responded, "That is our fire escape. However, many young people enjoy sliding down it for fun. We have had several fires here and devised this in the unfortunate event of a fire. Fire is always a concern for us in our buildings." Both men looked at the backyard of the institution. "We now have four water lines from the city in case of a fire."

Colonel Allen observed the two octagonal buildings that he had seen earlier. "What are those two buildings for? They are too small for a ward or office."

"Those are two remaining water closets; several were constructed when the three-story building was built around 1866."

"Were the water closets outside of the building?"

"Yes, it was the newest method of getting the water closet smell off of the wards. They were the best possible method at the time, but they are no longer needed. They are now storage rooms," stated Dr. Redwine.

"After the institution was connected to the Lexington water system and water was more available, bathrooms with running water were added inside all buildings. The octagonal buildings were the most modern at the time," added Dr. Redwine.

Colonel Allen was musing over what Dr. Redwine was saying while amazed over his knowledge of the facility and the patients. He wondered how long it would take for someone to become so wise about the institution; he also realized how much Dr. Redwine's experience was needed here.

After some time, they came down the stairway and stopped at the front of the Administration Building. "Sir, thank you so much for showing me around," Colonel Allen said. "I have learned so much." He slowly tipped his hat and shook hands.

Colonel Allen was leaving the grounds when he decided to drive his carriage around to the farm's barn in the back. The barn was past the original building to the back and on the right. He parked his carriage in front of the barn and walked in. There were three male patients grooming horses while others were bringing in crops for the kitchen. Colonel Allen noticed Reed interacting kindly with the patients. As he walked closer, Reed was directing others to load a wagon. He went over and greeted Reed while asking, "May I ask what they were doing?"

"They are loading sawdust into a cart," Reed said as they shook hands.

"Why sawdust?" asked Colonel Allen.

"There are sawdust beds in several of the wards, including Ward 15. They are used for patients who soil their beds. It reduces the smell and the need to change sheets often for agitated patients who must be confined to a bed."

"Oh, I remember seeing them on Ward 15. I didn't know what they were; they appeared to be boxes. Isn't that cruel to sleep on?"

"No, they are comfortable and cleaner than any other methods we have. I make sure there is a fresh supply each week within the institution and it is available to the keepers for their wards. Unfortunately, some keepers don't bother with the sawdust, and their wards smell badly."

"Oh, how interesting," stated Colonel Allen.

"And Mr. Champion always is very expedient with getting sawdust on his ward."

"You have a unique job. I wonder, is Captain Charlton Hunt Morgan still living?"

"Yes, he is in his late sixties and lives in the old Hunt house. He told me about his disagreement between the board and Dr. Chenault, the superintendent. Captain Hunt Morgan got caught in the usual crossfire with Kentucky state government. He had a government job with the US Revenue Department many years previously. It was a much more stable job than his asylum job; there was much less politics involved."

"And you are not concerned for your job?"

"No, I can always find another job. I would be sorry because I like this job, but so far, I have not had problems."

Colonel Allen shook hands with Reed and invited him to his home for supper. He gave him the address with the expectation that they would compare family histories in the future.

Colonel Allen returned to his office and prepared to present his investigation results to the grand jury. He was aware that this would be the first time that criminal charges would be brought against employees during the history of that institution. He believed that the legal process would be fair.

The presiding judge, Watts Parker, opened court in the Lexington Courthouse on October 2. He told the grand jury of local citizens, "You should decide whether the conditions of the asylum are as reported. If patients have been subjected to the reported cruel treatment, then no mercy should be shown to the guilty parties."

On October 17, the grand jury charged all four employees with the death of Ketterer. Three of the four employees never went to trial; the charges were dropped due to the difficult conditions of employees for the number of patients. Because R. R. Champion was the supervisor on Ward 15, he went to trial on October 24. After he testified, the jury dismissed all the charges against him while many praised him for his work. Colonel Allen gladly signed the papers on that day.

While the new Board of Control did not succeed in criminally charging employees with murder, they did succeed at focusing their blame on Dr. Redwine and the past Board of Commissioners. The new Board of Control continued the process of blaming the past without looking at the present problems of constantly changing employees. They showed no mercy for Dr. Redwine, even though he had tried to improve the facility for seven years.

Archives of the Kentucky Lunatic Asylum show that Dr. Redwine (1900–1907) was the tenth serving superintendent after Dr. Chipley (1855–1870). Of the previous superintendents since Dr. Chipley, Dr. Redwine was one of two employed with the longest length of time (the average length of time was 3.3 years) since Dr. Chipley. These statistics reflect the instability that citizens of Lexington had observed as they saw employees going and coming.

Colonel Allen became angry when he heard about the smugness that the new Board of Control members demonstrated in their criticisms. He asked his law partner, Henry, as they were leaving the courthouse, "When will the politicians stop interfering with that institution? While they use the facility for their own political purposes, they blame the dedicated employees. Why does the public tolerate it?"

"No one understands it. My father still writes about 'the spoils system of office holders' in his weekly letters to the paper. Yet, politicians just assume that what they do is always for the best. How naive. Actually, they do what is best for themselves," Henry said as they walked across Short Street to their office.

"I just have trouble with what I see; this is why I went into law instead of medicine; at least as a lawyer, I can try to challenge the politicians," Colonel Allen argued as he followed his partner.

"Yes, and we must continue to challenge or question those in power or it will never stop," added Henry.

Colonel Allen stated, "My father enjoyed the caring part of medicine but left when he could find no solutions. He never found a way to challenge the current politicians, so he moved on. As a lawyer, I can question the misuse of power in a court of law. It is a small part, but I have done it."

"Yes, Colonel, you have done your part, you made sure that one caring employee did not get caught in the political spoils system, a Mr. R. R. Champion. You may not have saved Dr. Redwine or the institution, but there is still one caring keeper who is able to work there," smiled Henry. "That was your part." They arrived at their office and went inside.

"Yes, Mr. Champion might be fired next year," laughed Colonel Allen as he hung up his hat. "Since he has no job protection, the next superintendent might not keep him. While the politicians blame their failures on the past, they need to look at themselves and how their political interference creates instability within the facility."

"That's true," Henry agreed as he was sorting through his mail.

"Is this only typical in Kentucky?" asked Colonel Allen as he continued with the subject.

"No, it happens in every state where political power is not challenged. While Kentucky has its share, other states have done similar things, within different institutions. Human nature is the same in every state, and it occurs where the desire for power is unquestioned," replied Henry Duncan.

"Has such political power controlled all of Kentucky's state institutions?" Colonel Allen continued.

"That has varied. Of the three early major institutions that I know about in Lexington, the Transylvania Medical School, Law Department, and the asylum, I believe the asylum has suffered the most severely in our time. The continuously changing of superintendents and employees has made it difficult for any stability there."

"Well, at least I did find some very caring employees in that first Kentucky asylum. The saga of the people and practices in those institutions need to be told," Colonel Allen said as he departed from Henry's office.

*   *   *

To summarize the importance of this opening chapter about Kentucky's first asylum, there were three changes that occurred in 1906. First, the Board of Commissioners, who ran the facility from its beginning, consisted of volunteer leaders from the local community and they met regularly at the facility. That board was replaced in 1906 by the Board of Control with paid political appointees having offices in Kentucky state government and control over all three state asylums. Since the focus was no longer on just one facility, the local citizens were very concerned. Yet, state officials claimed that improvements would come by treating all three asylums the same. This was symbolic of decisions that continued to be made for the facility.

Second, whereas the former Board of Commissioners assumed that employees were doing the best they could and death was a natural outcome of a patient's preexisting, chronic poor health, the new Board of Control took a more punitive approach. They began looking for scapegoats among employees when a patient died, bringing criminal charges against them. This drastic change resulted in four employees being legally charged in the 1906 death. Local citizens, as members of a grand jury, decided that the four employees were innocent because they worked on a ward with the most difficult and dysfunctional patients in the facility. While the local citizens recognized that the current employee/patient ratio of 4/50 was inadequate, the Board of Control insisted on firing the superintendent over that patient's death and established a pattern of blaming employees.

Third, Colonel Allen, as the local attorney general in 1906, was the first to conduct a grand jury investigation into the facility. He grew up knowing his father's difficulties as the first superintendent but came to realize the real care that had historically occurred in that facility. Although Colonel Allen was politically astute, he had difficulty accepting the political arrogance and control that he saw occurring within the first asylum, a sample of political conflicts within the facility.

These three changes were significant to the administration of that facility, while the prologue will start with chapter 2.

Sources for Chapter 1

Annual Reports of Eastern Kentucky Lunatic Asylum. *Legislative Documents*. Frankfort, Kentucky: 1881, 1883, 1892, 1900, 1901.

Annual Reports of the State Board of Control for Charitable Institutions. *Legislative Documents*. Frankfort, KY: 1907–1908, 1909–1911, 1911–1913.

Armstrong, David, and Armstrong, Elizabeth. *The Great American Medicine Show*. New York: Prentice Hall, 1991.

Bolin, James. *Bossism and Reform in a Southern City, Lexington, Kentucky 1880-1940*. Lexington, Kentucky: University of Kentucky Press, 2000.

Coleman, J. Winston. *The Squire's Sketches of Lexington* Lexington, Kentucky: The Henry Clay Press, 1972.

Collins, Lewis. *History of Kentucky, Vol. II.* 1924. Found in Lexington library. First published 1874.

Deese, Wynelle. *Lexington, Kentucky: Changes in the Early Twentieth Century*. Charleston, South Carolina: Arcadia Press, 1998.

Deutsch, Albert. *The Mentally Ill in America: A History of their Care and Treatment from Colonial Times*. New York: Doubleday, Doran, 1937.

Harrison, L. H. *Kentucky's Governors 1792-1985*. Lexington, Kentucky: University of Kentucky Press, 1985.

Lancaster, Clay. *Vestiges of the Venerable City: A Chronicle of Lexington, Kentucky*. Cincinnati, Ohio: C. J. Krehbiel, 1978.

Lexington Herald. "Grand Jury." October 17, 1906.

Lexington Herald. "Irregularities at E.K.L.A." October 2, 1906.

Lexington Herald. "Irregularities, Including Murder, at EKLA." October 2, 1906.

Lexington Herald. "Ketterer State Suit with Dr. J.S. Redwine." February 26, 1907.

Lexington Herald. "Sketches of Eastern Kentucky Lunatic Asylum." August 25, 1909.

Lexington Leader. "Asylum." January 24, 1897.

Lexington Leader. "Asylum Changes." June 1, 1900.

Lexington Leader. "Dr. Scott." January 30, 1897.

Lexington Leader. "Dr. Scott." February 4, 1897.

Lexington Leader. "Patients." July 3, 1898.

Lexington Leader. "Semi-Annual Inspection of the Eastern Kentucky Asylum." Lexington, Kentucky May 17, 1901.

Lexington Transcript. "The asylum Racket." October 1, 1886.

Lexington Transcript. "The Lexington Imbroglio." October 20, 1885.

Peter, Robert. *The History of the Medical Department of Transylvania University.* Filson Club Publications, No. 20. Louisville, Kentucky: John P. Morton, 1905.

Peter, Robert, ed., and William H. Perrin. "Data about John R. Allen." Easley, South Carolina: Southern Historical Press, 1979.

Scull, A. *Madhouses, Mad-Doctors, and Madmen: The Social History of Psychiatry in the Victorian Era*. Philadelphia: University of Pennsylvania Press, 1981.

Superintendent's Reports for Drs. Chenault, Clark, Redwine, Wiley, and Scott were found in the local history collection. Individual reports by each superintendent were originally filed in the Kentucky Archives, Frankfort, Kentucky.

White, Ronald. *A Dialogue on Madness: Eastern State Lunatic Asylum and Mental Health Policies in Kentucky 1824–1883*. Doctoral dissertation, filed at University of Kentucky, 1984.

Chapter Two

———◆━◆◆◆━◆———

1817–1823

Further south of Lexington on the Old Buffalo Trail, two men were riding north toward the Kentucky River, approaching the Fayette County line. The older rider was the sheriff of Fayette County; the younger one was a new deputy. They were returning to Lexington after delivering a message to the previous governor of Kentucky, Isaac Shelby, whose home and farm was near Danville, Kentucky, in Mercer County. Mercer County was on the Halls Gap extension of the Buffalo Trail.

The Old Buffalo Trail led to the small village of Lexington through the wilderness of Kentucky. The trail originated from the northern settlement of Limestone and continued through the north side of Lexington, which was the largest settlement in the county of Fayette, and went on to the southwestern part of Kentucky. The trail was a vital road for pioneers to move through Kentucky. By the year 1817, the trail had been in use for centuries by the Indians. It varied in width from twelve to twenty feet and became a major passage for commercial trade to the settlement. The trail through the growing settlement of Lexington became known as Mulberry Street.

"We head northwest after leaving Danville," the sheriff explained to the deputy, pointing up the trail, "and we go northeast after we are past Harrodsburg." He continued to watch the trail and observe the young deputy, who was very experienced with a gun.

"Yes, I see," the new deputy said, patting his horse. "I will learn. I see how the old path curves that way." They continued on their journey.

After leaving the governor's office in 1816, Isaac Shelby maintained political connections with the Fayette County officers, and different sheriffs often made trips to Danville to deliver messages to him.

Now, the younger deputy would be doing that job as the sheriff's duties required more time in the Lexington settlement.

"You say you are new to Kentucky?" asked the sheriff.

"Yes, I came from New England; my family has a farm there but I wanted to see the real frontier. So I moved here."

"You sure are good with a gun," added the sheriff.

"I have always practiced with my gun on the farm, but it was just for protection from wild animals, not Indians."

"We all had hoped Kentucky would be free from Indians by now," added the sheriff. "We can only assume that they have moved on since none have been reported in this area for a while."

"I like the woods, trees, and mountains. Being a deputy, I get out into the wilderness to see the county. It is really beautiful land, and the weather is mild here, compared to New England."

"Yes, Kentucky usually has mild winters. This is the 15th of January, and there is still no snow on the ground."

"Do you know what the message was that we delivered to Governor Shelby?" asked the deputy.

"Well, I'm usually aware of the message, since it is usually known in Lexington before I deliver it," added the sheriff.

"I did not know if it was proper for me to ask."

"Former Governor Shelby is usually notified of important events, such as when Governor George Madison died last year. That was not unexpected, though, he was in poor health when elected."

"I wonder why he ran for elected office when he was in poor health?" asked the deputy.

"Well, George Madison was a war hero, and he was elected for his heroism. The lieutenant governor assumed his duties. Isaac Shelby had already been notified when I delivered the message of his election last year, but most messages are out of respect to Shelby."

The sheriff puzzled over whether to trust this new deputy. He had not yet proved his loyalty to Kentucky. Special messages to former governor Isaac Shelby had become a tradition because he was so highly respected in Kentucky.

"So these messages are usually just public knowledge?"

"Well, not so much public, but they are not secrets that you will be expected to die for," said the sheriff.

"So have you delivered any really dangerous messages that you might get killed for?" asked the deputy.

"No, I've never had any attempts on my life except for the dangers of traveling through the wilderness."

The deputy continued pushing for answers; he asked, "Were the messages today as important as some of your others?"

"Well, I guess I can tell you about the messages that we delivered today," he said. After wondering about the deputy's insistence, the sheriff concluded that he was just one of those pushy Yankees. As they continued on their horses, the sheriff said, "One message was telling Governor Shelby about the incorporation of Fayette Hospital, the first hospital west of the Allegheny Mountains, in Lexington."

"Why does the settlement need a hospital?" asked the deputy.

"A public hospital is needed for those who have no money or family to pay for their care."

"Yes, but all this just for a hospital?"

"Well, it is important because Lexington is growing."

"I guess so."

"The other message," the sheriff continued, "was that John W. Hunt and other Lexington citizens have established the Lexington–Louisville Turnpike Road Company, the first in the state. The turnpike company will purchase a roadway such as this old trail, make improvements, and charge those who use the road. That will improve transportation around Lexington. So you see, the messages are not secret but they are important."

"So is that what most messages are like?" asked the deputy.

"Mostly, there is nothing serious. Your greatest danger is this land and the wild animals. But you are so good with a gun, you will be all right on your own," stated the sheriff. They stopped, unsaddled the horses, and walked on the Buffalo Trail, holding the reins to give the horses some relief as they continued on.

"I really liked seeing the settlement of Harrodsburg. I had heard of it in New England as the first settlement into Kentucky. Now, I have seen it."

"Well, it is really just shabby little cabins. There are no real brick houses there," commented the sheriff. "But have you ever seen such a fine house as Governor Shelby's?"

"Yes, there are brick mansions like that in New England. I could not believe it being in the wilderness, by itself." Both men moved more slowly on the trail.

"They call it 'Traveler's Rest.' I have been there several times, and each time, I am amazed at the beauty of it; it was built out by itself on a trail as a retreat for those traveling," stated the sheriff.

As they continued to travel northeast, they came upon the deep cliffs along the Kentucky River. It was slow going. But the views were beautiful, and both observed the area. The new deputy was in awe of the beauty of the place. This was his second time to view the area; the first time was at the beginning of this trip, and he still could not believe the unspoiled beauty of this place. He kept looking around. The deep cliffs around the river were undescribably beautiful.

The sheriff stated, "We need to walk the horses down these deep cliffs to the river, and then we'll wait for the ferry to take us across the river. Be careful, these cliffs are difficult, and we must stay on the path down to the Kentucky River."

The deputy was quiet as he carefully led his horse down to the bottom.

The sheriff gently spoke so as to not interfere with the serenity of the area. "I have always walked my horse down this path, even though he has been here many times. He can still fall. I've seen many an experienced rider fall because they misjudged the dangerousness of this path. We must continue slowly."

They walked down carefully with their horses behind, following each other. The river at the bottom was cool and serene with beautiful green-blue water.

"Yea, I see what you mean," stated the younger one as they reached the bottom of the cliffs. "This is really dangerous down these cliffs." The new deputy appreciated having the sheriff show him the way and said so.

The sheriff was always uncomfortable with compliments, so he continued, "That sure was a grand house, Isaac Shelby's, but there are many nice houses in Lexington." He looked at the high northern terrain of the cliffs on the opposite side of the river.

The deputy responded, "Yes, I have seen several brick homes and factories there."

The sheriff said, "Yes, there are three tobacco factories, four couch factories, several gun powder mills, and a lead factory for casting iron and brass in that small town."

"I also heard there's a university there?"

"Yes, Transylvania University has established a public school and seminary of learning. It has continued to grow with a law department and medical school. While both are small, they will grow into great schools," the sheriff stated proudly.

In the small settlement of Lexington, Kentucky, a university was established before 1817. A law department and medical school were formalized after specific libraries were purchased. Up to this time, the law department had had five successive professors to offer legal instruction at the postgraduate level, unusual for that time. While the law department's role in early American legal education was important, it was limited due to the small numbers of students; legal education was not a necessity in the frontier of Kentucky, but it would be later.

The medical school had followed a different course. The early medical school had two professors and that number increased in 1817 to six, with Dr. Benjamin Dudley becoming the mainstay of the department for many years. The first medical degree was awarded the following year. Classes grew from twenty to sixty. They met in the homes of the professors and at Trotter's storehouse on the corner of Mill and Main Streets.

"So will the ferryboat take us across the river again?" the deputy asked as they rested at the bottom of the cliffs.

"Yes, the ferry will return from the other side; we'll wait here at this landing. Kentucky has many rivers with ferry boats; you will get used to them." The river was absolutely grand and magnificent, and they stared at it silently for a few moments. The sheriff continued, "I always enjoy seeing this river."

Returning back to the previous conversation, the deputy asked, "When was Isaac Shelby's house built?"

"It was built when Kentucky was still part of Virginia. Oh, I remember that time, it was just four years ago and we still had problems with the Indians," added the sheriff.

"I read that Governor Isaac Shelby helped get rid of the Indians."

"I served with Shelby in 1813 when he met the British troops with the Shawnees on the Thames River. The Shawnee chief was killed and the British troops surrendered. That was when Shelby became a hero to Kentuckians. We would still be having difficulty with Indians if he had not succeeded. Now, all we have now to worry about are the politicians," the sheriff said, chuckling to himself.

Both men stood together, waiting quietly for the ferry. It soon arrived and they led their horses onto it, signaling to the ferry driver that they were ready. The deputy commented on how pleased he was to be in Kentucky. The sheriff was glad to hear that.

Both men sat in silence as they moved from one side of the river to the other. The water was so pure. They paid the ferry owner and led their horses north up a narrow trail through more deep cliffs. They soon reached the top and stopped to rest with their horses. They mounted their horses and continued on the Buffalo Trail toward Lexington. The sheriff was growing more comfortable with the new deputy.

The sheriff continued, "I started as a deputy like you after the war, because I knew how to shoot a gun and ride a horse. I didn't get much education living in the wilderness, but I can read and know that law and order is the only way a settlement can grow. Now that I have been promoted to sheriff, political and social connections have become more of the job. I'm not much of a politician but I like meeting people, talking to them, letting them know we are here."

The younger man chuckled and agreed. "I'm glad to be a deputy. I am really learning to like this land, it is beautiful and hilly." He continued to look around.

Both men were silent for a while, and then the younger one stated, "Do I see some buzzards over there, off the trail? See, over there near that larger tree, in the bushes?"

"Well, I think so." The older man stopped his horse, got off, and fired his gun into the ground nearby.

"Do you see vultures in the sky?"

"Yes, I do. I need to scare the snakes away through that thick brush, then we can go over to where they are settling."

"There must be something dead, there," stated the deputy.

"I would assume it is probably some dead animal that the buzzards are after, but we need to check into it since we are now in Fayette County. This is our area."

"I thought snakes were gone in colder weather; do you need to scare them away this time of year?" asked the deputy.

"Well, I just never take chances, just a habit. I guess that is why I'm still living after serving in several battles." The sheriff walked toward a tall tree where the buzzards were circling a dying woman. Her energy was spent as she cried out.

The scene under the tree was gruesome. Both men dismounted their horses, carefully and slowly, in disbelief. Blood was everywhere. They looked around, aware that there could still be others around who had done this gruesome act. They searched for other people with their guns pulled and found none except for the one woman at the scene.

At the bottom of the tree was a woman around the age of thirty. She was malnourished, barefooted, and partly clothed; she had a wild look of fear. She had been talking to herself, yelling, cursing, and tearing at her clothes. Her wild, frenzied manner was becoming more sluggish as death was approaching her.

The two men walked toward the woman, who attempted to run

from them but her strength was gone, and she could only whimper as they looked at her. The loss of blood was too much and death was obviously near. They could only watch in frustration as she was fast approaching it.

She looked at them, but she was not really there. She could only whimper, and then, there was no response. Some of her blood was still wet, but it was quickly drying. It was a gruesome scene.

Both watched in silence as she finally drew her last breath. They fired their guns again to chase away the vultures as the woman laid there. Her death came as a final relief to this bizarre scene.

The younger deputy responded, "Gosh, what happened to her? I see no gun, bullet, or weapon. She acted like a lunatic."

The sheriff responded, "She probably was." He stepped over to her and nudged her lightly with his heel. She did not move. "I guess she is dead. She must have pulled parts of her arms and legs enough to cause severe bleeding. I see no other reason for the blood." He continued to search the bloody scene for clues. "I cannot find any evidence that another person has been here. Just her; she did it to herself. I have seen this before."

They continued to search for any other person or animal having been around. The sheriff concluded, "She came to this location in some wild frenzy, manic behavior, attacking herself and finally bled to death." He went back to his horse and got a blanket, saying, "We need to pack up her body and return it to Lexington."

The deputy remained silent while surveying the scene. He had never seen such a scene. His lips became dry, and he had difficulty swallowing.

The sheriff continued to shoot into the air to scare away the vultures. "I guess they will lose their meal for now, but there will be more. I have seen too many of these deaths." He wrapped her body in a blanket. Picking up the blanket was easy, since the body was frail. He put the body wrapped in the blanket over his saddle.

The young deputy still had a sick feeling in his stomach and waited a few minutes to respond. "How do we know she came from Lexington? There are many small villages around." He tried to hide his queasy feelings.

The sheriff stated, "We don't know, but Lexington is the largest town;

someone might be able to identify her. She was poorly clothed and dirty; she was probably run out of town."

They were both silent until the deputy asked, "Why would someone do that to her?"

"If people cannot care for themselves, Kentucky law gives the settlements permission to force them out. They often go into the wilderness to kill themselves or be killed by wildlife." The sheriff's voice choked and cracked, betraying his feelings. "She was not bad looking either."

"Don't the people in the settlement know she could get killed in the wilderness?"

"Many settlements just run them out of town so as not to give them any public support. Everyone has to support themselves or else leave, that is the law."

The sheriff continued talking, knowing that his deputy was having difficulty understanding. "There are often many such people in the woods, and some do survive. Others are humiliated over not being able to care for themselves in the settlements and do not wish to survive." Both men continued silently toward Lexington. Both men contemplated their next steps as they got closer to civilization.

They saw the tobacco warehouses and carriages increase as they approached the settlement. The sheriff started talking about Lexington, saying, "The number of carriages here are twice the number of any similar settlement in the United States. Lexington is considered the largest and wealthiest town west of the Allegheny Mountains except for New Orleans, and it is the manufacturing center for the Western Country."

The sheriff continued, "I remember just ten years ago when Lexington had only about fifty houses, mostly frame and hewn logs. My parents moved here in 1788, two years before I was born. It was still part of Virginia then."

The young deputy stated, "I'm new to the area but I expect to make this my home. I like this area."

"Yes, it has been a good place for me."

The deputy asked, "Where do we take the body? Do we go to your office, the jail, or the undertaker?"

"I have always taken these bodies to the jail, first."

"That's on Short Street, right? Next to Luke Usher's Tavern?" asked the deputy.

"Yes," answered the sheriff, "the jail has always been on the northwest corner of Short Street since I have been here. The undertakers don't want these bodies because they can't make any money on them. Most families will not claim such a body; if they do, they have to pay for the burial."

"Why not?" asked the deputy. "They deserve to be buried too."

"Families usually never claim bodies of dishonored relatives. There is the shame and the expense. I will lock up the body until we can dispose of it; the cell will smell but the other prisoners will never know the difference. They all smell as well," responded the sheriff.

"So why are you even keeping the body since you don't expect anyone to claim it?" asked the deputy.

"I just want to make sure, but if nobody turns up in a few days, I will turn the body over to that Transylvania Medical School. They will take it. They are always looking for bodies to study."

"I heard that they are always asking for bodies; why?"

The sheriff sputtered and scratched his head. "For study, they say. They keep bodies to study and then dispose of them later."

Transylvania University's Medical Department included Drs. Dudley, Overton, Blythe, Drake, Richardson, and Brown, and the school anticipated more growth. Transylvania University was separated into an academy and a college. The academy was a preparatory department for students inadequately trained in the basic studies. The college consisted of liberal arts with further training in either law or medicine.

The curriculum was similar to those in eastern colleges. Besides a strict curriculum, the trustees paid close attention to daily schedules, examinations, and a student's behavior. At the end of each session, all students were to be publicly examined in the presence of the trustees. A great deal of emphasis was placed on public speaking, and seniors were required to present public orations.

The next day, the sheriff asked around town to see if anyone knew the woman they had found. He visited the homes of some major leaders of the city: Thomas January, Adam Rankin, George Trotter Jr., Thomas Pindell, and John W. Hunt. The first three were early settlers in the area. Pindell's father, Dr. Richard Pindell, had been a surgeon in the Revolutionary War and married Elizabeth Hart of Fayette County; he was a second generation in the settlement of Lexington. John W. Hunt arrived in the late 1700s as a young man to make his fortune, which he did. Each person listened sympathetically to the sheriff's description of the woman, but none knew her.

The sheriff visited Andrew McCalla, who ran the drugstore on Short Street, facing Cheapside. Andrew knew everyone in Lexington and most everything that went on in the settlement. He practiced herbal medicine for the majority of the local people. Most citizens preferred to visit McCalla rather than physicians, who were viewed as educated butchers or bloodsuckers, but certainly not healers.

The trustees of Transylvania Medical School believed differently. They and the professors viewed education as the only way to change a negative view toward physicians, and they worked toward that goal. Although McCalla believed in herbal medicines and did not trust the physician's medicine, he remained friends with those who believed differently.

The sheriff always enjoyed talking with McCalla. His memory of the past was very clear, and his participation in civic affairs was well known. He had helped many of the local lunatics by giving them herbs. The sheriff asked him if he knew the dead woman.

"No," answered McCalla. "I have not seen her in this area. It is a shame that there was no place for her care. Didn't you use to take some lunatics to the state hospital in Williamsburg, Virginia?"

"No, I never did, it was just too far to cross the Appalachian Mountains and fight the Indians. To take a lunatic there, the trip would require more than one sheriff, and that was too much time away from the settlement for two. The previous sheriff tried it but found it too difficult."

"Well, I am hoping to have a public hospital here in Lexington soon," McCalla said. "A group of local citizens has incorporated the Fayette Hospital this year to accommodate the lunatics and other distempered or sick poor."

"Yes, I have heard. Where will the money come from for the building?" asked the sheriff.

"We plan to have a lottery to raise money for the land, and other contributors will build the facility."

"Well," responded the sheriff, "I hope you can raise the needed money."

"Our city needs such a public charity for paupers and lunatics. That dead woman might have gotten the care she needed instead of dying in the woods." McCalla showed his usual enthusiasm for his projects.

"I wish you luck with that charity. It is certainly needed," the sheriff said, realizing he needed to leave.

The sheriff loved to talk to McCalla but he needed to hurry on. After excusing himself, the sheriff continued his investigation. No one had identified the dead woman by the end of the week.

Rev. Stephen Chipley was reviewing his sermon for this Sunday's service. He was the minister of a small but growing Methodist church, where some of the city leaders attended. His only son, William Stout Chipley, was seven years old and went with his mother, Amelia, to the church to meet in the church's study. Rev. Chipley and his son spent hours in the study while his wife went shopping.

The church study held many books that fascinated the young boy. Some of the books were difficult for his reading level but he occupied himself by flipping through the pages. There were many books of Methodist theology; one of his father's favorites was John Wesley's *Primitive Physic*. While this book was published in the middle 1700s, it was still prized by Rev. Chipley. It identified herbs for treating illnesses and discouraged the use of physicians.

Rev. Chipley often preached that medical care was better achieved by herb remedies, not by the care of a physician. But at this Sunday church meeting, Rev. Chipley was going to talk about caring for the unfortunates in Lexington. Lexington had followed the custom of "warning out," or making those who could not take care of themselves leave the community rather than providing for them. That custom was particularly disturbing to Rev. Chipley; he thought it was cruel and unconscionable in the wilderness of Kentucky. He had vigorously opposed this custom in his sermons. The discovery of the woman's body in the woods this past week was a sign to Rev. Chipley that it must be stopped.

The next morning, the sheriff returned to his office next to the courthouse. Two deputies reported to the sheriff that some citizens were concerned about bodies being taken from the local cemetery. These rumors included that a new physician at the Transylvania Medical College was having his medical students take bodies from the local cemetery to use in teaching. The sheriff knew that Dr. Dudley was supposed to be taking only bodies of paupers, but he wanted to talk to him. He would agree to provide unclaimed bodies for teaching to Dr. Dudley if he would agree not to bother the local cemetery.

Since the sheriff was satisfied that no one in Lexington claimed the dead woman found in the wilderness, he had decided to take the body to Dr. Dudley. He went to the jail and carried the wrapped body out.

Dr. Benjamin Winslow Dudley was chair of the Anatomy and Physiology Departments at the Transylvania Medical School. The school did not have its own building; they were using Trotter's Warehouse, on the corner of Mill and Main Streets, but they expected to soon have a building of their own.

In 1804, Dr. Dudley had journeyed to Philadelphia to study medicine at the University of Pennsylvania with Daniel Drake, John Cooke, and William Richardson. They all eventually taught at Transylvania Medical School. Dr. Dudley received an MD from the University of Pennsylvania and studied in Europe for four years of additional medical training. He returned to Lexington to invigorate the Medical Department at Transylvania Medical School. He was revered for his intellectual achievements by local citizens but known for his lack of common sense.

The sheriff carried the body into Trotter's Warehouse after greeting Dr. Dudley; the sheriff asked him, "Where do I put the body?"

"There, in the lecture room with the other bodies," Dr. Dudley said. "I'll show you, here. I can engage it for tomorrow's lecture." They walked down the hall. "I need as many cadavers we can get; this university and students are growing. There is a great need for trained doctors, and this university can only achieve that sacred duty if we have adequate numbers of cadavers from which to train them. What reward do you request for this?"

"Dr. Dudley, I'll bring you all unclaimed bodies, but sir, stealing from the cemetery is unlawful; local citizens will get upset with you."

"Common citizens don't understand the necessity of taking those bodies," he replied in an angry voice.

"Please," the sheriff said, "let me help you rather than you seeking your own sources." He continued, "Some of your sources have not always been legal or proper. If the rumors continue, I will have to do something official against you."

Dr. Dudley ignored the sheriff's comment and continued in serious thought. "I must have cadavers to lecture from; my responsibility lies in obtaining what is necessary to do my duty." The doctor viewed the body with interest. "What happened to her? She is so mangled!"

"I think she did it to herself. The way many of the unfortunates wander in the woods, you might have many more bodies. However, Andrew McCalla is trying to organize a hospital so these people will have proper care and live longer."

"Well, I hope he doesn't succeed, because that will cut into my supply for anatomy lectures. We must educate our doctors, and they must have cadavers to learn from. There are people in society who have limited abilities, and their highest calling may be to serve society with their own anatomy. They can improve our knowledge. Unfortunates are a drain on society, and such a hospital will be more of a drain. We are training medical doctors to cure people instead of using herbs like Andrew McCalla, who can only sustain them."

The sheriff was somewhat puzzled by Dr. Dudley's comments. "Sir, I'll do what I can, but you should do nothing illegal, okay?"

"Well, if you demand such an affirmation, I shall do what I need to do; I recognize that you are my best source. I thank you for your many kindnesses and your support of this university as it grows into a medical school where physicians can achieve training."

"Yes, sir, and I am pleased to help you," stated the sheriff.

"People like Andrew McCalla, who only use herbs for soothing, will die with the witch doctors. There are many new developments, such as phrenology, and these leaders are coming here."

Trying to maintain a friendly conversation and appear interested in science, the sheriff asked, "What is phrenology?"

"It is a science concerning the mind, and the medical school will have one of the leaders coming to teach here. This great institution will lead the nation in the most current scientific knowledge," Dr. Dudley stated eagerly.

The sheriff admired Dr. Dudley's enthusiasm but now suspected that many of the local rumors were true. Dr. Dudley had been stealing bodies from surrounding graves, indiscriminately, and that could cause trouble. As he was leaving the warehouse, the sheriff realized that he admired Dr. Dudley's knowledge but feared his ambition. The sheriff returned to his office.

In another part of the town, Rev. Chipley was adding books to his library. Dr. Benjamin Rush's latest book, *Medical Inquiries and Observations upon the Diseases of the Mind,* had been reviewed by him. Dr. Rush believed in moderate alcohol usage, which followed Rev. Chipley's beliefs. Rev. Chipley had often preached alcohol moderation to the frontier town of Lexington. Dr. Rush emphasized the use of depletion methods, such as bloodletting, purgatives, and emetics, such as calomel, but many of his patients died. Rev. Chipley favored using healing plants. He preferred Samuel Thomson's book and Hahnemann's work with homeopathic medicines, but that was opposite from the medical school.

Previously, on December 11, 1816, Mr. Handel had performed at the theater for the benefit of the new Fayette Hospital. Forty-eight citizens had contributed to the hospital, including Andrew McCalla, Thomas January, Rev. Stephen Chipley, Sterling Allen, and Richard Higgins. It was the following March of 1817 that they purchased what was called "the sinking spring property," with an immense subterranean volume of water flowing from a big spring in a wooded area off of Fourth Street and Henry's Mill.

A celebration for laying the cornerstone for the Fayette Hospital did not occur until June 30, 1817. A procession of local citizens marched from the courthouse on Main Street to the site. The sheriff and his deputies were there to lead the procession while judges of the circuit court and justices of the peace followed. The clergy, trustees, and professors of Transylvania University followed in their carriages. Other students of Transylvania University, trustees of the town, physicians, contributors, and others followed, some in carriages, some on horses, and some walked. Most people in Lexington were eager for a charity hospital where indigents could gain care, while others just wanted to rid the settlement of the unfortunates from the streets. That hospital was a real community effort, and the settlement had a parade to celebrate.

The sheriff started the procession, going west on Main Street toward the intersection of Georgetown Street. He pointed out to several deputies a large brick house on that street. "See the Sign of the Green Tree, the inn on the left? This inn has a good reputation and is often visited by wealthy visitors. You will rarely have trouble there. The visitors are respectable people."

Another young deputy, named Mcgowan, stated, "There are two other inns on this side of town, aren't there?" A large Mcgowan family was part of early Lexington and several served in local city positions.

"Yes, we just passed William Palmateer's brick inn, but it is not as well known as the Sign of the Green Tree. Palmateer's is smaller and caters to the more common people."

The sheriff and deputies continued on to Georgetown Street after leaving Main. They went north on Georgetown Street, where there were still several log houses, such as the Abel Headington house. Then, the older brick homes of Mary May and William Williams were sighted. Georgetown Street continued toward the junction of Henry's Hill and Fourth Street. The sheriff led the procession right on to Fourth Street, where they stopped; individuals got out of their carriages or off their horses and walked toward the spring, as the sheriff observed the local citizens.

The youngest deputy stated, "I didn't know Lexington had this many people. Everyone must have turned out for this."

The sheriff stated, "Lexington is really growing, and there are many educated people here; see the professors from Transylvania?"

"Yes," stated the deputy.

"The professors don't really associate with the other citizens, as they are busy traveling the world for new research. The students of Transylvania are from all parts of the states, mostly from wealthy families."

"Well, this is impressive."

"Then, we have our leaders, who are always trying to make Lexington more than a wilderness town; they want it to be like a big city. Then, we have just the common and simple people who could care less. So there is a real mixture of people here, as you can see."

The local newspaper, the *Kentucky Reporter*, reported that "a powerful and eloquent oration was given by Henry Clay Sr." He first moved to Lexington in 1797 to practice law. At this time, Henry Clay was serving his third term in the US House of Representatives and had brought fame as Lexington's first national figure. He was treasured for his statesmanship and colorful histrionics as a lawyer.

During the ceremony, three of Henry Clay's younger children were with him, as he was well known as a family man. His two older sons, Theodore and Thomas, ages fifteen and fourteen, were away at school in New York. It was a great day in Lexington.

The sheriff stood watching the crowd and noticed that Dr. Dudley was not present. One of the Transylvania students came over and spoke to the sheriff after the ceremony. That student appeared to be in his late teens and was a striking, good-looking young man, tall with dark blue eyes and gracious manners.

"Sir, I am John Rowan Allen from Green County, Kentucky. I am a second-year student at the Transylvania Department of Law. I heard from your deputy that you were in the Indian War with Governor Shelby?"

"Yes, I was."

"Then you might remember my father, General James Allen; he served with Governor Shelby."

"Oh, yes, he was a very brave man. I was so sorry to hear of his death during the war. We all depended on your father's advice."

"Yes, his bravery was well-known but disastrous to our family. However, I know he would be proud of me since I am studying law here at Transylvania."

"Your father was very proud of you. I had heard that General Allen had a family in Green County. I am glad to meet you."

"I am most pleased to meet you since I often hear of your dedicated work in carrying out the laws of this town," Allen said.

"Yes, and I have heard good things about the law department."

"Yes, I have many outstanding professors," said the young Allen. "I am most pleased to be studying there."

"Please call upon me if you should need my services," stated the sheriff as he left. *A most impressive young man*, the sheriff mused to himself, walking back to the crowd.

The Law Department of Transylvania University had earlier appointed James Brown to teach. He had graduated from William and Mary, was admitted to the Kentucky bar, and moved to Lexington in 1789. James Brown commanded the Lexington riflemen in 1791 and served as secretary of state under Governor Shelby. He was the first law professor until 1804, when he became secretary of the New Orleans Territory.

Henry Clay Sr. was appointed to the law department in 1805 and taught law for two years. He resigned, as his national political career kept him in Washington DC. Henry Clay Sr. remained a loyal friend to the Transylvania institution, and his political importance added to the reputation of the law department, even though there were fewer than nine students until 1821; legal education at the postgraduate level was not very popular. Young Allen was one of those nine students.

The sheriff noticed a man with several children surrounding him. He walked toward him, recognizing him as a short, quiet, well-mannered merchant of several stores within the settlement of Lexington. He was surprised to see so many children around him. "Sir, I have talked to you in one of your stores."

Shyly, he responded, "Yes, sir, I have had the pleasure to meet you. You visited one of my stores. I'm John W. Hunt, and these are several of my children." He pointed toward them as they were running around.

"Well, you have many active children. You are fortunate."

"Yes, I am fortunate. My wife is pregnant with our eleventh child, and I brought some of the older ones to view this important civic occasion."

Hunt reached for his ten-year-old son, John Wilson Hunt. "This one is so active and loud, but we have learned to contain him somewhat. My youngest, Francis Key Hunt, was born in February this year."

"Again, you are most fortunate to have so many children," responded the sheriff.

"Yes, I am. I built a home on Mill and Second Streets and hope you might consider visiting me and my large family."

"I would be honored, sir; thank you for your invitation." They shook hands and tipped hats. The sheriff was pleased for the opportunity to see so many Lexington citizens.

The following year, one of several banking houses in Lexington started failing, and construction on the Fayette Hospital was put on hold. Another firm, the Kentucky Insurance Company, which had been incorporated in 1802, also failed, resulting in a financial crisis.

The original contributors were still responsible for payments to the Fayette Hospital. Some asked for relief from their obligations on the Fayette Hospital, while others felt that such obligations needed to be fulfilled. The community continued to struggle with finishing the building.

As the Fayette Hospital remained unfinished, a lottery to raise more money for construction was initiated on October 9, 1819, but that was not enough money to finish the hospital. The building sat unfinished while the sheriff and his deputies checked on the one empty building.

In 1818, John Wesley Hunt was elected president of the Farmers and Mechanics Bank, and in the 1819 panic, his bank remained solvent. His reputation as a skilled and systematic business manager was established and continued for the rest of his life.

A promise of debtor's relief became part of the next Kentucky governor's platform. These promises were fulfilled by creating a new Bank of the Commonwealth. However, the Fayette Hospital remained unfinished.

Meanwhile, rumors of disputes circulated around town between three professors at Transylvania Medical School: Dr. Dudley, Dr. Drake, and Dr. Richardson. The sheriff had observed them arguing over Dr. Dudley's autopsy of a drunken Irishman who had been killed on the street. The sheriff could not understand the problem; the Irishman was just a drunk to him. At least that was how he saw things.

Dr. Dudley had performed his first operation of a lithotomy in 1817 (a surgical removal in the urinary bladder of a stone), and he continued to operate with great success. As his reputation grew, Dr. Dudley began to challenge anyone who would question his decisions, including other professors, such as Drs. Drake and Richardson.

Later that week, Dr. Drake was discussing this disagreement with the sheriff; he said, "I can't believe Dr. Dudley can be so childish. He says his integrity is being questioned and is now demanding a duel." While both doctors had grown up in the wilderness of central Kentucky, they had achieved fame as knowledgeable and respected local physicians. Dr. Drake saw no need to fight a colleague or take any risk with a duel.

"Have you tried talking to Dr. Dudley?" asked the sheriff. "He is a physician and should understand the dangers of a duel."

"Yes; he denies any problem but will not allow anyone to question him. He wants to have a duel over this issue, as if that would make a difference in our diagnosis. Can you stop this?" he asked the sheriff.

"No," the sheriff said. "It is not illegal to fight a duel in Kentucky. While a duel will not solve your problems, many still adhere to that old code. If both parties agree to a duel, I cannot stop it."

"Well, I'm not staying in Lexington with such a person around. Dr. Dudley is an ignoramus, a bully, and a liar. I'm disgusted with his medical politics." Dr. Drake stood up, shook hands with the sheriff, and left the sheriff's office. Dr. Drake made plans to leave town that day. The town was losing an outstanding physician.

The sheriff still believed that Dr. Dudley was too much of a gentleman to get involved in such a dispute. Yet, Dr. Drake had reasons to be upset with Dr. Dudley. The sheriff hoped that this duel talk would stop so that the parties could calm down and return to reason.

But before the sheriff was able to visit Dr. Dudley, he heard that there had been a duel between Dr. Dudley and Dr. Richardson, with the latter being severely wounded. Rumors stated that if Dr. Dudley had not intervened in an act of "surgical instinct," Dr. Richardson would have died. Both doctors returned to their teaching activities as if nothing had happened, while Dr. Drake left town.

The sheriff was disappointed in Dr. Dudley and told his deputies, "A real waste of educated people. How can they lead others while acting as children? Dr. Drake had more sense to leave town, but now the town has lost another good physician. When will those people learn to get along?" Everyone shook their heads in disbelief.

The sheriff heard the fire alarm go off early one morning in March of 1819. The pump fire engine was pulled by volunteer citizens to the county jail, which was on fire. Inside the stone building, it was completely destroyed. The jail had two lunatics inside; one had stolen some food from the market house on Water Street, and the other one had shocked some of the ladies with his behavior. Both lunatics perished in the fire. Immediately, plans were started for a new jail to be erected; Thomas B. Megowan was elected to be the new jailer.

By September 1818, the main college building was completed on the upper part of the college lot facing south toward town. It was an impressive structure—a handsome building with three stories with an ornamental cupola, affording many lecture and recitation rooms. One hundred students could be provided with board and lodging. It was a proud structure, and the townspeople admired it.

A few months later, excitement grew over President James Monroe's upcoming visit to Lexington on July 2, 1819. The sheriff was meeting with his deputies about the upcoming event. "It will be our obligation to escort people around," he explained. "I didn't know this was part of our job, but I'm told by the political bosses that if I wish to get reelected, I'm expected to do this."

He continued, "Of course, since I hired you, then you must help me. I'm not much at playing the political games, but as political factions develop, I need your support to do my job. Anyone have any questions?"

"Is it true that President Monroe will be staying at Sanford Keen's Postlethwait's Tavern? Will the tavern handle the whole traveling party?"

"Yes, all thirty-eight rooms will be reserved for the presidential party. It is the largest inn in town. The president is to speak at Transylvania University the next day, and we will escort them there."

"Will former Governor Shelby be escorted to town, or do we have to go to his home to escort him into the city?"

"We will be escorting the previous governor from Traveler's Rest into town. Two of you deputies have been there before and know how to find it, south of Danville. He will be staying with Major William S. Dallam on his farm, about five miles north of town. The second night, Major Dallam will have a party at his home for the president and other dignitaries, such as J. C. Breckinridge, Colonel Richard M. Johnson, General Percival Butler, General John T. Mason, and J. G. Trotter. Since the president will be visiting Trotter's home, we are expected to be there also."

The sheriff continued with the schedule, saying, "The third day, a large banquet is being given for the president at Postlethwait's Tavern by the owner's wife, Mrs. Keen, and more dignitaries are expected. Again, we are expected to be there all the time to greet people. We are expected to mingle around like gentlemen."

"What about our other duties?"

"You will be expected to do other duties last. I might hire new deputies for regular duties, but you know the citizens of Lexington and can make them feel comfortable; they should know that the law is there to protect them. Remember, you are representing a public office; make me proud. Such public support is important for the growth of this wilderness town."

When President James Monroe visited Lexington, the city proudly showed off for his visit. The sheriff was proud of his men.

The following March 3, 1820, the thirty-eight-room Postlethwait's Tavern and Keen's Inn burned down. The public house was replaced later by a more commodious three-story brick building, the Phoenix Hotel.

By March 15, the Transylvania Medical School lectures had ended for the year, and six more physicians received their diplomas. Dr. Dudley continued to be proud of his growing medical school.

By 1820, the population of Lexington had grown to 5,279. More lunatics were found dead in the wilderness, as they were rejected by the surrounding towns. The city leaders did not want to be responsible for their care. So they were often run out of town.

As a remedy, the State of Kentucky adopted a plan of boarding out lunatics to private homes; the expense came from the state, not the local cities. Each lunatic had to be adjudicated by a court of law, and if the family could not pay, then the State of Kentucky would pay a set amount for his or her care. This arrangement was viewed as progress in caring for the lunatics and unfortunates of the cities.

In 1821, the sheriff was surprised to be invited to Dr. Dudley's wedding. Many other Lexington citizens were present when Dr. Dudley married Anna Short, sister of Dr. C. W. Short. The bride was beautiful but shy and retiring from the crowd. Everyone was hoping she would help improve upon Dr. Dudley's social disposition, but she appeared to be lacking also. Others had observed her to be very compliant to his every demand, and they whispered among themselves their own disappointment.

The sheriff shook hands with Dr. Dudley and said, "I hope you and Anna have many good years together." Anna just smiled shyly.

Dr. Dudley replied, "I expect to," and pulling the sheriff away from Anna's hearing, he said, "Did you attain any cadavers recently? You know I'm really depleted at the medical school."

Surprised, the sheriff stumbled in words. "Sir, this is your wedding day, let's not talk business now."

"Well, I need to; I'm desperate. You can't always encounter all the cadavers I need. This requires my constant attention." Dr. Dudley rudely walked away.

Dr. Short came over to the sheriff and proudly said, "I'm so pleased to have Dr. Dudley as my brother-in-law; my sister has really done well. As you might know, Dr. Dudley ranks higher than any other man in the Western Country as a surgeon with so many important operations. I'm sure you know of his work, living in this city?"

The sheriff responded, "Yes sir, I've heard of his reputation," while he chose to ignore his growing disappointment in Dr. Dudley. He asked, "How did your sister meet him?"

"My sister met him at a medical meeting that we attended."

"Oh, that is interesting."

"I'm a physician from the southern part of Kentucky but have admired

Dr. Dudley for the past few years and encouraged my sister to meet him," stated Dr. Short.

"Well, I knew that she was new to this area of Kentucky, but she is still a Kentuckian and will be accepted here," added the sheriff.

Dr. Dudley had greeted other guests, including Robert Todd and his wife Eliza Parker Todd. As the dancing started, the sheriff started to leave.

He noticed Judge Richard A. Buckner with his family. The sheriff knew Judge Buckner from being around the courthouse and observed four individuals with him.

"Sir," said the sheriff, "nice seeing you here."

"Yes, weddings do bring out the best in us. Have you met my wife and daughter, Elizabeth?"

"No, I have not had the privilege. Mrs. Buckner and Elizabeth, I am honored. And is this your son?"

"No, my son is only eight years old, too young for such a nice wedding. This young man is Mr. John Rowan Allen from Green County. He has finished law at Transylvania and is working in my office until he passes the bar."

"Oh, yes, now I remember him. I met this young man several years ago at the Fayette Hospital ceremony. Your father was General James Allen, right?"

"Sir, that is correct," stated the young Allen. "I met you when the hospital was dedicated. Now, I am finished with school and learning law in the office of Judge Buckner. I have learned so much."

"I'm sure Judge Buckner is fortunate to have you; do you expect to stay in Lexington after passing the bar?"

"No, sir, I plan to return to Green County, where my family still lives, to practice law. They need me now that I am old enough to contribute to the family needs. My uncle, Mr. Sterling Allen, still lives in Scott County."

"Well, I wish you the best, and Judge Buckner, I will see you soon in the next court session. Mrs. Buckner and Elizabeth, it was my pleasure."

He excused himself to leave and went back to this office. One deputy was on duty.

"Who is Robert Todd?" the sheriff asked his deputy.

"Oh, he built the two-story house on West Short in 1813. It has at least eight rooms. They have several children and his wife is related to the Parker family. The Parkers are wealthy but the Todds are more modest."

"Is he associated with the medical school?"

"Oh, no, Mr. Todd is a businessman," stated the deputy.

"Well, the Todds are friends with Dr. Dudley and his wife. I'm not sure why except for business. Dr. Dudley is not usually very sociable. Yet I would assume that Dr. Dudley only associates with other physicians."

"Maybe his new wife is changing him," smirked the deputy.

"I doubt that she will ever influence him, but there still might be hope for him." The sheriff mused over the events of the wedding.

The deputy asked the sheriff if he had heard about the new doctor coming to the medical school, Dr. Caldwell.

"No," answered the sheriff.

"He is supposed be an expert on phren— something like that. It is supposed to be the study of the mind."

"Well, that Dr. Caldwell needs to study some of those professors there," said the sheriff. "Dr. Dudley can't seem to get along with anybody these days."

"I hear this Dr. Caldwell is equally as ambitious and difficult, and he is also considered very intelligent," added the deputy.

Dr. Charles Caldwell was recruited by Dr. Holley, the president of Transylvania Medical School. Dr. Caldwell had vigor, ambition, and intelligence; at age forty-five, he had reached an impasse in Philadelphia because of differences with his former mentor and chief medical figure in that city, Dr. Benjamin Rush. Dr. Caldwell was probably the most egotistical and self-assured man ever to teach in the Medical Department, but he was a prodigious worker, pouring out a torrent of written and spoken work. He loved speculative or theoretical subjects and delighted in debate or argumentation.

Dr. Caldwell was a dogmatic Philadelphian, who filled a valuable role as public relations man at the Transylvania Medical School. He purchased books and apparatus during a trip to Europe, which formed the core of the finest medical libraries in the country. He was often called the American father of phrenology.

In 1822, Transylvania Law School had existed for twenty-three years, with limited success at attracting students. It was continuing to grow as two well-established lawyers with prominent political positions were added.

That same year, Madison C. Johnson graduated from the law department at the age of fifteen. He was valedictorian of his class but he was considered by the university officials to be too ugly to march at the graduation ceremonies. He later succeeded at demonstrating his academic legal abilities over other lawyers.

While many believed that education in law would have been as much in demand as that of medicine, the old apprenticeship system controlled the field of law. Most lawyers, who themselves had been trained in the apprenticeship system, lacked enthusiasm for the academic method. The new law courses were often too general and diffuse, not practical for a man about to enter the profession. Only later did academic legal education show its advantages over the apprenticeship system.

The sheriff and a deputy were scouting around on Georgetown Pike, west of Lexington, a few months later when they decided to call upon Lewis Sanders at his farm.

Sanders had many fine cattle, sheep, horses, and hogs. His home was a two-story brick. He was sitting on his front porch as the sheriff and deputy approached. They greeted each other.

"We been scouting around," the sheriff said, "and wondered if you knew of any problems in this end of the county. I can't always get out this way."

"Nope, nothing much, things have been quiet. I'm getting my animals ready for the cattle show at Fowler's Garden off Winchester Pike."

"Didn't you have that show here at your place a few years earlier? In fact, didn't you start it here?"

"Yes, that was in 1816, but the show grew and my place was too small. It has been at Flower's Garden for several years now. Everyone has a chance to win prizes, and I hope to win this year."

"I'm sure you will with your cattle and horses," responded the sheriff as he continued. "The interest in horses is growing."

"Yeah, well, I have something new here. I have gained guardianship of four lunatics. The state pays me a monthly fee to feed and care for them as a keeper. They help me and my farm hands on the farm."

"How did you find out about that?" the sheriff asked; he was puzzled over the process.

"My neighbor in Scott County, Mr. Sterling Allen, has two lunatics, and he is their keeper."

"Are they any problem?"

"No, they are slow and must be shown how to do things, but once they learn, they are very helpful on his farm."

"So, you get paid a sum by the state?"

"Yes, I get a monthly sum for their care and get the use of their labor also. Some keepers are cruel to their charges, while others, such as Mr. Allen, will not be mean to them. He spends time teaching them."

"How do you become a keeper?"

"Well, it is really easy, just go to the county judge and tell him that you are willing to be a keeper. There are more lunatics who need keepers. When citizens realize they can make regular money by keeping them, then there will be more keepers. On a farm, their expenses are nothing, food is always around, and they can stay in the outbuildings. I wanted only male lunatics."

The sheriff said, "I have several unfortunates who stay in the jail to wait until they are adjudicated a lunatic by a state court of law. The jail in Lexington is now crowded as they wait for keepers to take them. I have never seen how it works on a farm."

"I got mine from a county jail, which was very crowded."

"Unfortunately," stated the sheriff, "the process for a keeper takes a while, and some cannot be kept in jail if they don't do anything illegal. I would like to see how yours are doing; can we meet them?"

"Sure, one is feeding the cattle, one is slopping the hogs, and the other two are in the tobacco field. I gave the dirtiest one the job of slopping the hogs. They all have their odd peculiarities; this first one is always talking to himself, another is a smoother talker, maybe a con man, the third one is very slow, and the fourth thinks everyone is plotting against him. At this time, they are living in the outbuilding, but two were fighting. We might have to put up another outbuilding." He lowered his voice so that they could not hear them.

"I would guess that would be expensive," stated the sheriff, lowering his voice as well.

"Yes, so I am still hoping that they will get along together. The one over there, he feeds some of the cattle."

"And this one?" asked the sheriff, without pointing but motioning to one near them.

"That one does a good job but he mostly talks to himself. When he is very angry or upset, he will talk to himself rather than face anyone."

"Hello," the sheriff said as he walked up to the first lunatic, "I'm the sheriff in this county; if I can help you, let me know."

He did not respond, and when Sanders tapped him on the shoulder and said, "This is the sheriff," he ran into the barn. Sanders coached him from behind the barn door and said, "This man is your friend, he will help you when you need it. Do not be afraid."

He came out looking fearful.

"I just wanted to meet you and tell you I'm a friend of Mr. Sanders and hope to be your friend. You are doing a good job here."

He smiled and started back to his work. He immediately started talking to himself, saying, "He will kill me, I can't believe him, he will take me away," as he was getting the feed ready.

Sanders smiled to the sheriff and said, "See, he talks to himself but it does not interfere with his work. We will go see the others; they are all very different."

The one slopping the hogs was resting against the building. He quickly jumped up when he heard the approaching horses and started to get the feed together.

Sanders approached this one and introduced the sheriff to him. This one recognized the sheriff from a stay in the Lexington jail.

He stated, "Sir, I'm doing much better than when you last saw me. Mr. Sanders has given me a good home, and I really show him that I can work."

Sanders beamed proudly. The sheriff noticed how filthy he appeared but his manners showed refinement. The sheriff wondered why he was a ward of the state when there were others much more disturbed.

The other two lunatics were in the tobacco field, plowing the land. It was hard work, and both were doing their best. The third one, the slowest of all four, was having problems, while the fourth one was busy working. A farm manger was watching them.

The sheriff stated, "I'm impressed with your use of them. At least they have a place to live. I hope things will work out. Well, we need to be going, sir." He shook hands with Sanders and motioned to the deputy to follow him, as they left on their horses. So this was the Kentucky boarding-out system at its best in the year of 1823 witnessed by the sheriff.

Dr. Caldwell had become well established as a lecturer at the Transylvania Medical College. He was considered the American apostle of phrenology and taught the subject in his medical classes. He wrote the first book published in America about phrenology, called *Elements of Phrenology*.

John W. Hunt and Richard Higgins had been appointed by the current governor to change the unfinished Fayette Hospital into a lunatic asylum. They had limited knowledge since there were few state-supported lunatic asylums. These two men had requested permission to attend Dr. Caldwell's lectures, seeking any knowledge available to them from the Transylvania Medical School.

"I hope we can learn more about Dr. Caldwell's ideas and be able to apply his knowledge within the lunatic asylum. We need any available scientific knowledge about the mind; as it is now called phrenology," Hunt stated.

"Yes, Dr. Caldwell has studied with Gall in Europe, so we can certainly learn from him," Higgins added as both men found a place to sit in the old warehouse.

"I guess all these other men," Hunt said, looking around the room, "are students in the medical school; there must be over a hundred here in this crowded warehouse."

"Yes," Higgins said. "This new science is popular with students. Did you know that the school has grown from twenty medical students in 1818 to now over two hundred just five years later?"

"Oh, here he comes," Hunt whispered. "I understand he obtained an MD twenty-five years ago but is now into phrenology research. He believes that phrenology has the answers."

Dr. Caldwell started his class, saying, "Gentlemen, I am here today to talk on the history and doctrine of phrenology." He proudly looked upon the audience, stopped, and looked around slowly. Then he resumed his lecture for over an hour.

He described the theory of psychology and the relations of the cerebral parts to the mental facilities. His subjects included the organology proper, the physiognomy and the cranioscopy, along with the temperaments, features, and attitudes. He looked at the audience and explained, "This is what we may properly term the phrenological systems of mental philosophy. Gentlemen, next week I will discuss the twenty-seven organs in detail. Do you have any questions? Then you are dismissed until my next lecture." He left the room.

Leaving the lecture, Hunt and Higgins were walking toward their carriages. Hunt stated, "I think we should attend more of Dr. Caldwell's lectures, maybe we can learn more. I hope more board members attend."

"Yes, I agree, he certainly is knowledgeable and a valuable source on this subject," Higgins added.

"Yes, this phrenology may help us with the asylum; any knowledge of what causes lunacy can certainly help," Hunt agreed. They were excited with their new knowledge but still confused as to how to apply it.

The sheriff walked to the Lexington Post Office, located at the home of Joseph Ficklin. He had some mail to pick up and he had not seen the postmaster for some time. He had heard that the postmaster was renting out a room to a university student.

They shook hands and greeted each other. "Sir, I hear you have a boarder with you, a student," the sheriff said.

"Yes," Ficklin answered, "a young bright student at Transylvania University. He will do well in life."

"It is good of you to offer a room to students, since there are very limited rooms in Lexington," added the sheriff.

"Well, this young man is from Mississippi; his name is Jefferson Davis.

He is hoping to get a commission to West Point after he finishes with Transylvania, so he might not be here long."

"More rooms will be needed as the university grows. It also helps the citizens with additional income from the students, of course if they don't cause any trouble," said the sheriff.

"Mr. Jefferson Davis has been no problem; I will miss him when he leaves," added the postmaster. The sheriff had noticed several new people in the town; a few were young enough to be students at the university. He always wanted to know who was new in town and why.

Later on, this Jefferson Davis would become the president of the Confederacy during the Civil War; he wrote often about his memories at Transylvania University and living in Lexington.

Sanders came into the sheriff's office several weeks later, stating, "Sir, there is trouble with my lunatics. One was found dead this morning."

The sheriff grabbed his hat and said, "Oh no; I will follow you to your place." He and Sanders arrived at the farm and went to one of the outbuildings. In the back of the building was the body of the slower lunatic. He had been beaten, and blood surrounded his lifeless body. The sheriff shook his head and wondered why anyone would bother to kill such a simple person. He walked around the scene and asked, "When did this happen?"

Sanders stated, "Last night; he was working yesterday. We feed them regularly at sundown and they go to bed. One of the other lunatics found him here this morning and ran to my house to notify me. I didn't expect this kind of trouble." Sanders appeared to be more concerned about his reputation than the dead person; he kept saying, "What will people say? Who will pay for his burial?"

The sheriff ignored Sanders, trying to understand how this could happen. He asked, "Does anyone check on them during the night?"

"No, they just stay in this building after they are fed. We never heard anything," Sanders stated.

"Do you know if there is any family, since the state was paying for his care?"

"I'm sure there is none; the court knew of none. Will I need to pay for the burial? That would cost more than I have made on him from the state. I really can't afford to bury him," Sanders stated anxiously.

"Actually, if you are not particular, I can give the body to Dr. Dudley at the medical school; they will bury the body after they are finished with it. Dr. Dudley will be happy to get the body, since there is no family to claim it."

"Oh, yes," claimed Sanders. "That will relieve me of paying for the burial."

"First, I need to know who did this," the sheriff said.

"Oh, probably the other lunatics; two of them are always talking about killing. They talk like that, many times," Sanders claimed.

The sheriff was not sure and wanted to seek his own answers. "Well, we need to see if there is a killer still around. We need to find that person." As the sheriff was thinking about what more to do, he asked, "Can I talk to some of your farm hands and the other lunatics? They might know something."

"Yes, just let me know if I can help," Sanders said.

The sheriff ended up taking the body to Dr. Dudley, who was very appreciative. The sheriff reported, "This body was in the boarding-out system, so he is not as malnourished as other lunatics have been." He hoped that the improved status of the lunatic would be appreciated.

"Well, yes, he is in better shape," Dr. Dudley said. "I was worried about this new boarding-out system, whether it would cut down on the number of lunatic bodies, but so far, it has not changed much. The bodies may be less dehydrated and malnourished now, but they are still around." Dr. Dudley thanked the sheriff as he was leaving.

The sheriff was wondering how someone could be so interested in healing through surgery but so indifferent to the needs of the other unfortunate ones. That puzzled him.

The sheriff returned to Sanders's farm to talk to the farm workers and others who might know something about the death. He talked to several workers, but the most interesting response came from the manager, who admitted that the dead lunatic was so slow that he would get angry with him. He quickly denied hurting him.

Other employees confirmed that the manager had a bad temper. The other two lunatics were afraid to talk to the sheriff. They ran and hid. The third one said, "The manager beat up him, he broke the plow on a rock. I am afraid of him."

After hearing this, the sheriff looked in the barn for the broken plow. There in the barn was a broken plow and a rock with blood on the ground. The killer had not even bothered to clean up the blood. "If that miserable manager did this, I will get him," the sheriff stated to himself. He continued thinking over and over, "How could anyone be so cruel to such an unfortunate person?"

He went to talk to Sanders. "Sir, what do you know about your manager? Did he want the lunatics on your farm?"

Sanders replied slowly, "He is new to this area and seems to know a lot about farming. He really didn't want to work with the lunatics and complained about them daily. Why?"

"I think he killed your lunatic out of anger for breaking the plow. I want to take him into town for questioning. Did you know that there is blood on the broken plow in the barn?"

"No, but what will I do for a manager? I need him," replied Sanders. "I can do without a lunatic but I cannot do without a manager of my farm."

"I'm afraid he is not what you think; if he would lose his temper with a slow lunatic, he is nothing. I will help you find a better manager who is kind and caring, not a hot-tempered person who easily beats up on someone as unfortunate as a lunatic."

Sanders agreed to let the sheriff find him another manager; they went to find the current manager, who later confessed to the killing.

The manager was locked up and tried in the Fayette County Courthouse. He was sentenced to one year for killing a lunatic. The manager stayed in the Lexington jail during that year and grew to despise the sheriff.

After his year in jail, the manager rented a farm in nearby Scott County and petitioned to become a keeper for several lunatics. Since the Scott County officials did not know of the manager's earlier abuse, he was given custody of several, and the income from those lunatics was sufficient to pay the monthly mortgage on the farm. The lunatics were poorly fed and barely clothed, and local citizens complained about their care.

The sheriff heard about what the manager was doing, but the farm was outside of his jurisdiction. This manager became typical of many keepers in the boarding out of lunatics. There was no one to protect them or oversee the care they were provided. The high expectations of the boarding-out system for the unfortunates were soon thwarted. Yet these keepers were the first paid Kentucky employees to care for them.

By 1822, the governor of Kentucky recognized the problems of the boarding-out system and criticized it as "expensive and not curative." Plans were developed to establish an asylum. The care was to be curative, and the Transylvania Medical School was expected to provide the necessary treatment. John Wesley Hunt, at the age of forty-nine, was appointed chairman of the board and administered the facility. He was a gentleman of great wealth and well respected. He was the first gatekeeper for the Kentucky system.

After graduating from Transylvania Law School, John R. Allen returned to Green County to practice law and was elected senator from his hometown. He was excited over the possibility that the state of Kentucky would lead other states in creating a second state asylum for lunatics. He was most excited that the lunatics of Kentucky would finally have a proper place for their care.

The idea of a full-time superintendent at the First Kentucky Lunatic Asylum was not even considered at this early date. Members of the board volunteered to manage with John W. Hunt as chairman, while the Transylvania Medical School provided the medically trained staff. A matron and steward provided supervision of the female and male wards as they planned for the first Kentucky Asylum.

Sources for Chapter 2

Acts Passed at the Second Session of the Thirtieth and the First Session of the Thirty-First General Assembly for the Commonwealth of Kentucky. *Public Documents*, 174–176. Frankfort, Kentucky: 1823.

Armstrong, David, and Elizabeth Armstrong. *Phrenology: Bone Head Medicine The Great American Medicine Show.* New York: Prentice Hall, 1991.

Caldwell, C. "Thoughts on Mental Derangement: Introduction to a Brief Course of Lectures on that Form of Disease." *The Transylvania Journal of Medicine, Vol.* 5 (1832).

Coleman, J. Winston. *The Squire's Sketches of Lexington.* Lexington, Kentucky: The Henry Clay Press, 1972.

Dain, N. *American Psychiatry in the 18th Century: American Psychiatry Past, Present and Future.* Charlottesville: University of Virginia Press, 1975.

Dain, N. *Concepts of Insanity in the United States, 1789–1865.* New Brunswick, New Jersey: Rutgers University Press, 1964.

Dain, N. *Disordered Minds: The First Century of Eastern State Hospital in Williamsburg, Virginia, 1766–1866.* Williamsburg, Virginia: The Colonial Williamsburg Foundation, 1971.

Foucault, M. *Mental Illness and Psychology* Los Angeles: University of California Press, 1987.

Kentucky Reporter, December 11, 1816.

Kentucky Reporter, October 9, 1818. These articles were found in original documents of Eastern State Hospital shipped to American Psychology Archives for preservation, Akron, Ohio.

Kentucky Reporter, March 15, 1820.

Klafter, C. *Reason over Precedents: Origins of American Legal Thought.* Westport, Connecticut: Greenwood Press, 1993.

Lancaster, Clay. *Vestiges of the Venerable City.* Cincinnati, Ohio: C. J. Krehbiel, 1978.

Mora, G. "The History of Psychiatry in the United States: Historiographic and Theoretical Considerations." *History of Psychiatry* iii (1992): 187–201.

Peter, Robert. *History of Fayette County, Kentucky.* Chicago: O. L. Baskin, 1882.

Peter, Robert. *History of the Medical Department of Transylvania University.* Louisville, Kentucky: John P. Morton, 1905.

Pusey, William. *Giants of Medicine in Pioneer Kentucky: A Study of Influences of Greatness.* New York: Froben Press, 1938.

Ranck, George W. *History of Lexington, Kentucky.* Cincinnati, Ohio: Robert Clarke & Co, 1871.

Rothman, D. *Conscience and Convenience: The asylum and Its Alternatives in Progressive America.* Boston: Little, Brown, 1980.

Scull, A. *Social Order/Mental Disorder: Anglo-American Psychiatry in Historical Perspective.* Berkeley and Los Angeles: University of California Press, 1989.

Shyrock, R. H. *The Beginnings from Colonial Days to the Foundation of the American Psychiatric Association: One Hundred Years of American Psychiatry.* New York: Columbia University Press, 1944.

Visscher, M. V. *Humanistic Perspectives in Medical Ethics*. Prometheus Books: 1972.

Wright, John D. *Transylvania: Tutor to the West*. Lexington, Kentucky: Transylvania University Press, 1975.

Chapter Three

1824–1829

The sheriff had kept a serious surveillance on the unfinished hospital building. It was a large brick building with separate rooms divided among three floors. He could see how it could be a nice building except that it needed painting and finishing. The money was not available from individual citizens to finish it. Now, the new governor of Kentucky was looking at finishing the building, giving the original investors relief from any future obligations, and using it for a state lunatic asylum. Many local citizens were delighted over this potential, while the sheriff continued to look for any problems within the facility.

This sheriff of Fayette County had settled in Lexington while others moved on as the settlement grew. He was one of many men who helped to settle the town; most of their names were undocumented. They were mostly soldiers from the Indian Wars who were good at handling a gun and helped to provide safety to the arriving citizens. While deputies were usually new to the area, if they stayed, they followed the sheriffs into keeping the peace in a wilderness of uncertainity.

The main road to Lexington, the Old Buffalo Trail, was enlarged to accommodate wagons; private contractors charged a fee for travelers using various parts of the road. Trade to and from Lexington had increased as the city became a major commercial market. As more people used the road to the small settlement of Lexington, sheriffs and deputies became more important to the community.

In early April 1824, the current sheriff was taking another lifeless body to Dr. Dudley at Trotter's Warehouse. This was a regular service that he provided, because he wanted to support the medical school and knew that it needed dead bodies to study. Also, the sheriff wanted to be able to reassure the citizens that Dr. Dudley was not taking bodies from their local cemeteries.

"Sir," he addressed Dr. Dudley, "this body is probably pretty pickled. The man was a frequent drifter at the local saloons. He got into a fight last night and was killed. There is no family, so I assume you can use his body." The sheriff laid the wrapped body down on a dissecting table and looked up at Dr. Dudley.

"Oh, yes," Dr. Dudley said as he started to examine the body, "this one will be most beneficial; it shows students the effects of alcohol upon the human form. Many of them have not observed such deterioration in humans."

"Well, alcoholics are pretty common around here; we have several bars."

"Yes, as you know, these frontier towns have a lot of alcohol consumption, and medically trained physicians must be able to diagnosis the ravages from that habit. However, I need any bodies attainable for my lectures. Since this medical school is growing, I must have more bodies from which to prepare our future doctors."

"Yes, sir," the sheriff continued, "I will do my best, but we cannot do anything illegal." He looked Dr. Dudley seriously in the face and knew that they had an understanding. Hoping to change the subject, the sheriff stated, "I also hear that your wife is pregnant with your first child. You are ahead of me; I've not even married yet. Congratulations."

Dr. Dudley appeared to relax and smiled. "Yes, the child will occupy my wife. I am so engaged here that there is little time for home. Again, thank you, and I understand our agreement." Both men started out of the old Trotter's Warehouse, excitedly talking about the plans to build a new facility for the medical school. Dr. Dudley left toward his home on

Broadway Street to check on his wife, while the sheriff returned to his office on Main Street.

Local Lexington citizens were happy to know that the new governor had agreed to complete the unfinished hospital and turn it into a lunatic asylum. The governor recognized that the current system of boarding out lunatics was wasteful and was without any curative results. He expected the new asylum to provide practical experiences for students at the Medical School in Transylvania University and to provide "cures" rather than just custodial care.

John Rowan Allen, as a young legislator from Green County, was eagerly listening to proposals about the first Kentucky asylum. Senator Allen expected to oberve the progress of the asylum throughout his years in office. He had contacted the asylum in Williamsburg, Virginia, and maintained contact with the keeper, James William Gault, so that he would be more knowledgeable in the needs of Kentucky's unfortunates.

The governor appointed John W. Hunt chairman, because he had proven himself throughout the region as capable at managing businesses. He established a Board of Commissioners with approval of the governor and conducted twice-a-month meetings at the Kentucky asylum. Board members were to have weekly contact with the asylum, hire the employees, order supplies, and petition the governor for necessary funds.

This Board of Commissioners was required to review each admission and determine who would pay for the patient's care. If a patient was sent to the asylum by a judge or jury, the State of Kentucky paid a fixed amount for him or her. If families were to pay for the care, they were expected to post a bond of five hundred dollars for expenses; they would be notified when additional money was needed.

In 1824, there were five original members on the board, which had started with eight in 1822. After two original members dropped out, John W. Hunt continued as chairman with Richard Higgins, John Brand, Richard Aston, and John Morton. Two of the board members were friends of John Hunt, and the other two were politically connected with the governor. A part-time superintendent was hired, Andrew Stainton (there is no indication that he was a physician), with his wife as matron. John

King was hired to be the steward with Andrew McCalla as the clerk and apothecary. Dr. James C. Cross, professor at Transylvania Medical School, was the first part-time physician.

Andrew Stainton had worked at an asylum before; he believed in maintaining order in the facility. He had wanted his wife hired as the matron so that he could control how the women's apartments were conducted. He had recommended King as steward to direct the men's rooms. He had no tolerance of others questioning his authority, as he often restrained patients.

Dr. Cross was different; he believed in experimenting with various medicines. He did not always believe in restraining a lunatic if other methods could work. Dr. Cross was well respected in the local academic community, whereas Stainton was not. They had an immediate dislike for each other.

Andrew McCalla was the only original hospital contributor to be employed at the institution. He was the local expert on herbal medicines and was often consulted by Dr. Cross. Many times, McCalla disagreed with Dr. Cross's use of calomel based on the teachings of Dr. Benjamin Rush. McCalla had observed that calomel had caused many deaths, and he distrusted the use of it. However, he respected Dr. Cross and followed his directions.

The first three lunatics admitted were named Charity, William and Ab; all three were unable to care for their most basic needs. By May 5, a fourth patient, Elizabeth, arrived from Bracken County; she had idiocy from birth and was considered to be incurable. These four had no family and were supported by the state.

By January 1825, there were around thirty-three patients; Charity had died in December and seventeen others were discharged as cured. Most of the care consisted of caring for basic needs.

Stainton and his wife left their positions after the first year; they had better offers from another asylum with "more promising patients." When they left, they said, "The Kentucky Asylum consists mostly of hopeless incurables."

Hunt, as chairman, called the usual bimonthly meeting of all board members to order. He listened to the cacophony of voices and cleared his throat; in just a few minutes, the meeting came to order. Chairman Hunt was fifty-two years old and one of the most respected citizens in Lexington. They met in a room off the central hall, since there were still empty rooms in the facility. He stated, "This building has rooms for one hundred patients; we had fifty-four at the beginning of 1826. If this institution is to meet its responsibility, one hundred additional rooms are needed to meet our goal of two hundred rooms. We have the money to start additional rooms on each side of this main building. The north and south sides of this building will be extended to include rooms on each side. Does anyone disagree with this plan, since the governor has provided the money for it?"

Everyone agreed and they were pleased that the Kentucky state government was supporting their facility. Then Hunt changed the subject, saying, "We need to find replacements for Mr. Stainton and his wife. Does anyone have any suggestions how to proceed?"

Richard Higgins asked, "How was Mr. Stainton hired? He was not a local person. He was also a difficult person to work with. His wife seemed to have no mind of her own; she only did as he said. I was not impressed by either one."

John Brand added, "They were always criticizing, especially Dr. Cross, who is more knowledgeable than them. Dr. Cross was using accepted medications as a physician, and they criticized him."

"Yes, I have heard some of that," stated the chairman. "He was recommended by the head keeper at the Williamsburg Public Hospital, Mr. Galt, who had hired Mr. Stainton and his wife at his hospital. I met them when visiting the Williamsburg Hospital two years ago to see how that hospital was conducted. I was hoping that their experience could help us."

"Why can't we find someone from Lexington, or at least from Kentucky?" Higgins asked. "Stainton was really not accepted in Lexington society."

The chairman responded, "Yes, I realized that he was not accepted but he had experience in a similar asylum, which I considered valuable. I thought they would both be good. Actually, all they did was to complain or find fault."

"Yes they did, and in the beginning, they were correct; things were not well organized," stated Brand. "They kept comparing this facility with the one in Williamsburg, which has been opened for years."

"We need to hire someone who is familiar with Lexington culture and not someone new to the area. We need a superintendent involved with the city and the citizens of our town," stated Richard Aston.

John Morton followed with, "Yes, I agree."

The chairman nodded his head and said, "Well, I guess we can prolong our search further and ask Mr. Andrew McCalla to fill in until we find whom we want. We need someone with previous experience in another asylum." All agreed.

"We also need someone from this area," stated Morton. "That is hard to find since there are so few who have the necessary experience in lunacy care."

The chairman stated, "We will wait and see if Mr. McCalla will continue to help us for a while. Now as you know, the physicians at Transylvania will rotate on a yearly basis. William L. Thompson will start his term this year."

They all nodded their heads.

"Also, our steward is asking for us to consider his wife for the position of matron, since Mrs. Stainton has left. Should we?"

Richard Higgins responded, "Well, he and his wife have tried harder to become part of the community."

Brand agreed and stated, "What do we know about her? Did she also work at the Williamsburg Hospital?"

"Yes," stated Hunt, "they both worked there. In the Williamsburg Hospital, individual officers were assigned to specific lunatics, whereas here, the matron and steward will supervise the keepers, who have more direct responsibilities."

"So our system is an improvement?" asked Brand.

"Yes, Williamsburg Hospital has had a more haphazard administration and is in the process of changing into more businesslike procedures, similar to here," added the chairman.

"So if Mrs. King is willing to adjust to our methods, we could use her. I think Mr. King has," added Higgins.

"Yes, I'm proud of our businesslike procedures here; I think our chairman has been largely responsible for that," stated Brand. "Our hospital is a model of administrative order. There are many private asylums that are not as good as our administrative management."

"Well, I agree, but the question is, do we hire Mrs. King?" asked Higgins. "I see no reason why not."

"Then, do we all agree?" asked the chairman.

"Yes, but is the salary competitive?" asked Morton.

"Yes," stated Hunt. "We pay equal to the Virginia asylum, which is also a state facility, and remember, employees will get their room and food, so their salaries can be used to build savings for their future."

"I think we all agree, let's hire Mrs. King," said Aston.

The chairman asked, "Is there any more business to be decided at this meeting?" No one said anything. Then he asked, "Does anyone have anything else for discussion?"

Higgins stated, "I do have an announcement; Dr. Charles Caldwell has another lecture tomorrow. He is an expert on phrenology and his knowledge can help us. We have been invited to attend."

"Yes, I agree, we can learn from Dr. Charles Caldwell's lectures," the chairman said, and then he adjourned the meeting.

Hunt was always the last to leave the building since he enjoyed visiting the lunatics. He saw King, the steward, and confirmed that the board had hired his wife.

"Oh, we are so pleased," responded King. "Since we live in this building, her more personal involvement will be an advantage. She sees the lunatics daily and can add her own talent with them. I will tell her; thank you, sir." King rushed out toward the front door.

As Chairman Hunt exited the front door, he noticed in the semicircle a lunatic being delivered by the sheriff of Fayette County. He welcomed the sheriff by saying, "Well, I see you have brought us another one. You can bring him in the front room."

After greeting Chairman Hunt, the sheriff said, "I'm not sure you will take this one, he is from Mississippi. He was found wandering with relatives traveling through Kentucky. They stated that he was traveling with them, fighting and walking away so they could not keep him with their group. I had to tie him up to bring him here." The dirty lunatic slid onto the floor and was unable to move. The sheriff looked to see if he was hurt and noticed that he was not.

"Mr. John King will see him to a room. I will ring the bell that will summon him," stated Hunt as he reached for a bell. "Is there any family?"

"Yes," said the sheriff, "one married daughter in Mississippi. He was going to Ohio to visit relatives but he was talking nonsense and threatening to hurt himself. She gave me her address."

"Well," observed Hunt, "I see he has no court papers coming from another state, therefore I will need to write the daughter in Mississippi and see what they want to do with him. They will need to send someone after him or pay for his care. He can stay until then."

The sheriff hesitated after looking around, "Sir, this is really a nice place here." He looked around the front room and into the hall. "You have sure done a wonderful job." He had not been inside the building since it was finished.

"Well, thank you, but I did not do it by myself these years. There is a board of citizens who have worked hard."

"Yes, I know, but you have a head for business, and the institution has benefited from your serious duty to it."

Chairman Hunt smiled shyly. While he had achieved so much recognition for his outstanding administration skill, he still showed a shyness coming from his limited background. Changing the subject, he stated, "By the way, I hear you are getting married this year. I couldn't believe it, you old bachelor. You have been the sheriff here for the past nine years, haven't you?"

"Yes, sir," he responded. "I'm thirty-six years old this year and had given up on any chance to marry. I am marrying Asa Blanchard's daughter. I have known the family for years and visited his silver shop often. Do you remember when his wife was killed by the Indians?"

"Oh sure, about ten years ago; how sad," nodded Hunt.

"Well, Asa Blanchard had four boys and three daughters, the oldest daughter being twenty years old and the youngest six years. Margaret, the oldest daughter, and I have been seeing each other for years but she would not leave the younger children until they were older. Now all children are able to care for themselves, and Mr. Blanchard has given his permission for me to marry Margaret."

"Yes, I know the Blanchard family, a good family, and he is one of Kentucky's best silversmiths. My wife, Catherine, has bought many fine silver pieces from him."

"It took me many years after being in the Indian Wars to settle down into marriage. Now that she is available, I decided I had better act quickly, before someone else found out what a wonderful person she is."

"Will you have a big wedding?"

"No, we will get married at her home with the family. We want our own place, and I've saved some money to buy one."

"That sounds great," beamed Chairman Hunt. He was always encouraging young people since he had seen his own children grow up.

"Yes, we plan to buy some land north of Edward P. Johnson, you know, Johnson's Grove on Mulberry Street."

"Oh, yes, he has several stagecoaches going over Kentucky into Ohio and Tennessee. He started here as a stagecoach driver."

"Yes, he is doing real well, establishing regular routes throughout Kentucky, and he carries the US mail from Ohio to Alabama. We are purchasing the land next to him."

"Well, I wish you happiness with your new life."

"I hope we can be as happy as you and your wife have been. You have been prosperous with twelve children; your marriage must be happy," added the sheriff.

"Yes, I have been most fortunate with a large family and many interesting events to occupy myself. There is never a dull moment at my home," added Hunt.

"Of course," added the sheriff, "a most interesting event happened last year, when Marquis de Lafayette, for whom Fayette County was named, visited in May. He stayed at the home of Major Keen on Versailles Pike. We escorted him into Lexington the next day. All the Revolutionary soldiers wanted to shake hands with the last surviving major general of that war, a real privilege."

"Oh, I'm sure," stated Hunt. "We have sure seen some real changes. I do need to go, although I enjoyed talking to you. Please do call on me sometimes and we can continue to talk."

They both left out the front door; Hunt got into his carriage and the sheriff climbed onto his horse. They followed the circle drive past the water spring, on out to Fourth Street. Hunt went east toward his home on Mill and Second Streets, and the sheriff went west toward Georgetown Pike, surrounded by woods.

The sheriff was picking up some wild meat from a farmer on Georgetown Pike for burgoo (a favorite wilderness meal to be served after a wedding). The meat had to cook for many hours. A variety of meat from different wild animals made the meal more delicious, and the sheriff planned to buy the best from surrounding farmers.

*   *   *

In 1827, Matthew Kennedy designed the first Medical Hall on the northwest corner of Church and Market Streets for medical students and professors, replacing the old Trotter's Warehouse. This two-story red brick building had four pilasters across the front and blind arches along the sides. John W. Hunt was a member of the trustees of Transylvania University who had commissioned the new building.

That same year, Mrs. Anna Short Dudley, being pregnant with her second child, died in childbirth, but the son lived. Dudley's first son, William Ambrosia, was now three years old. Several local people called on Dr. Dudley at his home to express their sorrow, as the sheriff and his new wife, Margaret, had done.

While the sheriff had seen Dr. Dudley on a regular basis when bringing bodies for teaching, he had become disappointed in him and tried to express this to Margaret. He tried to formulate his ideas later in their small home, saying, "I really thought he was a great guy, having performed so many operations and being known worldwide for his abilities, but he was just too, too … uppity, even with the other professors."

They both sat down at their modest kitchen table. Margaret got up to get coffee cups and encouraged him to continue speaking; he said, "Dr. Dudley is so smart and I admired that, but I have become very disappointed in him. He tolerates me because he can use me."

"I find him arrogant, don't you?" his wife asked as she reached over to pat his hand lovingly. He responded by giving her a kiss.

"Yes, although he was never that way with me, because he needs me; I find bodies for him to use in his teaching. Also, I am never a threat to him; I could never be what he is."

"Dr. Dudley is very competitive," stated Margaret. "While very insecure within his own self, he is a real giant to others. It is a real shame that he lost his wife, because we had hoped she would help him."

"I just feel so sorry for him," the sheriff said as he reached for his wife. "If that should happen to you, I just could not go on."

"Oh, me too, but I knew his wife, she was always very distant and shy. She was never really a part of his world. He had achieved fame before marrying her, and she was never really part of his life. She was just there."

"Yes, and I already had my job before you came along, and you had your own world of raising your sisters and brothers, but we have made a good life for ourselves, together," he said, smiling at her. They were in their own home and she was pregnant.

"Yes, but we have known each other a longer time. Dr. and Mrs. Dudley met at a medical meeting. They had the medical profession in common because her brother is a physician, but she did not achieve anything in her own right. There were many differences between them."

"Well, I really feel sorry for him."

The next few days, the sheriff asked around about Dr. Dudley, but few people had seen him except in his lecture room at the medical school. Dr. Dudley was isolated, and other professors noticed that he never stayed around the school, as he always had done before. While he took care of medical duties, Dr. Dudley was focused on taking care of his sons. The sheriff had found Dr. Dudley in his lecture room at specific times but he did not wish to be bothered unless there was a necessity. The sheriff honored his request.

Several months later, a man from Cincinnati entered the sheriff's office and asked, "Sir, can you help me? My son is badly sick. I have been told by the doctors in Cincinnati that a Dr. B. W. Dudley is the only one who can save him. Can you take my son with me to see him?" The son was in a carriage and moaning.

"Yes, we will find him," the sheriff said as he took the father and his sick son to the new Medical Hall. Dr. Dudley was in his lecture room, preparing for a lecture. He told the sheriff that he did not wish to be disturbed. But the sheriff insisted and carried the sick boy into the lecture room. Dr. Dudley could not resist examining the boy since he was in obvious pain. The worried father explained his concerns as Dr. Dudley examined the son very tenderly. The sheriff observed how Dr. Dudley went from his own self-absorption into a caring, healing nature.

The father explained, "Sir, I have no money, and I have been told that my son will die without your operation. I can only hope to pay you later. Just save my son, please."

After examining the son, Dr. Dudley stated, "Sir, you can worry about paying me later, but now, your son will be operated on. He needs it. I will move him into the operating area immediately." The doctor made arrangements for the operation, sterilizing all instruments and cleaning the operating room meticulously.

After the operation, Dr. Dudley returned to the father and said, "Your son will be fine after several weeks' rest. Don't worry about the bill."

"Oh, sir, thank you, I am so grateful!" the father cried as he made arrangements to transport his son out of the building as soon as possible.

Hours later and walking out, the sheriff followed Dr. Dudley to say, "That was sure a fine thing you did for that man and his son. I really want to thank you. I am surprised that you helped him because I know you did not wish to be disturbed."

"The boy needed the operation, and I am the best to do it."

"Yes, but you did it in such a caring and kind way," added the sheriff.

Dr. Dudley stopped for a minute and said, "Well, I've not always been so caring, but since I lost Anne, some things are just not as important and others are more important. I've done some hard thinking. But I don't want you to think I'm getting soft, eh?"

"Oh, no, I will not assume that you are soft, but you really did something good in there. I'm impressed. Please take care, sir." The sheriff tipped his hat and left the new Medical Hall.

The sheriff went home to his wife and explained what happened that day. He said, "Can you believe it? I never saw that side of Dr. Dudley; he really showed he cared about the boy. I was wrong about him; he can care, especially for those who need him." He took a sip of coffee after Margaret poured it.

She sat down and responded, "Maybe he has changed? Who knows?"

The sheriff thought for a minute and said, "Maybe, or just when he is doing his operations, he is an area where no one is equal and he can afford to be kind. I don't know which, but he is sure interesting. I just wish I had half of his knowledge, education, and ability."

Margaret responded, "You have done well with what you have."

"I sure would have liked to have studied to be a doctor. I never had a chance in the wilderness, since my family could not pay for any college education." They spent many hours talking about people that they had come to know.

The degree of doctor of medicine at this time required a student to take two years of lecture courses, unless he had been a practicing physician for four years, in which case he needed to attend only one year. All candidates had to be twenty-one or older, write a thesis on a designated medical subject, and pass two examinations, one before the faculty and one before the president and trustees.

Chairman Hunt called another meeting at the Kentucky asylum with members of the board. They now had a regularly assigned room on the first floor for the sole purpose of board meetings. Since the meetings were bimonthly, the chairman's office was placed in a corner of the comfortable board room.

John Morton started with, "I understand that the physicians here at the asylum charge medical students from Transylvania to attend lectures here. Is that correct?"

"Yes, that is correct. We do not pay them, therefore any money that the physicians can gain by lecturing students belongs to them," stated the chairman.

"My question: doesn't that interfere with the proper care of the patients? Does it hamper their care?" Morton asked.

"I haven't seen it; have any of you noticed anything?"

"Actually, I've noticed that some lunatics enjoy more special attention from the students," stated John Brand.

"Yes, I agree," Morton said. "Some get ignored, such as the less curable ones. Students are always looking at the more curable ones. I don't like that part of it."

"Yes, I have observed that too," stated Richard Higgins. "Students prefer the clean and talkative ones, not the dirty, nasty ones."

"Well, I hope John King will reduce the nasty ones here by running a more orderly asylum," Brand said.

"Yes, he is improving that," remarked the chairman. "Remember many of our patients come from filthy places or cannot care for their own basic needs. It is a difficult job." He stopped. "Does anybody have anything else for discussion?"

"Yes," stated Higgins, "I have a question about our cure rate in the governor's report, stating that we had seventeen cures in 1825. Mr. Chairman, how did you determine that number?"

"That was the number discharged for the year. Since we had thirty-three remaining in the facility at the end of the year, that gave us a recovery rate of nearly 50 percent," Hunt explained.

"But we had 94 admissions for the year of 1825, and 17 of that number is not 50 percent. It is much less," Higgins said.

"Most asylums figure the cure rate upon the number in the facility at the end of the year, not the total admitted. The Friends Asylum, which you know is private, has their recovery rate based on the number admitted, and they report one-third recovery rates for 1817–1819. The Williamsburg Hospital, the only other state-supported asylum like ours, has changed from using the number of admissions to the number in the facility at the end of the year. Therefore," continued Hunt, "I prefer using the number in the facility, which makes our rates equal to others. This is the practice now."

"But I have trouble," Higgins said, hesitating, "believing that we had seventeen cures. Most of the seventeen were private-paying families of the lunatics who did not want to pay for their care. They wanted to take them home instead, and I'm not sure that they were cured, they just left. Are we not playing games about this?"

"I agree, but when someone is discharged, they are considered cured. It actually means the hospital no longer must take care of them, so they are cured," argued the chairman. "That is the way things are calculated; it is the same as at all other facilities."

"Well, if that is the way things are done," Brand conceded, "but many times when the family had to start paying, they realize it would be to their advantage to take back their lunatic member. They take him or her home rather than pay. However, the family will still lock him or her in a closet and hardly feed him or her as before, but can we count them as cured?"

"Some families will retreat back to their previous ways of caring for their lunatic member. We treated them well here," Higgins said, puzzled. "But they become worse than before because the family does not properly care for them."

"If that happens," Hunt stated, "then it will not be long before the lunatic becomes uncontrollable and is readmitted here."

"Not if the family must pay," argued Higgins, "they can hire someone to care for him or her in a room."

"I can see your point, Mr. Higgins, but we can only do what we are doing, by creating the best state institution we can; we can't handle all family problems," added Brand.

"Also," added Andrew Aston, "we are following the trends of other asylums and their achievements. Remember, our financial support comes from the governor and legislators. They require good numbers, and we must show that." Everyone agreed to that comment, and the meeting was adjourned. These discussions were recorded by the chairman in the yearly reports, and they reflected the problems of the time.

Several months later, the sheriff was talking with his deputies about the legislative bill passed in 1828 that prohibited the importation of slaves into Kentucky. "I'm afraid that there are several families who will end up fighting over that issue," he said. "There is also an emancipation organization in town that is very vocal. We need to be careful not to get into these disputes. Our job is to keep peace and order."

"But, sir," raised a deputy, "what if one of us wants to oppose these laws of protecting slaves? Can we have an opinion?"

"You let the court decide the issues, not us. You are to keep the peace. Law and order is your job, not deciding issues. Citizens need to see you as being faithful to your jobs and their good. You need to keep your opinions at home, not on the job."

Senator John R. Allen continued to correspond with the keepers of the Williamsburg asylum. He had heard that their asylum was so overcrowded that another was being opened by 1828. He marveled at Virginia's commitment to caring for their lunatics and vowed to see that the Kentucky asylum was given adequate support from the legislature.

In January of 1829, Hunt called the bimonthly board meeting at the asylum. It was more than a regular meeting due to certain items. All five members attended: J. W. Hunt, Richard Higgins, John Brand, Richard Aston, and John Morton.

Hunt opened the meeting by saying, "Andrew McCalla has been serving this institution since the beginning in several capacities, as part-time superintendent and apothecary, but he is just too feeble to continue. We need to find someone else to fill those positions. Mr. Morton, do you have any ideas?"

"No, I had hoped that some of our resident physicians would be interested in the job, but they cannot devote full time to the position. They prefer teaching and traveling."

"There are others who feel the job is not a challenge," stated Brand. "They have no interest in a position here."

Aston added, "Some of the physicians will not consider the position if they have to answer to a board. They feel that they should make the decisions instead of answering to a board of lay people such as us. This is a growing opinion of many physicians."

"Also," stated Higgins, "Dr. Charles Caldwell would be excellent but he travels around lecturing too much to devote himself to another full-time duty. I wish he would take the position, but he is busy organizing phrenology societies in the larger cities and publishing some of his larger works."

Brand protested, "I'm not sure Dr. Caldwell would be good. He has good ideas but is not good with practical matters."

The chairman may have agreed with Brand but instead changed the subject by summarizing the proceedings, saying, "As I see our discussion, we all agree that we need to find a full-time superintendent and a local person who can work with the medical school. None of the medical school professors will take the position. We can only continue to search."

The chairman introduced another problem: "Our facility has ten acres of land, while many other asylums are expanding their operations into more farm land. It becomes a good occupation for the lunatics. Should we petition the governor for more land? Do we need to follow this growing trend?"

"Yes," stated Higgins, "if the lunatics can work on a farm and grow their own food, we can cut the amount of money that is required by the state to supply them food. It can also occupy their time while here."

"Can some of them work enough to maintain a farm," asked Aston, "or will this be more of a drain on the budget?"

"All the asylums that have farms have been able to cut their expenses by doing their own farming. Remember, the employees live at the asylum, and they can supervise the whole farm and food gathering. I think it is a good idea," stated Brand.

"We will petition the governor," concluded the chairman. "Another item that we should discuss is a fence in the back to contain the excited male and female lunatics. This provides room for the more agitated lunatics to expend their energy rather than restraining them in their apartments. It gives them room to spread."

"Yes," added Brand, "several private asylums have fenced areas for their more disturbed patients to wear out their energy so that they become calmer later."

"Do we need to petition the governor for money to pay for the fence?" asked Higgins.

"No," answered Chairman Hunt, "we can handle that construction from our repair fund. Buildings need to be approved by the governor, but I assume a fence would be part of repairs. Should we do it?"

"Oh, yes," said Brand. "Think of the fresh air that the most disturbed patients will be exposed to. While better lunatics can walk around the grounds for necessary fresh air, those confined by restraints often do not always get fresh air. Many are locked away and never see daylight. This way, they can get fresh air in the fenced-in area." All agreed, and the meeting was adjourned.

On March 9, 1829, the sheriff was sitting in his office next to the courthouse on Main Street, talking to his deputies. That morning had been quiet, and they had wandered outside, milling around with others at the courthouse.

Gun shots were heard on West Main. The sheriff immediately jumped up and went for his gun. All headed in that direction.

A crowd had gathered in front of the old State House on West Main. This was the office of the *Kentucky Gazette*, the local newspaper. The sheriff quickly arrived and found the editor, Thomas R. Benning, severely wounded; Charles Wickliffe was standing over him with a gun. The sheriff carefully eased over to Charles and said, "Just calm down, and we will talk about this; let me have the gun." Charles dropped his gun and walked out of the newspaper office.

Others in the crowd scrambled to help Benning, the wounded editor. He was carried to his home, and two doctors, including Dr. Dudley, were called to help with the injuries. The sheriff and his deputies followed Charles Wickliffe, who had walked toward the jail, waiting to be arrested.

"Sir, we will need to arrest you," the sheriff said. "Do you have any other guns on you?"

Charles responded, "That scoundrel deserves to die, he defamed my father; no, I have no other weapons. Just take me inside the jail. I would do it again if I could."

After Charles was placed in a jail cell, he asked the sheriff, "Will you notify my father where I am?"

"Yes, we will," said the sheriff. "I have already sent a deputy to your father's home at Glendover. Did he know you were planning to do this?"

"Actually, no, I did not plan to draw a gun, but I knew that I had to defend the honor of my father. That editor had printed antislavery slander about him. I had no choice."

Robert Wickliffe had been a senator from Fayette County for years and had been a leader of the pro-slavery factions in the area. The next day, the sheriff learned that Benning had died; Charles Wickliffe would be charged with murder. Local citizens were taking sides in the conflict.

Benning's funeral was held the following day. Those against slavery attended the funeral, while those in favor stayed away, dividing the small town. Lexington was no longer a settlement town unaffected by national conflicts.

The sheriff talked to his wife that night about the incident; he said, "Can you believe how this has divided the town? Most minded their own business, but now, everyone is taking a side." He sat down at their table, and Margaret got coffee cups ready as they continued to talk.

She responded, "Isn't this just some of the rich families in the county? Obviously, the Wickliffes are wealthy slaveholders, but most in Lexington do not own slaves, do they?"

"Well, that was true before this murder, but many citizens believe that it was just cold-blooded murder. People who have never cared about slavery are now agitated that Kentucky's oldest newspaper editor was killed." The sheriff took a sip of coffee.

"I heard that Mr. Benning did not have a gun on him, whereas Charles Wickliffe is claiming that he shot in self-defense. He had the only gun, so how is that self-defense?" Margaret asked while taking a sip of coffee.

"That is true; Mr. Benning had no gun and was trying to get away when Mr. Wickliffe shot him. They had been arguing but Mr. Benning had no protection. Mr. Charles Wickliffe said he was defending his father's honor."

Margaret stated, "I have also heard that Mr. Henry Clay Sr. will be defending him; I wonder what kind of defense he will present. Many citizens saw Charles with the gun, and there is no dispute that he shot Mr. Benning, so how can it not be murder?" She sat shaking her head.

"Yeah," said the sheriff, "and Henry Clay says he has never lost a case; this one may be different. I just can't see him defending someone who is a cold-blooded murderer. This is really bad for the town." He looked at his coffee cup.

"It sure is; even old friends are against each other. This slavery issue is really getting bad. Many did not take sides until the murder, and now citizens see things changing. I am sure glad we have each other and agree against slavery."

"Yes, me too, but my main concern is to keep the peace and make sure no one tries to take Mr. Wickliffe out of the jail. I am keeping three night guards on at the jail. I will do my best to make sure he goes to trial for this cold-blooded murder."

"He is only a boy, twenty-one years old; how sad," observed Margaret.

"Before, arguments were just among the professors, such as when Dr. Dudley did not want his opinions questioned. Now, it is different. The old families of Lexington are divided, and the townspeople must decide between them."

The trial of Charles Wickliffe occurred on June 30, 1829. All of Lexington turned out for it in the old three-story courtroom. Masses of people and newspaper writers made it difficult for the sheriff and his deputies to make their way into the courtroom.

After the district attorney rested his case, Henry Clay addressed the jury for two and a half hours, claiming that anyone had a right to defend himself. He showed his reputation for forensic eloquence. The jury stayed out only five minutes, and Charles Wickliffe was set free. This victory for the slaveholding class in central Kentucky continued to widen the gap between the two factions.

As the sheriff directed the crowd out of the courtroom, many citizens expressed shock. They had observed the oratorical skills of Henry Clay and knew that Robert Wickliffe was a powerful man, but not to the exclusion that Charles should get away with murder. The sheriff noticed their disbelief and disappointment as the crowd passed out of the courtroom. Yet, they could only respect Clay for his outstanding legal skills.

Later, the sheriff returned home, exhausted, and saw his wife tending to the food. Margaret had already heard the news. He said, "I just can't believe the pro-slavery forces in this town are so strong that a man can kill someone and be set free. I just can't."

"Well, Lexington is different," stated his wife.

"And do you know that Henry Clay, who is such an excellent lawyer, has two sons who are constantly in trouble? If he is so eloquent, why can't he raise decent sons?"

"Well, I've heard that both Thomas and Theodore drink too much," stated his wife.

"Yes, they were in jail in Washington DC and have had trouble settling down to any vocation. Both had excellent educations, but they spend their time drinking and living off their father. They are a disgrace to such a fine man."

At the next board meeting of the asylum, a report by Dr. Samuel Theobald was presented; the doctor also wrote for the *Transylvania Journal of Medicine* and had served as the resident physician for the first Kentucky asylum in the past year.

The chairman read the report:

I wish to emphasize the importance of medical and moral means in the care of lunatics. I have used a theoretical base of parental government in this institution. The keepers are expected to act as loving parents who expect the lunatic to conduct proper behavior or to perform certain tasks equal to his or her functioning. If the lunatic does not do as expected, the employees are to take away certain privileges, such as desserts or recreation, in a caring way. If a lunatic cannot be controlled with parental government, only then will he or she be restrained with a cold bath, shackles, tranquilizer chair, or straitjacket.

The chairman interrupted his reading and said, "I have observed Dr. Theobold's work here; he has been most helpful in caring for our lunatics. He has some good ideas."

Hunt returned to reading the report:

This great institution will improve the possibility of more cures, if there are three distinct divisions created for each sex. One division will consist of those who can care for themselves and have some propriety of conduct. The second division will have apartments for those with less good conduct and require more care. The third division will house those needing the most care. Those lunatics who can improve their conduct will seek the first division apartments, while those unwilling or unable to improve will associate with similar habits in the third division. I make these suggestions for your consideration. It was signed by Dr. Samuel Theobald.

"Do we wish to consider Dr. Theobald's recommendations?" asked Hunt. "It is true we do not have any organization among the lunatics."

"How can we organize into three divisions?" asked Higgins. "We have a center building of about a hundred apartments with fifty more on one side and fifty more next year. Must we use the center apartments for division one, and the other two on each side?"

"Oh, no," reacted Aston, "we have more lunatics in the third division; therefore, the center building is larger and should contain them."

"We can't follow Mr. Aston's suggestion," stated Brand. "The front door will open into the worst cases of the third division, those who cannot care for themselves."

"Of course, you are correct," stated Aston. "Those entering the building will immediately see the worst cases. That would be very embarrassing to the public and to our cause."

"Actually, that would be correct," followed Higgins. "Instead, we might house the males on the right side and females on the left. The whole third floor, including the additions, can care for division three; the whole second floor, including the two additions, will care for division two; and the first floor could be used for division one. The first floor can continue to be the main eating area for the neater lunatics. For the untidy ones, food can be delivered to their areas. The basement will continue to provide additional housing for the keepers and storage."

"Yes, that will work," stated Hunt. "It will also leave the big hallway on the first floor for socials. The doors in the center section can be opened up for air ventilation during the summer, and the first floor hall is best for socials."

All agreed to the plan. The chairman adjourned the meeting and walked out with the other members. He stopped to meet the newer lunatics.

The dinner bell was ringing to announce the assembly of lunatics into the main dining room. Hunt observed the food and cleanliness of the table. He watched blissfully and left, pleased with the progress he observed.

By the end of 1828, the Transylvania Medical School had 151 students. On the night of May 9, 1829, the large Administration Building, four stories high, caught fire. Cassius Clay, a student on the third floor (who would later become a famed abolitionist), was awakened by the flames and escaped, calling out for help. The other students and professors living there barely escaped with their lives, but no one was killed.

Fire equipment, the sheriff, deputies, and citizens quickly gathered as the fire spread from the top to the bottom of the building. Great effort was made to keep the fire from spreading to the other buildings and homes on Mill and Market Streets. Some people tried to save the college library on the second floor by tossing books out of the windows, but the law library, all six hundred volumes, went up in smoke. Most of the scientific apparatus was saved, but several hundred dollars' worth of scientific manuscripts, collected over many years, were lost. The whole building was a total ruin within two hours, and the whole town felt the impact. Individuals expressed remorse while school leaders made plans to rebuild.

Several months later, on the morning of October 9, Sterling Allen met with Hunt at the asylum. As he walked into the front door, Mrs. King greeted him. "I'm here to see Mr. John W. Hunt," he said softly, tipping his hat to her. She smiled and showed him into a room off the hall.

Hunt was sitting at a desk, absorbed in papers, when he looked up and greeted Allen. "Mr. Allen, I'm so glad to see you. I've heard good things about your farm in Scott County. Please sit down."

"Yes, we have been fortunate with the land there. It is very rich land for raising horses. And I've heard about your capable leadership here; this is really a nice place," Allen observed.

He sat down across from Hunt, ready to discuss a difficult problem with him.

"As you know," Allen started, "This is not a social call; in fact, my wife does not agree with what I am considering. I needed to talk to you since you handle such problems."

"Yes, I understand you have a lunatic, named John and nicknamed J. J., who has been working on your farm for several years."

"Yes," Allen said, choking, "he is actually part of our family. I took guardianship of J. J. and his sister several years ago under the keeper's law. They are slow but friendly. They were both abandoned by their family on our farm."

"You certainly were generous," stated Hunt.

"Well, we took them in, and they do simple work on the farm. For the last few years, the state paid me a sum for their care, but we always treated them respectfully. No one is allowed to harm them."

"Now, if I recall," responded Hunt, "they were on your farm when you had a social last year. My family and I attended. They were not shy and helped with making the burgoo and serving the food to guests."

"Oh, yes, they appeared to be happy; my children always played with them. They were part of the family. Even my nephew, John Rowan Allen, the senator from Green County, developed an interest in them," Sterling said.

"Well, what can I do for you, sir?" asked Hunt.

"I need your advice about putting him into your institution here. We cannot continue to provide for his basic needs."

"Yes, we can provide for him here."

"It started when the sister died; J. J. just stopped doing anything. We gave him time to get over her death, but he just continues to be unwilling to take care of his basic needs."

"Oh, I was not aware that she died; did it happen recently?"

"It was three months ago; she died in a stupid accident, falling down an old well shaft. After her body was recovered, J. J. could not believe she was dead. Now he just sits and stares into space. My wife took him into the house, hoping he would improve, but he did not respond. We cannot continue this way."

"And your wife, you say she disagrees with putting him in here?"

"Yes, but if she sees him getting better care than we can give to him, she might be more willing. She has heard bad things about other places that care for these unfortunates."

"Yes," said Hunt, "he needs to come here. You will need to petition the county judge for the proper papers to admit him. I suggest you bring your wife here to visit. How old is J. J.?"

"I think he is thirty-six; he was sixteen when we got him and his sister about twenty years ago. They really were part of our lives. We hate to lose him after losing her. They both had a winning smile, even after their family left them. I will do as you say; thank you, sir."

Hunt walked out with Sterling while patting him on the back and assuring him that his wife would like what she saw at this asylum. As they were walking out the front door, Sterling noticed several carriages on Georgetown Pike, hurrying from Scott County toward Lexington.

Sterling said, "Those same carriages were out on Georgetown Pike this morning as I went by. I hope there was not another duel out there. There have been some duels earlier near Captain Henry Johnson's place about six miles out."

"Well, I hope not. We have some real agitated people now," stated Hunt, getting into his carriage. "I hope to see you soon, and we will welcome J. J. into the asylum."

As Hunt proceeded on Second Street toward his home, he noticed a crowd of people around Glendover, the home of Robert Wickliffe on Second Street and Jefferson. He stopped his carriage and saw the sheriff coming toward him.

"Is there anything wrong?" he asked.

The sheriff responded, "Yes, Charles Wickliffe and George Trotter have fought a duel, and Mr. Wickliffe has been seriously hurt. I'm afraid it is fatal. He was brought to his father's home."

Hunt knew that both men were good friends at one time; he asked, "What happened?"

"Since the death of Thomas Benning, Mr. Trotter has taken over the editorship of the *Kentucky Gazette*; he has been making insinuations about Charles Wickliff murdering Mr. Benning. They have been planning a duel for several weeks. I knew nothing about this. As usual, Mr. Wickliffe had to defend his honor."

"How foolish; they are both in their early twenties, aren't they?" Hunt asked sadly.

"Yes, and both came from well-established Lexington families. When will they decide that dueling, although legal, will never settle things, except to kill?" the sheriff asked.

Hunt went on to his home on Mill and Second Street to tell Catherine, his wife. He could only feel sad for the father, Robert Wickliffe. Hunt was proud of his twelve children and his wife. One daughter was married to Calvin Morgan in Huntsville, Alabama, and had a growing family. His sons were doing well; one attended the medical school, and another was studying law. A third one was interested in local politics and the family business. The others were learning to manage his farms. He stated out loud to himself after resting in his home office, "Oh, what a sad day for Robert."

The funeral services were held the next day at the Wickliffe home, where a large crowd of friends and relatives was in attendance. While there continued to be speculation and ugly talk about young Wickliffe's death, most agreed that the whole affair was conducted on a highly honorable basis. No charges were filed against Trotter.

Trotter ignored the unfavorable talk, believing that he had fought the duel honorably and bravely. He wrote in his paper, "I do not approve of dueling but to the host of scoundrels, if they wish to experiment upon my cowardice, they can be accommodated."

The sheriff was relieved to discover that no one sought to "accommodate" Trotter, who continued on as editor of the *Kentucky Gazette*. The sheriff had hoped that the two sides would settle into some compromise without more bloodshed.

In November, Sterling Allen brought the proper papers to admit their lunatic, J. J., to the asylum. Mrs. Allen came and was very sad, crying into a handkerchief. She had hoped that she could help him but he was unresponsive. J. J. was pathetic, lifeless, and unresponsive to any conversation with Hunt. John King took J. J. to the top floor, housing the most difficult patients. Hunt explained to Mr. and Mrs. Sterling, "J. J. will be placed in the third division; as he progresses, he can move toward the lower floors with more privileges. This asylum is organized into a parental government to give more privileges as they progress."

Mrs. Allen asked, "Will he be beaten? Many asylums do that and he can usually be persuaded if one talks to him when he is his usual self. I don't want him to be beaten."

Hunt responded, "We must restrain those who are fighting or agitated, but J. J. is neither at this time. Our physician will examine him and determine how he should be handled. We have weekly dances here in the hall for those who can attend. If J. J. is able, he can come to them. Maybe you both might wish to come?"

"Yes, we will come, it might be fun and maybe J. J. will come to the dance if we are here. He used to enjoy dancing," responded Sterling.

"We will have a band to play music and refreshments will be served to all. Only the lunatics who dress and behave appropriately in the previous week are allowed to come. If you can wait until the Thanksgiving parties start, then maybe J. J. will be feeling better and be able to attend," stated Hunt.

"Yes, we will plan to attend several parties here at the asylum during the holidays," Sterling stated as they started to leave.

Senator Allen from Green County came to visit J. J. in the asylum. Senator Allen had visited Sterling Allen's home often as a law student at Transylvania and had become acquainted with the two lunatics on his uncle's farm. He wanted to visit J. J. while taking the opportunity to view the asylum, which he had supported as a legislator.

While waiting in the entrance of the original building, he noticed the cleanliness and quietness of the facility, unlike many asylums of the time.

Seeing Hunt, he stated, "Sir, I am Senator Allen; Mr. John W. Hunt, I presume?"

"Yes, I am."

"I am so pleased to meet you. Your reputation follows you as a capable leader in one of our finest state institutions."

"Well, thank you but we also have an excellent Board of Commissioners."

"But you have achieved a great deal with this institution. It has grown under your able leadership."

"Well, I have heard good things about you. You have supported many requests for us in the legislature and with our requests to the governor. We thank you for your support," stated Hunt.

"But I'm just doing my job for a good cause."

"I understand you have an interest in our lunatic J. J., from Scott County?"

"Yes, he lived with my uncle, as you know, and I had met him then. I'm so sorry he had to come here but it was best for him. I'm just glad this place was available."

"He is improving, and we will see him later. I understand that you would like to view our facilities?"

"Oh, yes, the building is impressive."

"This original building has three floors with an additional one in the basement," stated Hunt.

"How many patients can you accommodate?" asked Senator Allen.

"It first accommodated one hundred in individual rooms, and we added fifty rooms on one side of the building; next year, fifty more rooms will be completed, giving the institution a total of two hundred rooms. Our expectations were to handle two hundred lunatics."

"Are you full?" asked Senator Allen.

"No, but we are not able to return lunatics to families as fast as we would hope. We are equal to similar institutions," he said, as they walked down the wide hallway.

"This is so clean; how is it kept so neat and clean with such lunatics?"

"The more disturbed and dirty ones are on the top floor, and if they improve, they are moved to another area. Mr. and Mrs. John King are excellent at maintaining the clean facilities. They have been in our employment since 1825."

"You have a farm here also?"

"Yes, as you know, the legislature has approved money for land that will be used for farming, occupation, and fresh air. We also have a fence to protect those most disturbed and allow them fresh air." They reached the back of the original building. "Here, we will go up the stairs to the next floor," Hunt stated proudly.

They walked through the second floor as Senator Allen looked around. The windows were tall, giving plenty of fresh air into the hall with individual apartments. They walked back to the stairway and walked up to the third floor, where they met J. J., the one who had lived with his uncle.

J. J. was pleased to see his visitor, and Senator Allen spent some time with him in his room. After saying good-bye, the senator left to rejoin Hunt in his office, saying, "He is much better. He told me he likes working on the farm."

"Yes, but he still does not take care of his appearance; the farm is where he does not have to have proper grooming."

"He has improved from when I last saw him; at least he recognized me," observed Senator Allen.

"Hopefully, he will take more interest in his dress and can attend the weekly dances," stated Hunt.

"Yes, he was very neat at one time and maybe he will get back to his past neatness," observed Senator Allen.

"Would you like to see our kitchen?" Hunt asked. "It is outside on the right of the building; food is brought through the basement and distributed to three dining rooms. It is an efficient system."

"Yes," stated Senator Allen.

"We need to go back to the stairs, down to the basement, and outside. Of course, the kitchen is away from the original building to reduce any fire hazard." They observed several employees and a few lunatics preparing food. "These lunatics have to demonstrate clean habits before they can work here," added Hunt.

"They appear to be very helpful," added Senator Allen.

"Yes, many are able to learn well and we teach them ways that will help them outside," added Hunt.

"That is really remarkable."

"Would you like to see our other improvements to the grounds?"

"Yes, if you have time,"

"I have time today. We can walk around to the side of the kitchen; over on the right is our spring house; it has a pump house and cistern where water is available for the kitchen and washhouse next to the original building," Hunt explained.

"The trees and grounds are beautiful," stated Senator Allen.

"Thank you, there are two privies on each side of the original building and two airing yards, one for males and one for females. These facilities are the most efficient way for the more excited ones to expel their manic energy rather than restraining them."

"Yes, I can see that," uttered Senator Allen.

Hunt continued to show Senator Allen the institution; he proudly explained about how the lunatics were expected to demonstrate good behavior as they are moved from the upper ward to the lower ones. "The more trustworthy patients are given privileges to work on the grounds."

Hunt observed the grounds.

"I have some statistics that I have compiled; do you wish to hear them?" asked Hunt.

"Why, yes," stated Senator Allen.

"For the years from May 1824 to September 15, 1829, there were 137 men and 77 women admitted here, for a total of 214; 47 died here, 43 were discharged as cured, 6 were discharged as improved, and 16 more discharged as unimproved. Eleven of them eloped. I'm pretty proud of those 43 who were cured."

"Yes, that is better than other similar facilities," stated Senator Allen. He was most impressed with Hunt's nurturing efforts as a gatekeeper.

The Kentucky Lunatic Asylum was showing potential to take better care of the unfortunates of the city. The Transylvania University with its medical and legal departments were still teaching students and gaining recognition for quality education. The newest Transylvania building had been lost after a fire but classes were held in homes around the growing town of Lexington. Transylvania University was still considered a tutor for the west by some.

Yet, Lexington was becoming a city divided between the citizens.

In the late 1820s, the Old Buffalo Trail was incorporated into a Maysville, Washington, Paris, and Lexington Turnpike Company. A sixty-five-mile road between Lexington and Maysville was built at a cost of $426,000, which included thirteen toll houses and six covered bridges. This was the first major attempt to provide a better road for travel in Kentucky. While water transportation was developing in other American cities, Lexington had no major river port for water transportation and was limited to the Old Buffalo Trail.

Sources for Chapter 3

Act to Carry into Operation the Kentucky Lunatic Asylum. *Senate Journal*, (1824): 137–138.

Adams, Joan Titley. *The Eastern State Lunatic Asylum, 1824–1844: A Reappraisal of Its Early History*. Unpublished at University of Louisville Medical School.

Coleman, J. W. *Famous Kentucky Duels*. Lexington, Kentucky: The Henry Clay Press, 1969.

Coleman, J. W. *The Squire's Sketches of Lexington*. Lexington, Kentucky: The Henry Clay Press, 1972.

Hunt, John W. (1824–1830) *Reports of the Kentucky Lunatic Asylum*. Available in Lexington Archives Lexington, Kentucky.

Kentucky Reporter. March 15, 1820.

Kentucky Reporter. January 16, 1828.

Klafter, C. *Reason over Precedents: Origins of American Legal Thought*. Westport, Connecticut: Greenwood Press, 1993.

Ramage, J. A. *John Wesley Hunt, Pioneer Merchant, Manufacturer and Financier*. Lexington, Kentucky: University of Kentucky Press, 1974.

Theobald, S. "Some Account of the Lunatic Asylum of Kentucky." *Transylvania Journal of Medicine* 2, no. 4 (November 1829): 500–511.

Visscher, M. *Humanistic Perspectives in Medical Ethics.* Prometheus Books: 1972.

Wright, John D. *Transylvania: Tutor to the West.* Lexington, Kentucky: Transylvania University Press, 1975.

Chapter Four

1830–1839

In the early part of January 1830, John Brand was talking to Richard Higgins in the office that they shared. Brand was currently fifty-five years old, while Higgins was sixty; both were remembering their early days in Lexington. They had come to the settlement as young men to make their fortunes, and they did.

"This city has been a good market for us in our business. The growing frontier needed our products," commented Brand.

"Yes," Higgins responded. "We have profited from selling hemp and cotton yards overland between Philadelphia and Natchez among large markets. Lexington has become the center of westward expansion and overland trading since 1812. We have done well as partners, and so have many citizens of Lexington."

"But," responded Brand, "I'm concerned that Lexington may lose its advantage to cities like Cincinnati and Louisville as water transportation improves. Lexington is not near any water, and we can lose trade to water transports."

"I had hoped that President Jackson would support an improved roadway system for more overland shipping," Higgins stated.

The northern part of the Old Buffalo Trail from Maysville through Lexington had been proposed by Henry Clay Sr. in 1830 to extend the

Cumberland National Road through Kentucky, creating a national road. The Old Buffalo Trail needed to be improved to be able to handle more transportation. The bill was passed by Congress but vetoed by President Andrew Jackson. As a result, commercial trade to and from Lexington became slower on the Maysville–Lexington Toll Road.

Brand said, "The president vetoed the Maysville Road Bill. Many of us local merchants saw that bill as the last hope for Lexington."

"We will not be able to keep up with the demand for products if the roads cannot carry them. The roads are too muddy several months of the year. Lexington may be doomed from a lack of future growth," Higgins said; he was very concerned.

"Maybe not; did you know that John Hunt and other merchants are considering a railroad project? It may be a feasible way of moving our products and create new trading markets to keep Lexington as a thriving community," Brand said enthusiastically.

"Yes," stated Higgins, "I had heard that and even talked to John Hunt yesterday about his plans."

"Everyone is in favor of a railroad, but they want the railroad to go through their town. The citizens of Frankfort cannot imagine a railway from Lexington to somewhere on the Ohio River without it going through Frankfort. There have been heated debates between citizens and the newspapers as to which towns the railway will follow, so nothing is settled. We must act soon, however," added Brand.

"They forget the purpose of the railway," argued Higgins. "Lexington needs to be able to ship products out or else our commercial businesses will die."

Brand held up the local newspaper, the *Kentucky Reporter*, and read, "All the hemp factories in Lexington sent over one thousand wagon loads of its products to Louisville last year and imported large amounts of sugar, coffee, tea, and iron by wagon." He set the paper down and said, "Now, the railroad is our only hope. They will be forming a group of stockholders, which I hope we can participate in. The books will be open for five days to allow individuals to buy a subscription."

Brand, Higgins, and Hunt did indeed buy subscriptions at the stockholders' meeting on March 6, 1830. Other stockholders included Dr. B. W. Dudley, and the remaining $400,000 was subscribed by Elisha Winter for himself and his wealthy associates. Henry Clay Sr. was numbered among his wealthy associates, but Clay Sr. was away at the time and was placed on the list as a rather heavy subscriber.

Another meeting at Postlethwait's Inn in April was presided over by Clay, who emphasized that "the project will succeed." The route from Lexington was to be started at the earliest possible date. Citizens from Louisville subscribed $200,000 so that the route would go into Louisville. The railroad was the major discussion throughout the year.

*   *   *

In October 1830, Brand arrived in his carriage at the asylum to attend the regular bimonthly meeting. Hunt still was chairman of the asylum board, with three of the same original members, Richard Higgins, John Brand, and Richard Aston. A new member, T. P. Hart, father-in-law of Henry Clay, replaced John Morton.

Brand could not help but reflect upon his own contributions to this asylum. It started with one square building and now was enlarged to provide care for all those who needed it. He was proud of his part in its success. He usually anticipated these meetings, but things were different today. He needed to talk with his friend.

Brand had arranged to arrive at the asylum at the same time as Hunt, the chairman, his closest friend and business partner. After greeting each other, they approached the front door of the asylum and waited for the matron, Mrs. King, to unlock the door and admit them to the facility.

John King, the steward, greeted them and escorted them into the committee board room, usually used for serving meals for the more able lunatics. Both men observed the cleanliness of the room and set the room for their meeting. They complimented King for keeping a clean house.

"We expect to be here for nearly two hours; can you keep the lunatics out during our meeting?" asked Hunt.

"Of course, the lunatics who can understand will take the responsibility of guarding the door and be rewarded for helping me. I will see to that," responded King, who politely excused himself and shut the door to the two board members.

King proudly reminisced to himself about how he and his wife were the longest keepers of this institution. They had gained a repetition for fairness and kindness in these well-paid positions. Mrs. King conscientiously saw that all the female patients had adequate clothing and were appropriately clothed in their apartments before allowing them into the halls. Warm clothing was always provided when needed. John King checked regularly on the men and saw that their needs were adequately tended. He followed the care methods of Dr. Theobald, who called it "parental government."

Parental government consisted of giving rewards to lunatics who did as was expected. If a lunatic could not be controlled, only then was he or she restrained in shackles or straitjackets. He prided himself in being a fair keeper to the ones in his charge and viewed himself as using the most progressive methods. King periodically checked on those in restraints and assured them that freedom was possible when they could control themselves. Some other asylum keepers were more into punishment, while King was known as a kind one. The Kings took their work seriously, but they had one fault that would later result in them losing their jobs.

After the door closed to the board room, Brand anxiously stated, "Mr. Hunt, I have something dreadful to discuss with you, something you should hear from me rather than from talk in the town." He was visibly shaking.

"Oh, do sit down and tell me," responded Hunt. "I can't imagine anything so bad."

"My daughter, Elizabeth, is being prevailed upon by Theodore Clay to marry him. He is very demanding and follows her everywhere, and she cannot escape from him. He has a bad temper, and my daughter is more interested in Mr. Higgins's son, Richard, than Theodore Clay, who will not accept her refusal."

"Well," observed Hunt, "I can see that you are concerned. I have known Theodore Clay all his life, and at one time he was a promising young lawyer. More recently, I have heard of his unsteadiness in jobs and indifferent morality. However, a good wife and marriage can help him, especially someone like your daughter."

"Certainly," stated Brand, "and my wife and I had given Theodore permission to see her. However, it has not been the usual courtship; he has been unreasonable and obsessed with her. He is easily irritated. I'm very concerned for my daughter."

"Yes, I have heard he gets irrational at times; I'm so sorry."

"My concern here," Brand said, taking a breath to relax, "is that Richard Higgins Sr. will attend this board meeting today, and his son is seeking to court my daughter."

The difficulty was that Theodore Clay was demanding and threatening to Brand's daughter. Both Higgins and Thomas Hart, grandfather of Theodore Clay, were board members. Hart could see no wrong in his grandson and could not understand why Brand's daughter was refusing to court him. This was all the talk in the town.

These families were part of the early society of Lexington, and they were all involved in caring for the asylum. Brand was uncomfortable with the other members knowing that the younger ones were being torn apart by social gossip and criticism.

Hunt listened. "Why did you not handle the Clay boy yourself rather than letting your daughter become the town talk? Lexington is still a small frontier town, and respectable families usually handle such matters themselves rather than adding to the town gossip. You are certainly a well-respected family."

"Oh, I know now that we did not handle this properly, but Elizabeth is my only daughter, unlike you, who has many daughters," stated Brand. "We wanted her to decide first, but now, Theodore Clay will not accept her refusal. As you know, the Clay family is highly regarded here in Lexington, and Theodore has always been unable to do anything wrong."

"Yes, Henry Clay Sr. is well respected; however, there have been many times when Theodore and his brother, Thomas, have shown their bad habits in Lexington," stated Hunt.

"Others," added Brand, "tend to look the other way because of their respect for Henry Clay. Just this October, Theodore returned from St. Louis after having consumed all his money and he is now living on his father's goodwill. The Clay family is hoping that marriage will settle him down; therefore, they are encouraging it for both sons, just to settle them down."

"I remember Theodore as a lad; he gave a 4th of July oration, mostly due to the influence of his father and family," stated Hunt. "I'm sorry for your concerns, but we have patients to see and decisions to make for the next two weeks. What does all this have to do with the meeting?"

"I wanted you to know that we may develop conflicts. We are all loyal to our families and may have difficulty reaching common agreements."

"Mr. Brand, I see your point, but our duty is to this great institution. Thank you for telling me about this potential problem; as chairman, I will try to keep out individual prejudices when deciding what is best for this institution."

"And sir, I want only what is best for this institution, that is why I am telling you this," apologized Brand.

"We will talk of this later. Let's now prepare for the other members."

Hunt greeted the arriving members. The meeting continued with a general discussion about plans to build a separate building for the most disturbed patients. The governor had approved funds for a new building as a way of separating the more disturbed from those who could improve. Every member agreed.

After the meeting, Hunt and Brand left the room together. Both men stopped in the hall to observe the lunatics sitting and lying on the floor with clean shirts and pants; their hair was neat. Hunt talked to another one mopping the floor and praised him for his work. They proceeded toward the entrance.

Hunt whispered to Brand on the way out, "Remember when he was admitted? That is J. J. from Mr. Sterling Allen's farm. His conduct and manners have improved. He is now boarding in the tidy apartments on the first floor. He attends the weekly dances and participates with others."

"I understand Mr. John King depends upon him to keep the floor clean," added Brand.

"Yes, such improvements are what we are achieving here. I am so proud."

"I agree, but why must we continue to add more buildings? Last year, we had thirty-five patients leave but admitted more. Is this typical of other facilities?" Brand asked.

"I know of only a few similar institutions."

"Do they keep adding buildings like us?" asked Brand.

"Yes, all the asylums are adding. The need is so great and the demand has never been met."

"So, you think that when the demand is met, then the need for more rooms will decline?" asked Brand.

"There are only a few state-supported asylums in the United States. But Virginia has opened its second state hospital, while South Carolina has opened one. There are many more private facilities, but I do not know much about them; they usually have more private funds," responded Hunt.

"The private ones do not take our type of lunatics either," stated Brand.

"Yes, they take the ones who have a paying family or some other income. We take the ones who have no money and the state pays," added Hunt.

"All this is very interesting. I would like to know about the other asylums. Are they adding more building, as we are?" asked Brand.

"I shall seek advice from the medical professors at Transylvania Medical School as to your question," Hunt said as he boarded his carriage. "You can call upon me tomorrow afternoon at my home, and we can discuss all your concerns." Hunt shook hands with his friend.

The next afternoon, Brand called upon Hunt, and they sat near the roaring fireplace in his parlor. Across from the fireplace was a desk and bookcase, giving the room the appearance of an office. Two of Hunt's sons, John Jr. and Charleston, passed through and greeted Brand. Both sons were attending the Transylvania University, one in medicine and the other in law. All twelve of Hunt's children were at home, reflecting a much busier household than Brand's.

"John Jr. and I visited the medical school with professors this morning at the Medical Hall," stated Hunt.

"I am eager to know what they told you."

"Dr. Cross is still a professor there and remembers when he was our first physician at the asylum.

"Oh, yes," answered Brand." I remember him."

"I discussed your concerns about our growing need for more buildings. Dr. Cross claims that there is little known about other institutions, and state care for the insane is such a new idea that there are no answers. He did confirm that all such facilities are adding buildings."

"I can believe that," stated Brand. "We are real pioneers in the area of state-supported lunacy care."

"We know that the private hospitals do not take the pauper lunatics, whereas the state asylums do. The paupers are more hopeless cases and have less chance of a family taking them home."

"Therefore, we need to add necessary buildings for them."

"Yes, all are adding buildings," responded Hunt. "However, several of the professors are interested in bringing students to visit our Asylum."

"Why?" asked Brand.

"Students are viewing our Asylum as a source of learning rather than just being a place of shame. I'm so pleased."

"That all sounds so very good!" Then Brand changed the subject by saying, "Do you think Mr. Thomas Hart and Mr. Richard Higgins will stay on the board? They both appeared to be uncomfortable yesterday, and neither one asked anything about my family. I could sense a distance."

Hunt responded, "I think they will stay. Both are very committed to the work of the asylum and smart enough to realize that families will work out their own differences."

"I hope so."

Hunt continued, "Mr. Thomas Hart is very good with his political connections, and he can always find some source of money. We need him on the board to influence the governor and obtain financing for the institution. He volunteered to provide food for Thanksgiving and Christmas dinners since the state treasury will not pay for such items."

Brand nodded his head and said, "The patients will enjoy that."

Hunt continued, "Mr. Richard Higgins is a businessman who is valuable to the board for his knowledge about construction. They both are dedicated to this institution so I think all this will pass; I hope so."

"I'm so sorry that the disagreements between our young people have led to this," Brand said.

"Have you considered writing to Henry Clay?" Hunt asked his friend. "I know he has just finished his term as secretary of state and is considering a run for the presidency, but he is very concerned about his children and he is reasonable."

"Well, his wife, Lucretia, daughter of Thomas Hart, stays here at Ashland. I have considered talking to her," answered Brand, "but she denies that anything is wrong with her children."

"Yes, I know Lucretia Clay is that way. However, Henry Clay is not and has expressed concerns to me about his two oldest sons," stated Hunt.

"Theodore is obsessed with my daughter; is that lunacy? We deal mostly with the pauper lunatics, but Theodore has had the best of opportunities; can this be lunacy?"

Hunt leaned over to Brand and whispered, "I did talk to Dr. Charles Caldwell about Theodore Clay's behavior and asked him if this was lunacy."

"Well, what did he say?" asked Brand. "I know Dr. Charles Caldwell is well versed in the theory of phrenology."

"Yes, and I wanted to know if his knowledge could explain such behavior," added Hunt. "This was a personal interest for me since I am uncertain if Dr. Caldwell can explain anything with his phrenology theories."

"Well, did you find out anything?"

"He sees the Clay son as being destroyed by alcohol usage. Dr. Caldwell believes in temperance with alcohol, and for some people, such as Theodore, where alcohol usage has always been a part of his life, he sees alcohol as causing his erratic actions and lunacy. Since we deal with the more unfortunates of life, we don't often see those who have had excesses in their life, such as Theodore Clay."

"I'm not surprised," stated Brand. "We all know that alcohol usage is common in that family, but most members never reach Theodore's level.

Alcohol usage is really very common in the early settlements, especially among ignorant people, but excessive alcoholism among the more educated is something we rarely see."

"Well, phrenology believes in reform through self-knowledge; however, Theodore and his family are unwilling to see that anything is wrong. Phrenology can only help those who are willing."

"Would it help me and my family?" uttered Brand.

"No, not unless this is your problem, but you must consider strongly writing your concerns to Mr. Clay; he is a very reasonable person. He is concerned for his family and needs to know about his son's behavior."

Brand thought for a minute. "Well, I could try writing him and seeing if he has any suggestions; it might work."

"I think he would be willing to listen to your concerns."

"I have suspected that Theodore Clay is insane; he is so preoccupied over my daughter." Brand shook his head in disbelief. "But Theodore is not the usual kind."

"Well, Theodore Clay certainly had every opportunity in this world. Have you considered talking to the sheriff? You and your family might need protection, and the sheriff needs to know this."

"Yes, I will do that."

"The sheriff will know what you need to do to protect your family, if Theodore gets worse."

"Well," responded Brand, "we might need that protection. I do have two sons who might be helpful."

"Gratefully, we are no longer a frontier settlement where we have to defend ourselves with a gun," added Hunt.

"Thank you so much for discussing this with me; I must leave." Brand stood up and reached for his hat. "I need to check on our Spring Street hemp store."

Hunt added, "I remember when there were no other stores in that area except ours. Now there are four?"

"Yes, that is correct; the town has surely grown. Well, I hope to see you later," Brand said as he shook hands with Hunt and left.

Brand did visit the sheriff, who assured him that Kentucky law had a provision for protecting citizens from dangerous lunatics. If twelve homeowners determined a lunatic to be dangerous, the court could commit him or her to an asylum against his or her will. Brand felt better knowing about the legal protection, whereas previously, individuals protected themselves with their own guns.

There are many letters in Henry Clay's collection, published and edited by the University of Kentucky, but none from Brand. There are other letters in Clay's collection about his son Theodore, which this author examined. (see references at the end of this chapter.)

One letter from Henry Clay, dated October 31, 1830, to his third son, Henry Clay Jr., stated "my regrets and disappointment are so great in respect to your elder brothers, Thomas and Theodore W. Clay." He described their behaviors and said, "Thomas is at home [and has] been in two debauches and the last threatened his life … also Theodore."

Henry Clay Sr. may have been aware of the Brand family concerns when he wrote, "On the subject of a certain young lady … [Theodore] is, we all begin to fear, quite deranged. He seems to be doomed to misery and to render wretched all around him."

The Fayette County Court records show that Brand contacted the clerk of the court on September 29, 1831, and said he "considered his family in danger of Theodore Clay, provided that he is not taken in custody and confined." Brand sent his daughter to stay with relatives in Mississippi for her own protection.

The county sheriff was summoned to impanel twelve good and lawful men to determine if Theodore W. Clay was a lunatic. The panel decided that he was a lunatic and should be confined to the local asylum. Citizens on the panel included Dr. Charles Caldwell, Colonel Leslie Combs, Robert Wickliffe, and John Postlethwait.

The sheriff took Theodore Clay to the asylum, and John King, steward, provided him with a room. The town was shocked that Henry Clay did not seek Theodore's release, but the Brand family was relieved.

On October 22, 1831, the first part of the railroad was laid. The local citizens of Lexington were pleased, and a procession was formed on the Transylvania University Campus with General Combs as marshal.

Following General Combs with his aide on horseback were local military companies, Governor Metcalfe, officials of Lexington, faculty and students of Transylvania University, and stockholders of the company. The procession moved in a circle around the university lawn to the location of the first rail. President Winter handed Governor Metcalfe a hammer, and he proceeded to drive the first spike.

Immediately after the rail-laying ceremony, Dr. Caldwell addressed the group. While Dr. Caldwell often used his lectures to discuss phrenology, he spoke on this day with polished and eloquent phrases of the railroad's advantages to Lexington and the adjacent countryside. He acknowledged that competition with the steamboat provided other cities with newer and swifter modes of transportation, but he predicted that the railroad would gradually restore prosperity to Lexington. Then Dr. Caldwell ended by saying, "May we hope to put into active operation once more our time-honored medical college and attract a creditable number of students." He was always an ambassador for the Medical School of Transylvania.

Dr. Caldwell's speech was viewed by the young Dr. William S. Chipley, who had graduated from Transylvania Medical School the previous year. He admired Dr. Caldwell's knowledge and had studied with him to learn practical applications of phrenology.

After leaving the ceremony, Hunt remarked to Higgins about Dr. Caldwell, "He talks about phrenology theory but never seems to get around to really using it to help people; it is just rhetoric. I've lost interest in his opinions. Of course, he is right about the railroads, but I'm not sure of his other ideas."

"Dr. Charles Caldwell is a great man, he published an important book, *Elements of Phrenology*, a few years ago," argued Higgins. "He is just one of those people with theories and no practical application."

"But of what value is phrenology if it cannot be applied in a way that is helpful?" asked Hunt.

Higgins responded, "This phrenology has great potential for the future; just wait and see."

Hunt was thinking about more pressing business needing his attention. Calvin Morgan, his daughter's husband in Huntsville, Alabama, was having difficulty paying his taxes, and they were losing their farm. Hunt offered Morgan management of one of his farms in Lexington if they would move to Lexington. Their son, John Hunt Morgan, was named for him, and Hunt wanted to spend time with him.

Another of Hunt's sons, Charleston, was running for mayor of Lexington. In 1832, Charleston became the first mayor of Lexington as the city was incorporated with a Board of Councilmen installed. The population had grown to upward of seven thousand citizens. The sheriff, now forty-two years old, swore in the new mayor.

This same year, Robert S. Todd purchased a fine Georgian house at 574 West Main Street. Originally it was the Sign of the Green Tree Inn. One daughter, Mary, lived there until she visited her sister in Illinois, where she met a young Abraham Lincoln. The rest is documented history.

The next year, after being committed to the asylum, Theodore Clay wrote to his father, "In my letter which I wrote last week, I did not speak of getting out of this. I believe I am at a loss to know how I am to be released from this place. I have no expectation that in the press of business which must crowd upon you, time will allow you to answer my insipid and useless letters. ... I suppose you could have more weight than anyone else. My greatest wish is to simply earn my living and enjoy a portion of the good things of life. They have just elected Charleston Hunt lord mayor of the town. I have no news to offer you; but that our friends are well as I feel myself to be; and not to be too pertinacious, anxiously desirous of having something to do."

At the end of January 1832, in another letter from Theodore to his father, he wrote, "I received your favor and the documents in 3 parcels and return you my sincere thanks. ... This attention during your variety of engagements which must oppress you is as grateful as unexpected to me. I have executed your request for Dr. Jordan and he says he intended to have written to you. ... The concern you and my good mother feel for my welfare, and the disposition you express to lend me aid, was secure in the belief you had. ... I need not stop to say that a prejudice perhaps natural exists in Lexington, for which also perhaps I can account, and which I confess myself both unable and unwilling to undertake to stem, if I have the option. A footing of equality as I think myself entitled to was fully communicated to me in one way or another will not be awarded to me. The plan you suggested of going on your land in Illinois has occurred to me: but some security in bank; or a small loan of $2,000 would make such a retreat acceptable to me."

Theodore's letter continued, "I think Dr. Jordan informed me you were good enough to assume the little sums I owed in Lexington. I would be glad if convenient, you would send me a copy of *Elliott's Almanac* for 1832."

On January 29, 1832, Andrew McCalla died at an advanced old age. He had succeeded at establishing the asylum and contributing several years in the apothecary. His wisdom, knowledge, and dedication would be missed by the asylum board members. He also had knowledge about natural curative methods different from the newly trained physicians.

In February 1832, Henry Clay wrote to Hunt as chairman of the asylum board, stating, "I have to thank you for your friendly letter respecting Theodore Clay. [As a concerned father, Theodore's] condition has been a cause of inexpressible regret and anxiety to us. I am happy to learn from you, as I have from others, that there is some improvement in his situation. Dr. Jordan has mentioned to me that exercise on horseback would be beneficial to him. I have left at Ashland [his home in Lexington] a grey horse that he rode. Will you do me the favor to send for that horse and have it kept, at my expense, at the hospital for his use?"

*   *   *

Hunt was called to the institution on the night of March 6; someone had died. As he hurried into the front door, John King greeted him sadly. "I knew you would want to know, J. J. from Scott County died tonight. Remember, he had lived with Mr. and Mrs. Sterling Allen for years and they visited him often."

"Oh, yes, I remember," stated Hunt. "He was doing so well here, helping with the cleaning. He had gotten better. This is horrible; where was our protective custody?"

"We found him dead in the dining room."

"Oh, how horrible," Hunt said, sitting down in a near chair. "What happened?" He felt so bad after being the one to recommend J. J.'s admission here. "How could this have happened?"

"Several lunatics were in the dining room and they got into a fight. As far as I know, he did not fight. He was beaten by two others who go around threatening ones who will not defend themselves. The two that I suspect are now locked up."

"Oh, poor J. J.; yes, I agree, he would not fight," observed Hunt. "I just can't believe you did not hear something happening."

"I was busy with another patient. You know, Theodore W. Clay; he is always demanding answers. I was talking to him when the fight occurred."

"What about the two that killed him?"

"They are just real crazy and there is nothing we can do. Keeping them locked up is all we can do; they should stay locked up," replied King. "I was worried about telling the sheriff that there has been a death here. I would have sent for him but waited until you got here."

"Yes, you were right," stated Hunt. "I hope this information does not get to the newspaper. Mr. and Mr. Allen will be notified. They have been coming to some of the weekly dances to see J. J. I would hope that they will understand."

The sheriff was called and he followed with the usual questions of how it happened. The incident was explained to the sheriff and the Allens. All were sad, but death and lunacy were commonly associated. Hunt had hoped to change that common association, but even he had discovered that a well-managed facility cannot prevent every death.

On April 9, 1832, Henry Clay Jr., Theodore's brother, wrote to his father that, "Theodore visited me today at Ashland with Dr. Jordan, who attends him. He looks better than I ever saw him before. The necessity of placing him where he is was certainly a melancholy affliction for all of us; but it has long existed and he is now in better health than he has been for a long time."

Theodore Clay wrote his father on May 20, stating, "I wrote to you some weeks ago stating that I found myself unpleasantly situated here [at the asylum]. ... Far from desiring to remove obstacles, they seem inclined to increase rather than to remove. And I feel no reason why I should be subject to the will of others and not a free agent. I have written a respectful request to the Commissioners and they have given me not an answer. I expect therefore that Justice will be done to me and hope that it will be speedily."

Henry Clay Jr. wrote to his father in June of that same year, "You write inquiring about Theodore. You say that his letters to you are perfectly rational. Theodore has not yet recovered his rationality on all subjects. I will first give you Dr. B. W. Dudley's opinion and afterward my own. According to that worthy man and excellent physician, Theodore is deranged upon two subjects, love and ambition. The first can only be cured by time, the second by humiliation. By humiliation he means that Theodore should be treated by all as an ordinary young man incapable of self direction. ... Dr. B. W. Dudley thinks that Theodore has already had too much liberty in the use of a horse, and that we have done wrong by sending him the political periodicals, as it would seem to show evidence for his opinions. He doubts as I do, whether Theodore will ever be a useful member of society, for he has not been before."

Henry Clay Jr. shared his own opinions with his father: "The other day Theodore left the asylum and came to Ashland: he was with me a night and part of two days: while he was there he convinced me that he was not restored. We [other family members] were about to have a meeting of the Commissioners, for the purpose of entrusting him with me until your return. But my own conviction and Dr. B. W. Dudley's strenuous assertion persuaded me not to make the proposal. Theodore is again in the asylum, and I hope that all our friends, especially you and my mother will so restrain your feelings as to permit him to return there."

Henry Clay Jr. stated, "But after all the humiliation and misfortune is in his insanity and not in his residence at the asylum, which is but the mode of his recovery. I write my opinions sincerely and frankly. Affection for you and for Theodore has equally inspired my words."

On December 13, 1832, Theodore's sister, Anne Clay Erwin, wrote to her father that "Theodore went home the day after you left, and although Mama is now fully convinced that he is deranged, he has so far conducted himself quietly and she is much happier than if he were anywhere else."

In 1832, Senator John Rowan Allen ended his terms of representing Green County. He had taken care of the family's holdings and completed his responsibilities to them. He moved to Lexington and married Elizabeth Buckner, daughter of Judge Richard Buckner. He decided to practice law with his father-in-law and study medicine at the Transylvania Medical School. He had observed how many lunatics were bled according to Dr. Benjamin Rush's directions. Many had died, and for others, bleeding did not help them. As a lawyer, he often questioned this practice and decided to study medicine himself to assess the value of using bleeding methods with lunatics.

*   *   *

On June 3, 1833, the Asiatic cholera came to Lexington. During the next three to four weeks, fifteen hundred people became sick; they died at the rate of fifty to sixty a day. Businesses were closed and many people fled the city. The sheriff and deputies checked with local citizens to see if they needed help.

Dr. Dudley told the sheriff how he stayed in his home and preserved his two sons from the disease. He explained how during surgery, he noticed that any water could be a source of contamination and he learned to use only boiled water. He applied that same information to his family during the cholera epidemic. They stayed in their home, and none became sick.

By the middle of July, the plague had left 502 people in the city dead. The asylum lost thirty-three lunatics during the epidemic. An orphan asylum was founded on West Third Street to care for children whose parents had died from cholera. Dr. Richard Pindell, husband of Elizabeth Hart, died taking care of the sick. He had been a surgeon in the Revolutionary Army. Major Thomas H. Pindell, Dr. Pindell's son, was one of the first contributors to the Fayette Hospital. After serving in the War of 1812, he became a respected merchant in Lexington. His son, Richard Pindell, became an attorney, was appointed commonwealth attorney, and later became the second manager of the asylum.

Early in 1833, Henry Clay Sr. was presented a private traveling coach by admiring friends. This was his personal traveling coach to use between his home in Lexington and the nation's capital. Edward P. Johnson served as driver for the private coach until additional drivers were hired. Mr. Johnson had developed a regularly scheduled coach line over Kentucky; his office was in the Phoenix Hotel.

* * *

In December of 1833, Henry Clay Jr. wrote to his father, "The Commissioners have taken Theodore once more under their protection. The decision to recommit Theodore was mainly his sister, Anne; he had become too dangerous to have in the house. Theodore's face is pale and emaciated and his mind is filled with suspicions and conspiracies. We ought never to resign hope, and the discipline of a Hospital is the best remedy for this disease."

During 1833, Transylvania University published a Catalogue of the Officers and Students at all three schools: the medical, law, and Morrison College. The medical school had 260 students, with 105 from Kentucky. There were 39 medical students from Tennessee, 25 from Alabama, 20 from Virginia, 19 from Mississippi, 11 from Georgia, 10 from South Carolina, 7 from North Carolina and Illinois, 5 from Ohio, 4 from Missouri, 3 from Indiana, 2 from Louisiana, and 1 from Pennsylvania and Florida, showing the wide geographic areas that this school influenced.

The faculty had been increased to take on the additional numbers of students. Those of the faculty were Rev. Benjamin Peers, president; Dr. B. W. Dudley, professor of anatomy and surgery; Dr. Charles Caldwell, professor of the institutes and clinical practice and medical jurisprudence; Dr. John Cooke, professor of the theory and practice of medicine; and Dr. William H. Richardson, professor of obstetrics and the diseases of women and children.

Other professors included Dr. Charles W. Short, MD, professor of materia medica and medical botany and dean of the medical facility; Dr. Lunsford P. Yandell, professor of chemistry and pharmacy; Dr. Robert Peter, librarian of the Medical Library; Daniel Mayes, professor of law; and Madison C. Johnson, secretary to the Board of Trustees, with Robert Wickliffe as chairman and John W. Hunt, along with fourteen other Lexington citizens on the board.

The Law Department had fifty students, with about thirty-two from Kentucky. This 1833 catalogue also identified the students in Morrison College and its preparatory school. There were thirty-two students, with all but four from Lexington.

Young Chipley had lost interest in Dr. Caldwell's theory of phrenology and left Lexington after completing his medical degree. He had observed so many internal problems at the Transylvania Medical School that he moved to Georgia to establish a private medical practice.

The railway from Frankfort, Kentucky, to Lexington was completed on January 31, 1834. Previously, President Winters had to make an eloquent appeal to the citizens of Lexington to pay their subscriptions so that there was sufficient money to pay for reaching Frankfort by train. The *Kentucky Gazette* stated, "It is with a sigh of relief that this much on the railroad has been accomplished. Construction on the railroads had been stopped so long at Frankfort that it became known as the Lexington and Frankfort Railroad Company."

*   *   *

On January 1835, the Board of Commissioners at the Kentucky Lunatic Asylum had their regular meeting. The board consisted of the same members except for John Morton, who was replaced by Rev. Stephen Chipley. Chairman Hunt started the meeting by giving a full report of last year's activity as follows:

"We had at the beginning of the year 83 lunatics with 54 being received, 19 were discharged, 5 eloped, 21 died, leaving 93 now in the house. Since we have opened in 1824, there have been 502 admitted, 219 discharged or eloped, and 190 died. Anyone have any questions about these figures?"

Brand asked, "How many are here from this county?"

"Well," the chairman said, "I count eleven remaining from Fayette County, whereas those from surrounding counties are five more."

"So that makes most of them from this area?" asked Brand.

Chairman Hunt responded positively, as he looked over the room for other questions.

"How many out-of-states do we have?" Brand asked. "I'm assuming that they all pay privately?"

Hunt recalculated the list of lunatics and announced, "There are seven from other states and all are privately paid. They are from states that do not currently have a state hospital. One is from Ohio, which is in the planning stage of opening a state asylum."

The newest member, Rev. Chipley, asked, "How many lunatics of the first two years do we still have?"

The chairman replied, "As you know, each lunatic is assigned a number in sequence to being admitted. Theodore Clay was the 388th to be admitted, and even when he was placed on home leave, he returned using that same number."

"Theodore was admitted in 1832?" asked Rev. Chipley.

"Yes, he was; therefore, in answer to your other question, Rev. Chipley, there are six remaining from the first two years, and number 73 is the last of that six, the 73rd admission was in 1825."

Rev. Chipley said, "Elizabeth, from my church, was admitted on May 4, 1824; she is now the oldest admission in this institution, right?"

"Yes, and Mary, Polly, and Allen were also admitted in 1824," answered Hunt. "The other one admitted in 1825 was Obesance. On December 30, the 448th admission was a male from Lewis County."

Brand asked, "Sir, as I recall, in the early days, a majority of those were idiots?"

"Yes, Mr. Brand," stated the chairman. "I have previously calculated those with a diagnosis and currently we have fifty-six with the disease of mania, fifteen with the disease of idiocy, seven have epilepsy, two have mania a potu, two with peurperil, one with dolore, and another is here as the result of a fall. The larger number of mania shows we now have the more treatable ones."

"Remember," replied Brand, laughing over what he considered silly, "after the first year, Mr. and Mrs. Stainton left the institution because they claimed it was full of idiots and incurables?"

"Oh, yes," stated the chairman, "I remember those days. Now we have more treatable patients," He turned to Rev. Chipley and said, "Sir, we are so glad to have you here with us on this board. I understand your son, William S. Chipley, is practicing medicine in Georgia?"

"Yes, he is there as a physician, having finished from our own medical school. While I do not have much respect for physicians, I do believe Dr. Cross is an exception. I believe in herbal methods and distrust most doctors."

"Well, your son had the best medical training at the Transylvania Medical School," added Chairman Hunt.

"Yes, if my son follows some of the most knowledgeable professors at Transylvania, I will be pleased. He is now twenty-five years old and must make his own decisions. He enjoys living in Georgia, but there are still Indians there."

"We do need well-trained physicians," added Brand.

"However," continued Rev. Chipley, "I did know several of the early lunatics such as Elizabeth, Polly, Allen, and Ann, who used to wander around town. They appear to be satisfied staying here, while I see Polly and Ann are working in the women's department." He continued standing to make his opinions known.

"Yes, they are," added the chairman.

"I am most pleased with their progress," continued Rev. Chipley as he started to sit down. "One question I have, if I should ask, what are the diseases such as mania a potu, peurperial, and dolore?"

Laughing, Chairman Hunt said, "Reverend, you need to know that we do not determine the names of diseases; we are given information that comes to us from the court records. We have laughed about some of the names of diseases because we have often wondered what some of them mean. As you, we really have no idea. It really makes no difference in how they are treated, it is just a medical thing."

"Also, many of the local physicians do not agree upon what the names mean. We all have questions," added Brand with a smirk. Other members shared a grin.

The chairman called a halt to private comments and asked, "Are there any other problems we need to discuss?"

"Yes," stated Thomas Hart. "I would like to know when we will be hiring a full-time superintendent. We need someone who has the medical knowledge to direct this facility; many other asylums are hiring full-time superintendents now."

"Yes, we all agree," stated the chairman. "However, no one at the Transylvania Medical School is interested. We have asked for several years. There is one who might be available in a few years, Senator John R. Allen."

"Yes," stated Brand, "he has moved here and married into the Buckner family, a well-respected legal family."

"Senator Allen has developed an interest in caring for lunatics. If you remember, he kept up with one of the lunatics killed a few years back. His uncle, Sterling Allen, had cared for J. J. until he was admitted here. Also, as a senator from Green County, he had an interest in the care of lunatics when he was in the Kentucky legislature. He gained some political and financial support for us in the past."

"Sterling Allen was an original contributor to this facility," added Rev. Chipley. "He was such a caring person."

"Yes, both sides of his family have had a long involvement with this institution, and he has visited here many times. He is now going to Transylvania Medical School to learn to be a doctor."

"He will be good," stated Brand.

"Yes, he is certainly our best prospect at this time. There are no others interested," stated the chairman. He recognized Brand for a question.

"I understand Dr. Benjamin W. Dudley, as chair of anatomy and surgery, had earlier proposed to move the Medical School of Transylvania to Louisville. That town is growing faster than Lexington due to it being on a major waterway. Is it true that the faculty agreed and they are making plans to do so?" asked Brand. The other members responded to the news in shock.

Chairman Hunt responded quickly, knowing it was a surprise, "Currently, Dr. Dudley has deserted the cause. Four of the six members of the faculty have been blamed for that movement. Dr. Charles Caldwell was the most active and is expected to be dismissed. Drs. Yandell and Cook will not be reappointed next year. Dr. C. W. Short, brother-in-law to Dr. B. W. Dudley, has already joined the medical school in Louisville."

"So," said Richard Higgins, "the rumors are true; we will be seeing some changes with the Transylvania Medical School next year?"

"Yes," said the chairman. "We will wait and see." He looked around at the bewildered faces. The chairman knew more but he had an obligation to let the Transylvania Medical School announce the details. "Are there any more things to discuss?" he asked. "Then, I will adjourn this meeting." Each person was feeling apprehensive about the future of the medical school.

On December 28, 1836, the mayor of Louisville petitioned the legislature to move the Transylvania Medical School to that city. The petition was rejected, but a second medical school was created in Louisville. There would now be competition between two Kentucky medical schools. Dr. Dudley was reappointed to be chair of anatomy and surgery at Transylvania Medical School. The Louisville Medical School was more promising because of its location.

In 1837, Hunt presided over a meeting of the Board of Commissioners at the Kentucky Lunatic Asylum, although he was now sixty-four and had lost his wife in October of 1835. He was still an able leader and sought to add any new scientific advances. He wrote regular reports about the institution and always presented his yearly report to the board. He presented the following information:

There are 113 patients and some of the grounds were fenced at a cost of $1,442.69. We have added a firehouse to the wash-house where a fire engine is stored and a workshop is provided for patients.

We have added an iron-and-drying room to the wash-house and built a cistern to supply the fire engine. We have erected a new building in the back to care for the more disturbed ones at the cost of $6,018.06. Is there anything else we should discuss?

The chairman was showing an unusual slowness with his sitting and standing while opening the meeting up to further discussion.

Higgins asked, "Sir, is Dr. J. C. Jordon still our resident physician?"

"No," answered the chairman. "He never was a resident physician. He was hired by the Clay family to accompany Theodore Clay while here at the institution. However, the Clay family is now declining to support Dr. Jordon further. Dr. Jordon helped McCalla out as a clerk at this facility in the past, but he is not interested in full-time employment here."

Hart, grandfather of Theodore Clay, asked to respond. The chairman granted him the time, and he said, "The Clay family is discouraged over any improvement in Theodore and feels that extra financial expense is wasteful at this time."

"We are so sorry," Chairman Hunt said as he pushed to express his regrets.

Hart continued, "My daughter, Lucretia Clay, has finally accepted Theodore's lunacy and the family can rarely afford the extra expense of a private physician regularly. Theodore does require an attendant with him when out on the grounds or he will run away."

"Yes, it is such a sad situation," replied Brand. "He had so much potential at one time. Theodore has graceful manners and a flow of conversation that renders him an object of interest to all visitors, especially the medical students. We feel remorse for your daughter's family." Other members of the board supported his comments.

Hart continued, "The family is following the recommendations of Dr. B. W. Dudley, that Theodore be given less liberty and more confinement. Dr. Jordon is no longer needed, and the asylum has a right to discharge him." His hurt over his grandson was obvious in his face as other members felt his grief.

After some silence, Rev. Chipley asked, "Who is our resident physician?"

"Actually, the staff of Transylvania Medical School have continued to alternate since no one wants the position on a full-time basis," stated Chairman Hunt.

"Well, I think that is best since many of the educated physicians do not want to deal with lunacy. I'm not sure their medicine works with lunatics either," added Rev. Chipley.

"I'm sure your son as a physician might not agree," said Brand. "Dr. Caldwell's phrenology has many good claims."

"Oh," added Rev. Chipley, "my son has all those educated ideas of new medical cures. That is similar to phrenology, which has never been useful at this asylum, although Dr. Caldwell has been given many offers to apply it here."

"Dr. Caldwell claims that our lunatics are too uneducated for phrenology," added Chairman Hunt. "However, I'm not sure that is correct. Dr. Caldwell is good in theories but short on application. He never applied it."

Rev. Chipley asked to be heard as he said, "I still believe in herbs and physical activities as best for comforting our most disturbed patients. I'm most pleased with the enclosed fencing near the building where the most disturbed can walk off their excessive energy rather than always restraining them."

Chairman Hunt smiled at Rev. Chipley and said, "Sir, I also have an educated physician son, and I understand what you say. The physicians can only care for medical problems, and sometimes, that is very limited." Then he recognized Higgins.

Higgins said, "I was so excited about Dr. Caldwell, who had psychological knowledge about the mind, but he really had nothing to offer here at the asylum. He was a real failure here."

"Dr. Caldwell did write an article published in the *Transylvania Journal of Medicine* in 1832 titled 'Thoughts on Mental Derangement, Introductory to a Brief Course of Lectures on that Form of Disease,'" said the chairman. "The whole seventeen pages emphasized his belief that the knowledge about madness is found through an acquaintance with the study of phrenology." He recognized Brand.

"Did his article specify any causes of madness?" asked Brand.

"Well, he stated that the difference between madness and other maladies arises from the difference between the organs in which they are seated," summarized the chairman.

"What does that mean?" asked Brand.

"As I understand it," continued the chairman, "if they were interchanged, such as the organ of madness that constitutes the seat of madness, with the seat of peripneumony, then it becomes peripneumony. His proof is when diseases of the thoracic and other organs pass into insanity, and insanity into them," commented the chairman.

"Dr. Caldwell did make specific remarks," added Higgins, "about mental derangement. The mere change in the condition of the faculties of the mind, from that of health, does not constitute the real malady."

"He sees the external evidence of the disease lying within the form of a morbid condition of the brain; that to him is what constitutes madness," added the chairman.

"Dr. Caldwell concluded that when an organ is healthy, its functions are healthy. External causes will excite diseases, such as mental derangement, in those who are predisposed to it. As a phrenologist, he sees insanity as a disease of the mind, having no connection with any abstract spirit," finished the chairman.

"Have his theories of phrenology been useful elsewhere?" asked Brand.

"Yes," stated Higgins, "the more educated public are interested in applying it to their lives and in the raising of their children. There is a proposal for a monthly publication, which is exciting. However, I agree, it was not useful here."

"I assume that we will have more problems if the medical school leaves Lexington," Brand said. "We depend upon that school."

"I know there is still talk about the school moving, but I don't see that happening. There will be a second one in Louisville," added the chairman. "Transylvania Medical School is too much a part of Lexington to move."

"Yes, a second medical school will satisfy the people in Louisville, but not ours," stated Higgins. "It will split the number of students."

"Is Dr. Caldwell leaving?" asked Brand.

"Yes, I have heard that he is. Is there any other discussion? If not, I will dismiss this meeting," concluded the chairman.

Dr. Caldwell wrote an article that was published in the *Louisville Journal*, "A sketch of the rise and fall of Transylvania Medical School." On May 19, 1837, another article followed in the *Lexington Observer & Reporter*, where he was severely criticized for the first article. He was dismissed from the Transylvania Medical School in Lexington and moved to the Louisville Medical School, where he became one of the leaders. He filled the same chair of medicine and clinical practice as he had done previously in Lexington. He continued with lectures on phrenology, with most of his adherents being medical professionals.

Phrenology became popular in lectures, as did what was called "cranio scopic" examinations by two brothers, Orson and Lorenzo Fowler. In 1838, they established the *American Phrenological Journal,* which became a national phenomenon. This was the first real attempt to provide any theoretical basis for understanding human behavior. Yet it was never applied adequately to the care of pauper lunatics. Phrenology was the early psychology of the time.

*   *   *

Senator John R. Allen married Judge Richard Buckner's daughter, Elizabeth, and returned to practiced law with his father-in-law while attending the Transylvania Medical School sessions of 1834 through 1838. While he had spent eight years as a Kentucky senator and eagerly followed the developments of the Kentucky Lunatic Asylum, he became concerned with the lack of medical care for those in the asylums and with the practice of bloodletting lunatics.

Bloodletting was common in medicine up through the 1800s, but bleeding as a treatment of lunatics was started by Dr. Benjamin Rush in Philadelphia. Since they were trained by Dr. Rush, most of the Transylvania Medical School professors practiced bloodletting at the Kentucky asylum.

Senator Allen felt that he could not criticize that practice without first being a physician himself. He attended the medical school and soon met Dr. B. W. Dudley.

Dr. Dudley did not believe in bleeding lunatics because he had never observed any improvement from the process. While he did not openly oppose bleeding, he never used any procedure unless he could observe the benefit. He developed a respect for Senator Allen with his prior experiences as an attorney and senator. Allen gained respect for Dr. Dudley as he attended his lectures and shared his dislike for the practice of bleeding lunatics. They were looking for other solutions.

*   *   *

Later in 1839, the chairman finished his usual visit to the asylum and observed the sheriff coming into the building. At this time, the sheriff was forty-eight years old, and they both had become old friends. They had had many discussions about Lexington in the earlier days.

Hunt immediately recognized from the sheriff's seriousness that this was not a social call. After exchanging courtesies, Hunt motioned for him to go into an office off the hall.

"Sir, I have some serious business to discuss with you," stated the sheriff. "This involves your steward, Mr. John King."

"Please, how can I help?" Hunt asked with a surprised look.

"Henry Clay Jr. has asked me to investigate reports that Mr. King is selling Theodore Clay's clothes. I need your help."

"Y—yes, you certainly have my help, but I cannot believe that about Mr. King, this must be a mistake," Hunt said.

"Henry Clay Jr. is asking to have a servant who knows Theodore Clay's wardrobe visit the asylum and determine if he has any items missing."

"Well, Theodore is always claiming that someone is taking his clothes, but then he also claims physical abuse by his family. With him being a lunatic, we would never believe him."

"Yes, I can understand that, and I do not believe what Theodore says, but there is other information that may confirm this suspicion. Do you remember Mr. Edward P. Johnson?"

"Oh, sure, he is the stagecoach owner here in Lexington," stated Hunt. "He has been very successful."

"Well, he observed for the last few months several trunks with Theodore Clay's name being sent to a Cincinnati clothing marketer."

"Oh, my," responded Hunt.

"Johnson became concerned and while in Cincinnati, he found out that the money from the clothing marketer is being deposited into a bank account for Mr. John King. Johnson mentioned this to Henry Clay Jr. after returning to Lexington. Clay Jr. acknowledged that Mr. John King has never been given any permission to do such a thing and came to me yesterday with this information, asking how to proceed."

"Why didn't the Clay family come to me?" asked Hunt.

"They want proof about the story. I think they want to bring criminal charges against Mr. King if an investigation proves to be correct," responded the sheriff. "The Clay family does provide exquisite clothing for all members, and Theodore is included in that part of their life."

"I just have trouble believing this also; what can we do?"

"I will send for the servant to come tomorrow, and we will wait for proof that clothing items are actually missing."

"Yes, Theodore has his own apartment; therefore, if the servant knows what he had in clothing, then we can determine if Mr. John King has actually taken those items."

"Also, you might look more closely at the asylum books and see if there are some large amounts of items taken by Mr. King; he might have been helping himself to other things."

"Yes, I will, but I just cannot believe this of Mr. King."

"Yes, I know what you mean," stated the sheriff. "But let us wait until tomorrow. I will visit you this time tomorrow and then we will know."

They agreed upon that plan.

The next morning, King was walking through the hallway and noticed a servant in the apartment of Theodore Clay. Theodore was outside, discussing his views of the world with those who would listen to him. King stopped and questioned the servant, realizing that the servant was there to examine Theodore's clothing. King, with a new feeling of panic, allowed the servant to continue but went immediately to find his wife.

Motioning for her to come quickly from the clothing room, King stated, "We must hurry, the Clay family has sent their servant to examine Theodore's clothes. We must leave before they find what out what is missing."

"We can leave now before anyone discovers that we have left."

"We have enough money in Cincinnati to last us for several years. Theodore Clay does not deserve any of that money, it is now ours to enjoy," claimed King.

"Theodore Clay is just a spoiled child," stated Mrs. King.

"I feel sorry for the pauper lunatics, but Theodore Clay has always been given too much. All that money is wasted on him. Now we can enjoy it." They rushed downstairs toward their apartment in the basement.

Not hearing their talk, Chairman Hunt stopped them in the main hallway and asked, "May I see you, Mr. King?"

"Y—yes, I was just helping my wife do a chore into Lexington; can I see you after we return?"

"Is this the end of your shift?" asked Hunt.

"No," King responded, "when an item is needed for the asylum, my wife purchases it and I escort her to town."

"Well, I am asking that you delay that chore at this time."

"Yes, sir," King said, as he was thinking fast about his escape. "I was actually on my way to an emergency upstairs that I must help with; let me see you after that, sir."

"Well, I should not interfere with emergencies," the chairman said, "so, please see me after you are finished."

By that afternoon, Hunt had determined that King and his wife had charged items that were not needed at the asylum. He went to their apartment in the basement and noticed that all their personal items had been removed. They had moved out. He was so disappointed to conclude the obvious. He just did not want to believe their crimes.

By the time the sheriff came back, Hunt had determined more inconsistencies in the asylum books.

"Sir," stated the sheriff, "Mr. John King has sold several expensive clothing items belonging to Theodore Clay. We know that now, and I am here to arrest him. I have a warrant for his arrest."

"I'm afraid Mr. and Mrs. King have already left. Their apartment has been cleared of all personal things," replied Hunt.

"How did that happen?"

"Mr. and Mrs. King have not been seen since this afternoon. I suspect they saw the servant in Theodore Clay's apartment."

"I will send a deputy to Cincinnati to find them. Hopefully, they will be caught. Do you know that many people who work in asylums commit crimes and move on to others? They are often not caught. They are able to hide within different asylums without being noticed in most towns."

"But," protested Hunt, "Mr. and Mrs. John King were so good with the lunatics. They seemed to care about them."

"Well, I can't understand that, either. Did they have any trouble with Theodore Clay, maybe more than with the others?"

"Yes, I did observe that Mr. King resented all the attention and special privileges that Theodore Clay received. He often stated that Theodore was too spoiled and received too much money. But I had trouble believing that he would steal from Theodore or any other lunatics."

"How long have Mr. and Mrs. King been working here?"

"Since 1825, around thirteen years," stated Hunt. "They served well for a while, but what happened to change them?

"Some people do change after being well respected when they have the opportunity to be dishonest, I'm sorry to say."

"I do remember that Mr. John King stated that he came from a very poor family and had to work hard even as a child. He resented Theodore Clay's wealthy family."

"He was probably jealous of Theodore."

"That was his flaw; I do remember that there were times when Mr. King did not want to give Theodore proper consideration for attending the weekly ball when Theodore had been appropriate in gaining that reward."

"So there were some indications with him?"

"Yes, there were some; I had to intervene several times. Mr. King must have been jealous of Theodore's money. I was just so blind to that."

"No, you are such a nice person, you just did not think that Mr. King was not so nice," surmised the sheriff.

"Well, I'm so disappointed in Mr. and Mrs. King."

"I will notify all the authorities and see that they are arrested," stated the sheriff.

"Well, I guess we have seen several problems in our years here. Do you remember when this institution was first started?"

"Yes, it was at the parade to the sinking springs when I first met you with some of your children," responded the sheriff. "I remember meeting Mr. John Rowan Allen, a law student at Transylvania University, who later became Senator Allen and now is studying to be a physician at the medical school."

"I remember you led the parade, with the professors at the medical school. We all had big hopes," stated Hunt.

"It was just a frontier town, and we were so relieved to be rid of the Indian problem. Now, we have many beautiful brick homes, including yours," said the sheriff.

"Well, I hear you have a nice brick home next to Johnson's Grove, where there are other nice homes," added Hunt.

"But you are ahead of me with having children and grandchildren," added the sheriff. "I have only three children and have no grandchildren yet."

"Yes, I am most fortunate with having twelve children and many grandchildren, and I had a good wife, may God rest her."

"My children are just now getting old enough to consider going to college. You know, I never had a chance to get much schooling, but all my children will go to college if I have anything to say about it," replied the sheriff. "In this town, education is possible. Maybe one of my sons will go the Transylvania Medical School or Law Department; I hope so."

"I also never went to college, but my children did as I know what you mean," echoed Hunt. "I moved to this frontier town as a young man to make my fortune, and I did. It had the best opportunities for me, and I was blessed, regardless of never having a good education."

"You have done the best you could with all your many abilities. I also admire Dr. B. W. Dudley, who used his abilities for helping people. Yet do you remember the duels that several of the medical professors had? I could never understand killing for honor, but today, the fighting has changed. Are we any more civilized?"

"No," answered Hunt, "and people still do not care for the unfortunates of society. Can you believe I am now sixty-six years old? I need someone else to take over this institution, but we cannot even get a physician to take over regularly. There are many who wish to propose ideas, teach, and observe, but none are willing to give the consistent attention to regular, and sometimes boring, duties. I cannot find a successor."

"Your dedication and attention to duty has always been a credit to your character; it will be hard to replace you," followed the sheriff.

"And you have certainly made your mark in Lexington the last twenty years," added Hunt. "This was a lawless town when you came, and you have given the citizens a respect for law and order."

"Yes, I am proud of that," added the sheriff.

"Many men in your position move from town to town, but not you. You have stayed to your duty and succeeded."

"I have a great family that has helped to sustain me, and this town has continued to grow with me," saidd the sheriff.

While both men continued to discuss the early days of Lexington, they had also witnessed a local process of committing dangerous persons into the facility as part of a national trend in many asylums. While the legal process is really a history worthy unto itself, for Kentucky this was significant not just because of the famous name. It was also a community process requiring citizens to identify insanity at a time when it was still unclear.

Sources for Chapter 4

"A Catalogue for the Officers and Students at Transylvania University" *Transylvania Journal of Medicine.* (1833).

Clay, Henry Jr. Parts of letter written to his father, Henry Clay Sr. Copies were given to this author when conferring with Dr. M. Hay. Later, the papers were added to what had been published under *Papers of Henry Clay Sr.*, Vol. 9.

Clay, Mary R. *The Clay Family.* Louisville, Kentucky: John P. Morton, 1899.

Clay, Theodore. Parts of letters written to his father, Henry Clay Sr. Copies were given to this author when consulting with Dr. M. Hay. The papers were published later as *Papers of Henry Clay Sr.*, Vol. 9.

Clay, Thomas H. *Henry Clay.* G. W. Jacobs & Son: 1910.

Commonwealth of Kentucky v. Theodore W. Clay. September 1831. File #746, Fayette County Circuit Court.

Eastern Kentucky Lunatic Asylum Report, January 17, 1833.

Hopkins, J.F. & Hargraves, M.: Vol. 1-6: Zeager, W. & Hay, M. Vol. 7 & 8: Hay, M. Vol. 9, *Papers of Henry Clay, Sr.*, Lexington, Kentucky: University of Kentucky Press, 1959-1984.

Hay, M. Conversations about the papers of Henry Clay, January 1988.

Kentucky Statesman, October 15, 1858.

Lancaster, C. *Vestiges of the Venerable City: A Chronicle of Lexington, Kentucky.* Lexington-Fayette County Historic Commission Cincinnati, Ohio: C. J. Krehbiel, 1978.

Lexington Transcript. "John M. Clay Obituary." August 11, 1887.

Maj. Thomas Hart Pindell. *Lexington Fayette County Historic Commission.* Lexington, Kentucky: Paddock Publishing, 1981.

Maysville Turnpike Road Committee Report in Library Special Collections and Archives Frankfort, Kentucky: Kentucky Historical Society, 1826–1827.

Neely, M., and R. G. McMurtry. *The Insanity File: The Case of Mary Todd Lincoln.* Carbondale: Southern Illinois University, 1896.

New York Times. "The Son of Henry Clay," May 19, 1870.

Observer & Reporter. March 28, 1833.

Observer & Reporter. "Doctor Charles Caldwell and His Hostility to the Transylvania Medical School," December 28, 1836.

Observer & Reporter. May 19, 1837.

Peter, Robert. *The History of the Medical Department of Transylvania University.* Louisville, Kentucky: John P. Morton, 1905.

Sapinsley, B. *The Private War of Mrs. Packard.* New York: Paragon House, 1991.

Wright, John D. *Transylvania: Tutor to the West.* Lexington, Kentucky: Transylvania University Press, 1975.

Chapter Five

1840–1854

In this part of Kentucky, the Old Buffalo Trail was renamed the Maysville–Lexington Road; it allowed settlers to move inland to early Kentucky settlements. It was now a privately owned turnpike; toll gates charged five cents for horseback riders and seventy-five cents for a stagecoach. While Henry Clay Sr. had gained approval in the 1830s for government money to purchase the Turnpike Road Company, extending the road to the Cumberland National Road, President Andrew Jackson vetoed the purchase. However, by 1840 money became available to expand the turnpike of the Old Buffalo Trail to be part of the Cumberland National Road. The section through Lexington continued to be called Mulberry Street.

However, it was the railroads that really increased commerce trade to Lexington and helped the city to grow. Railroads were completed from Lexington to Louisville and Frankfort, Kentucky. They were owned by private companies with local people such as John W. Hunt on the board.

A second Medical Building was completed in 1840 on the northwest corner of Second Street and North Broadway. The first Medical Building at Church and Market Streets contained one large lecture room for chemistry classes, a chemical laboratory, and a sizable anatomical amphitheater for preparing and dissecting bodies. The second Medical Building was bigger, with three large lecture rooms, a library, a museum, five dissecting rooms, and a private office for each instructor. Into this new building was moved the fine medical library and apparatus accumulated by sizable purchases here and abroad.

Nothing was lacking to make a fine medical school in the small settlement of Lexington. However, the school was struggling, as fewer students attended. Newer medical schools, including the Louisville Medical School, were drawing students away from the older Transylvania Medical School.

Senator Allen often talked with Dr. Dudley in his office in the new Medical Building. Dr. Dudley encouraged Allen in his methodical and legalistic approach against bloodletting. His thesis would need to be defended before all the Transylvania professors. Such a defense required many hours of preparation and was necessary for graduation.

A knock interrupted their thoughts. "Dr. Dudley, sir, I have another body for you," stated the old sheriff.

Dr. Dudley opened the door and said, "Yes, I see you have been so kind; where is the body? I certainly need one for tomorrow's class."

"The body is in the dissecting room; it was another drunk who got into a fight last night. I took two drunks to jail last night, assuming that both were just passed out. This morning, this one was dead. I don't know why he died, but he has no family and no one will pay to bury him."

"Well, anybody can be expedient from which my students can learn," responded Dr. Dudley.

"I left it in the dissecting room, which is where you usually put bodies in the old Medical Building" stated the sheriff. "This new building is nice, sir."

"Yes, you are correct. I really appreciate your diligence in such matters. You have been so useful in getting bodies for this school. I really discern your favors. I only wish there were more. Oh, have you met one of my outstanding students, John R. Allen?" asked Dr. Dudley.

Allen stopped his writing and stood up; he said, "Yes, sir, I recognize the sheriff from the past. We met at the dedication of the asylum, years ago when I was a student attending law school there."

"Yes, it has been some years ago," the sheriff said as he shook hands with Allen.

"Sir, I think it was when I was a student in the Law Department. As you might know now, I have married Judge Buckner's daughter and returned to study medicine," said Allen. "You also knew my father, who was in the war with the Indians."

"Yes, I did know your father, General James Joseph Allen. He was a great man," added the sheriff.

"Now, my wife and I live in a house on Mulberry Street, just north of downtown. The house is big enough for children, and my wife is expecting our first. She is busy setting up the house while I pursue the study of medicine."

"I remember your wife as part of the Buckner family, a fine family; we are glad to have you returning to Lexington," added the sheriff.

Allen nodded his agreement, "Yes, I am happy to be here."

"Your father-in-law, Judge Buckner, is a well-known lawyer. I understand his son has also studied law; you are joining them?" The sheriff observed how handsome and confident Allen had become. He was no longer the young and inexperienced boy of the past. He showed the unusual charm of a well-bred intellectual family.

He replied, "Yes, I am helping with the Buckner law firm but I will leave when I finish medical school. I studied law earlier because my family needed the legal skills to manage their affairs after my father was killed in the 1812 War. Now that I have met my family obligations, I can fulfill my dream of studying medicine." He stopped to control his excitement, and then he continued, "This medical school is so exciting to me. Finding answers to human suffering is the highest calling I can have." Allen remembered his manners and ended his conversation by saying, "Sir, I am most pleased to see you again," as he returned to his previous writing.

"Yes, sir, I agree," choked the sheriff. "Doctors can do a great deal of good." He pointed to Dr. Dudley and continued, "This is one of the best." He looked at him. The sheriff had developed a deep respect for Dr. Dudley, who appeared to ignore the sheriff but was obviously pleased as he continued with his paperwork.

"Well, I must be going, but call upon me if you ever need my services," the sheriff said, tipping his hat to both men and looking at Dr. Dudley. "I will continue to help you, Dr. Dudley, with finding bodies as I can legally do so." He walked out and shut the door.

"How old is that sheriff?" asked Allen. "It seems that he has been a part of Lexington a long time."

"Yes, he has been here a long time. He is in his fifties and has several children. He knows everything that happens in this town," replied Dr. Dudley. "I need to go see the body he brought and determine what state of deterioration it is in. Since alcohol is a common problem in this frontier, the effect on the body will be a good lesson for my students. Do you wish to come?"

"No, sir, I need to return home. As you know, my wife is expecting our first child, and I need to make sure she is comfortable."

"Well, take care of her; when I lost my wife, it devastated me. I now raise my two sons alone," added Dr. Dudley. "My work saved me, but my sons have needed a mother."

"And you have done well with your sons, sir; until we meet at your next lecture."

Allen left from the Medical Building on Second Street and Broadway and went toward Mulberry Street. His carriage moved slowly on this day, as the dirt streets were still wet from the last rain. He noticed the home of John W. Hunt on Mill Street as he continued on Second Street. He had visited Hunt several times to discuss the conditions at the Kentucky asylum.

Allen arrived at his home on Mulberry Street. His wife had friends visiting: Mrs. Elizabeth Duncan and Nancy Brand. Elizabeth Duncan was married to Henry T. Duncan, and Nancy was wife of George W. Brand. They all welcomed him home as they continued to talk to his wife, Elizabeth, who was visibly pregnant. Nancy Brand was also pregnant.

After the women left, Elizabeth sat down with her husband in their living room, decorated with the Buckner family leftover furniture. They were young, just starting out, and the family had contributed to their home. Elizabeth was always interested in the old Lexington families and wanted to keep her new husband informed; she said, "Can you believe that

Cassius Clay will be running against Robert Wickliffe Jr.? Those two are always fighting against each other over the slavery issue."

Allen, hoping to stay out of local family discussions stated, "This slavery issue is tearing families apart. While both men have valuable issues to consider, the continued contention between them will cloud the issues. Yes, it is sad for the families caught in the middle. I understand that Cassius and Robert Jr. were friends as children."

"Yes, they were. Robert's brother, Charles, was killed over the issue years ago, and now it continues. Cassius Clay is fighting against the repeal of the 1833 Negro Law, whereas Wickliff is fighting for it. I have also heard from Mary Jane's family, the Warfields; they are opposing Cassius Clay and secretly fighting against him. Mary Jane and her children are siding with her family. It is so sad that such families are split," added Elizabeth.

"Yes, that was partly why I got tired of the law, which became a way of dividing people, not healing them. When people are fighting for their opinions, it divides them and there is no end," Allen said.

"Yes, dear; I'm happy for you. But remember, Mary Jane knew when she married Cassius Clay that he was a passionately against slavery. She was just a foolish girl at the time and never realized that these issues could separate families. As the Warfields lean toward slavery, her husband is passionately against it."

"Well, I remember you advised Cassius not to marry Mary Jane when we were living at your family's farm. I remember we had a party for many of Lexington's single young people, and both Cassius and Mary Jane were there. You advised Cassius against getting involved with her."

"Yes, I did, but Cassius was so set on his passions for Mary Jane, and she was such a playful girl. Now, she has several children who are always spoiled by the Warfields, and Cassius is without the loving support of his family. He might be more understanding if he had a loving family."

"Well," added Allen, "I am passionate against the abuse of the insane but giving speeches offers limited chances of improvement. I want to be part of the process that cares for the unfortunates in society with the best improved medical care, not just one who passes legislation or talks about it. I'm happy studying medicine."

"Yes, you are sensible to work within a system to change things. You are educating yourself in medicine to disagree with the practice of bloodletting rather than arguing or dueling with someone about it. You are more sensible, which is one of many reasons I love you," said Elizabeth. She rose to see that supper was started.

He followed her into the dining room, stating, "We can have a good life in Lexington with me as a physician, here. But I'm afraid this issue of slavery will only get worse, and some of those people are your friends." Allen took his medical books to the table to study.

Elizabeth just smiled and corrected him, "They are *our* friends." But she reminded herself that he was still the tall handsome figure with dark blue eyes and gracious manners that she had fallen love with in her father's law office. She did not puzzle over why her husband was changing from law into medicine, because he always needed a challenge. Law had been a family expectation for John to fulfill, and he did that. Then, he became a senator, and the challenge was gone after eight years. Now, he was seeking a different challenge in medicine, and she could understand that. She was most happy to have married him and still be in Lexington with her old friends.

*   *   *

John W. Hunt had continued chairing the bimonthly meetings at the Kentucky asylum. By 1840, his business partners, Richard Higgins and John Brand, had been replaced by newer board members due to their age. Yet, Rev. Chipley and Hunt had continued on the board, even though they were very elderly and frail. Both men were determined to provide proper leadership to the institution, so they continued with their duties, hoping to find replacements that would care about the facility as they had.

The chairman announced that there were 142 patients in the facility at the close of 1840. A three-story building was being completed on the back of the original building, providing separate rooms for those who became sick and separating them from those who were not. Other details were discussed, and then the meeting was closed. After the meeting, Hunt followed Rev. Chipley out to his carriage.

"Rev. Chipley," he asked, "how is your son?"

"He is actually doing well. As you know, he finally graduated from Transylvania Medical School and stayed here in Lexington for a while. He was upset over the difficulties between the medical school and Dr. Caldwell. He had placed so much confidence in Dr. Caldwell and then was disappointed over him leaving Lexington." Rev. Chipley sat on a bench within the semicircle of the grounds and motioned for his driver to come around with his carriage.

"Yes," replied Hunt, "Dr. Caldwell was a disappointment to many. He spent several years building up the Transylvania Medical School and abandoned it when the one in Louisville was opened. I understand he is still there. I wish him well, but he was a very difficult and self-assured person."

"Well, my son William felt Dr. Caldwell was brilliant with all the phrenology theories and took every course that he taught. His confidence in Dr. Caldwell was shattered when he left everything here that he had previously supported. Dr. Caldwell's quick turn-around really disappointed William. My son and I tend to disagree over many new medical ideas, and he did not follow my ideas. He did with Dr. Caldwell." Rev. Chipley reached for help getting into his carriage.

"Dr. Caldwell disappointed many people but he seems to have hurt the young ones the worst," Hunt stated with empathy. "We older people have seen many disappointments and may even become immune to such." Hunt helped his friend into the carriage.

"That is true, and the controversy between Dr. Caldwell and the medical school hurt my son. As a child he observed the medical school grow and always anticipated attending it. While I have always had poor expectations of physicians, my son saw things differently and idolized them. Problems within the medical school shattered his respect for Dr. Caldwell, so he moved to Columbus, Georgia."

"William took issue with Dr. Dudley around his time of graduation, didn't he?" asked Hunt.

"Yes," he said, telling the carriage driver to wait for a minute. "William did not like Dr. Dudley's article about a procedure that he used. William considered the excessive cutting of bodies unnecessary and challenged him."

"Yes, now I remember, I witnessed that challenge," said Hunt. "Here was William, a student physician, going before the Board of Trustees, questioning Dr. B. W. Dudley, who had long been associated with the medical profession. William was brave."

"Well, I worried about that. If you remember, he defended his thesis in 1832 but he did not graduate until 1840."

"Well, some of the requirements changed, and William had to take more courses. While his thesis was completed in 1832, he was determined by the board to need more courses before getting his degree in 1840. While defending his position with Dr. Dudley, he was later vindicated by the board. He gained a great deal of respect for his willingness to defend his strong convictions," added Hunt. "Dr. Dudley was willing to accept the challenge of William's ideas."

"Yes, that was my William," Rev. Chipley said, sitting back in his carriage. "When William feels he is right, he will stand and not move."

"Is he teaching in Columbus?" asked Hunt.

"Please excuse my need to sit down," Rev. Chipley said, "but as you know, I have poor strength and must sit. No, William is not teaching. He is practicing medicine in that area. He really loves the people and even tells me that he treats Indians."

"Well, you are most fortunate to still have your son," Hunt said sadly, "as you know, I lost my physician son. I need one to care for me, now."

"Yes, so do I, but as you know, William is our only living child. I miss his discussions with me. We always debated the differences between medical and herbal cures. When he was younger, he thought my herbal cures were all wrong, but as he developed into a physician, he started seeing some of the benefits to them. Now we can discuss the differences as adults. I do miss him."

"Well, my old friend, I too must be going," Hunt said as he started to leave.

"Yes, I should be going, my wife will worry about me if I am too long," Rev. Chipley said, waving.

Going home in his carriage, Hunt was feeling so weary, wishing someone would relieve him of the burden at the asylum. There were always citizens willing to donate their time to the board of Transylvania University. The asylum board was different, as no one wanted that much responsibility for lunatics, except for those who might exploit it for their own gain. As chairman of the board, he was always begging for money since the State of Kentucky only provided for needs that were proven. While he had been good at bargaining for funds, it was a hassle that many did not wish to encounter. Then, the ugly head of politics was always a consideration, which he could handle, but he was growing weary of it. He often wondered to himself, *Will there not be someone who can take this responsibility from me?*

The next year, Hunt was reading his usual periodicals. He especially liked the *Boston Medical and Surgical Journal* that his son had made arrangements for him to receive before his death. The *Journal* would periodically review different medical facilities. Hunt enjoyed seeing what other facilities were doing. It was in the April 21, 1841, issue of the *Journal,* that there was a review of the Kentucky Lunatic Asylum. Hunt was surprised, since he had not been contacted by the *Journal.* He was considered the most knowledgeable person, but he knew why: he was not a medical doctor, and his opinions did not count to them. He decided to ask Allen, as a past senator who understood politics and as a current medical student, to review the article.

* * *

Mrs. Elizabeth Allen had delivered a son, whom they named after John R. Allen's father, James Joseph. The son, however, died within the year. They planned on having more children.

It was several weeks later that Allen was asked to visit Hopemount, Hunt's home. The next day, Allen arrived at Hopemount and knocked on the fan-shaped door; the butler led him into the modest but elegantly decorated house. Hunt came into the room, and they shook hands.

Allen said, "Sir, I am most pleased to see you; you wish to seek my advice?"

"Yes, please come into my office. As you see, my home is now quiet, but it had been full of activity with twelve children around in the past. Although I would prefer the previous activity of children, I must take what is available. The good side of this is we can talk more easily."

"You asked me if I had access to the April *Boston Medical and Surgical Journal*. I did find a copy at the medical school and read the article about the Kentucky asylum," Allen stated as he sat in a nearby chair.

"That article really bothered me; no one in authority talked to me. However, I realize that I'm not a medical doctor, so they would not necessarily talk to me. I still consider myself the most knowledgeable of this asylum." Hunt trembled with anger. He was not one to show anger except by trembling.

"Of course you are, but you have to understand their methods; they only talk to medical doctors. I discovered that when, as a lawyer, I could not understand the overuse of bloodletting. While I was a lawyer, no one would listen to my medical opinions, but now that I'm becoming a medical doctor, some authorities are listening to me. You are in similar circumstances."

"We have always had difficulty getting full-time medically trained physicians, and now, with my age and the other old members of the board, new board members are needed. I just cannot find them. Have I failed?"

"No, you have not! We just need to try different ways to find good keepers and people to manage them. Let us look more at the article and maybe consider some of the recommendations," consoled Allen.

"The main criticism stated in the article is that economy and security were the only matters within the asylum. Well, I would say yes, that is all I know. The fact that there is no full-time physician who can look at the medical cause or length of derangement previous to admission is true." Hunt felt hopeless to realize that after all these years, he was no longer regarded as a competent leader. He was not used to that. He was seeing his life's work at the asylum failing because superintendents were becoming required, and he could not find one. This article was the first indication to him of that inadequacy at the asylum.

Allen looked at Hunt, who smiled back and stated, "Sir, we have to do something. I will talk to people at the medical school."

"I have done that for years. The physicians are always sympathetic, but no one will consider the full-time position," Hunt said. "I will bring up this report at the next board meeting, but all the members are like I am: we have tried for years, to no avail. We have looked for a full-time physician who is experienced in such matters, but no one is interested."

"Well, something must be done," said Allen, rising from his seat to shake hands. "You and I must put this asylum into the new advanced knowledge of our time." Allen began to leave. "Sir, I will get back to you. I will talk to some political friends too." He continued to puzzle over the situation on his way home.

The next few months, Allen talked to friends about the needs of the asylum. All agreed to discuss the problems, but no one was willing to accept the medical or board member positions. He was talking to his wife about the problems of the asylum.

"Well, why don't you take the physician's position after you finish school in the next two years?" asked his wife, who was pregnant with their second child. "By then, we should have several children."

"Elizabeth," he said tenderly, "I have yet to finish my courses and defend my dissertation. I would love such a challenge, but they need someone now. They want someone with experience in lunacy care."

"Well, you could propose yourself and build up the Board of Commissioners before you finish. It will probably take that long to find members to be on the board anyway. Also, good citizens might be more interested if they knew that you would be joining it."

"Now, Elizabeth, I don't think I have that much influence upon people. I have friends, but there will not be a lot of people flocking to the board because of me. Remember, the Board of Commissioners is unpaid, and they must be individuals who believe in the cause and can afford to contribute their time."

Elizabeth set at the table for dinner as she said, "Your stability, medical knowledge, and desire to do good will attract members to the board. While John Hunt attracted members to the board in his time, his time is over, and citizens are less willing to donate time to the cause. He is still a good man, and the asylum is fortunate to have him, but his time of maximum influence is gone. That is reality, sad but true."

Allen was always amused by his wife's insight and bluntness. She was right, and he knew how much he needed her. Aware of her pregnancy, he asked, "Are you all right? I mean with the baby?"

"Of course, I hope to have many more babies. This one has been kicking some. Besides that, you know I'm right about Mr. Hunt. He needs your help. Actually, the asylum needs your help."

"Yes, I will go back and talk to Mr. Hunt." Allen did go back and talk to Hunt, but he never mentioned his consideration about the job as physician. He was just not ready to commit himself until he was sure he could complete his medical degree within the next two years.

Allen still had to defend his dissertation, which he knew was unpopular with most of the remaining professors. He knew it had taken Dr. William Chipley eight more years after he challenged Dr. Dudley to get his medical degree. Therefore, Allen was not sure when he would graduate.

Allen was studying an article by O. S. Fowler in the *American Phrenological Journal*. He was amazed with the range of subjects that the phrenologist had written on, including education, memory, matrimony, love and parenting, religion, and temperance. All were problems of the general public. He decided to subscribe to the *Journal*. He remembered meeting Dr. Caldwell during his years in the Transylvania Medical School. Dr. Caldwell had written several articles for the *Journal of Phrenology*, and when he left Lexington, he had disappointed many citizens. Many of the current medical professors rejected Dr. Caldwell's theories and the subject of phrenology. Therefore, Allen did not mention his current interest in phrenology to members at the Transylvania Medical School.

Allen had noticed that Hunt was developing a dependency upon him for advice about the asylum. That bothered him, as he was still a medical student and unqualified to give medical advice. While Allen lacked medical experience, he obviously had more knowledge of insanity than other physicians. He not only had the growing medical knowledge, he had a legal perspective that other fully trained physicians did not have. However, he was uncomfortable giving advice to Hunt.

*   *   *

In the fall of 1842, Allen was asked to meet Hunt at the asylum. John arrived at the original building and asked the steward for Hunt. He noticed a familiar-looking young man in the adjoining room but was distracted by Hunt's haggard appearance.

"Sir, you asked for my service?" Allen said, knowing that Hunt was weakening from worry and concern about the asylum.

"Yes, please, I need your legal opinions. Please come into this next room, where we can discuss it." Allen followed Hunt into an office with two chairs and a desk. The windows looked out into the airing yards of the asylum in the back of the original building. The airing yards had been a source of pride to the chairman and board members as alternatives to restraining the more disturbed patients. The airing yards were fenced areas, separated by sexes, giving the most disturbed patients opportunity to exercise off all their excessive energy without hurting anyone.

They sat down into the two chairs while Hunt asked, "Did you recognize the man in the front room?"

"He looked familiar, but I did not get a good look; who was it?"

"That is John M. Clay, son of Henry Clay Sr. As you know, his brother Theodore has been here at the asylum nearly ten years. John is having the same symptoms as Theodore, who was court committed to this asylum. My legal question, sir, is should we follow the same process?"

"What are the symptoms?" Allen asked. "I understand Theodore was threatening the Brand family over their daughter's lack of interest in him. Is that true with John?"

"Well yes, there is another girl in town involved, but the family succeeded at keeping John away from her. The family is not fearful, and John is more aware of his own danger. He has seen his brother and recognizes the symptoms more within himself. He is now only threatening to kill himself."

Allen continued, "The legal question for a court commitment involves if the person is considered to be dangerous to someone else. Is that so?"

"No, not to another person, just more to himself, but he is willing to refrain from harming himself at this time," added Hunt. "Henry Clay Sr. will be arriving later, and I needed your legal advice on how to proceed with this admission."

"I understand. Henry Clay Sr. is one of the best legal authorities around," added Allen.

"Yes, so I did not wish to be so ignorant in front of him. I knew he would know the law, and your legal opinion will be helpful for me. Thank you for your service to me," added Hunt.

"Mr. Hunt, as a physician-to-be, I have some other questions about this case; has John M. Clay been drinking?"

"He denies it, and of course he does not smell, so I cannot tell. There is alcohol that does not smell, and I know the Clay family buys the expensive brands of alcohol that are difficult to smell."

"How did he end up here at the asylum?" asked Allen.

"The sheriff found him on Main Street, threatening to kill himself because his girlfriend would not marry him. The sheriff talked to him and brought him here. This was last night."

"While I am not familiar with this specific case, I would bet that John has been drinking too much. I know him and his family."

"Yes, you might be right," added Hunt.

"I would recommend that John M. Clay be given time to sleep off any alcohol and see if his father is willing to take him home. If John can see his brother and realize how alcohol has hurt him, he might change his alcohol habits," analyzed Allen.

"Yes, all the Clays have a habit of drinking in excess; some can handle the alcohol, while others have not been able to," added Hunt.

"The difference that I understand from Theodore, is his alcoholism led to him becoming very threatening and dangerous to a family, leading to a court commitment. Hopefully, John will not follow that direction if he sees what might await him," Allen stated confidently.

"Yes, your ideas have helped me to know what to do. I will discuss the matter with Henry Clay Sr. when he arrives. Thank you so much."

Allen left the asylum and followed the case of John M. Clay through discussions with Hunt. Hunt was pleased that Henry Clay Sr. was eager to bring his son home and keep him out of the asylum. Henry Clay Sr. insisted that his son never drink in downtown Lexington; all his drinking was limited to home, where family members could restrict his behavior. While Henry Clay Sr. did not expect abstinence from his sons, he had learned, from experience with Theodore, that drinking at home would not embarrass the family in public. John M. Clay agreed to this stipulation and moved into the family home, Ashland, with his parents. Living at Ashland was a haven for John, as daily responsibilities were handled by his mother and servants. He never returned to the asylum, except to visit his brother.

Allen was asked to come to the asylum again. He was busy with his dissertation and could not go at first. He just did not feel that he had the time to spare. After thinking about the problems that Hunt had, he changed his mind and hurried over. He arrived in the front door, asking for Hunt, and noticed many of the lunatics were having supper. Hunt approached him.

"Sir, you sent for me?" asked Allen.

"I need your medical opinion; yes, I know you are not yet a physician, but I trust your opinion more than any of these new doctors at Transylvania Medical School. None of them care like you do." He led Allen into a dark room, where a filthy person was tied to a bed. He had come to the asylum as violent and fighting, and the family could not handle him.

"Do you recognize him?" asked Hunt.

"Isn't that George Trotter, the editor of the *Kentucky Gazette*?"

"Yes. He has been sick and confused. The family brought him here, not knowing what to do with him. He had to be tied to the bed to control him. We do not know what to do with him; he once was a competent person."

"Do we know how long this has been going on?" asked Allen.

"No, but you remember that he killed his boyhood friend in a duel; remember the duel with Robert Wickliff Jr., when both were twenty-one years old?"

"Well, yes, but that was years ago."

"Could killing his childhood friend make him insane?" asked Hunt.

"Well, let us look at other causes; he did continue as editor for many years. So how old is he now?"

"Nearly sixty; he does ramble on about the past; could this be remorse over that?" asked Hunt. "We don't usually see educated people become lunatics."

"I see your problem. I will do some tests; you might call in other physicians. His confusion looks more like some physical deterioration or old age rather than remorse. We need to make him as comfortable as possible."

Trotter was taken to a room where his friends could often visit him, but he did not recognize them. Allen continued to visit him and determined that senility was causing his confusion. He could find no other solutions except to provide common liquor to help keep Trotter comfortable in his room until his death. There were no other solutions that offered any better results.

*   *   *

The summer had come, and the sheriff was doing his usual duty at the courthouse. Henry Clay Sr. was defending his cousin, Cassius Clay, against battery charges. Cassius had delivered a heavy blow to Samuel M. Brown during a debate between Robert Wickliffe and Garrett Dabis at Russell's Cave Spring. Cassius took issue with the Wickliffe faction, and Samuel Brown struck him with a club. Cassius Clay responded with more force.

Cassius was acquitted for defending himself, while Henry Clay Sr. kept his record of never losing a case. The citizens of Lexington only shook their heads as the sheriff continued to observe the crowded courtroom.

That night at the kitchen table, the sheriff was talking to his wife about the Cassius Clay case. "Can you believe that Henry Clay Sr. has never lost a case? He really knows how to say things so that his client is always a winner. I only hope he is on the right side; as you know, Henry Clay Sr. is considering running for president next year."

His wife, Margaret, put down cups for adding coffee.

"Well, he sure is well respected in Lexington," she stated. "That Clay family is really something, though. While Henry Sr. is so well known, his cousin Cassius has his strong pro-slavery ideas; his son Theodore is a hopeless lunatic; and the other sons are not much better off. They all have excessive drinking problems. What a family. Henry's wife stays at Ashland and Cassius Clay's wife hides at the Warfields' home." Margaret continued sipping her coffee.

"Yes, neither one has done well with their families," answered the sheriff. He reached for his coffee cup and sipped.

"I did visit with Elizabeth Allen, whose husband is finishing the Transylvania Medical School. Dr. Allen will be accepting the superintendent's position at the asylum in January. The asylum has needed a full-time physician for a long time. Elizabeth is just glad to remain in Lexington," as Margaret continued their conversation.

"That is good to hear; I have known him for several years. I knew his father in the Indian Wars. Lexington is fortunate to have such an outstanding person to live here," added the sheriff. Hearing about the news delighted him.

"I understand he has been helping Mr. John W. Hunt for some time. Mr. Hunt is just too old to continue with his duties, but no one else would help," said Margaret. "Mr. Hunt has resisted others from misusing the asylum and now, he has Dr. Allen, who is trained and able to do the work."

"That is such good news," added the sheriff.

Margaret continued with her information, "Also, Mr. Richard Pindell, an attorney and longtime friend of the Buckner family, has agreed to be chairman of the Board of Commissioners, relieving Mr. Hunt of his responsibilities."

"Well, I'm surprised; the chairman's job has been so thankless."

"Dr. Allen was able to encourage Pindell into the job. It seems that Richard Pindell's father was financially saved by Hunt in the panic of 1837, and Richard is still grateful. The asylum will now have a chance to become more progressive with both of these two people leading it."

"Well, I am pleased that the institution will continue with able leadership. I shall go visit Mr. Hunt to thank him for his dedication to the asylum all these years," stated the sheriff. "Mr. Hunt and I really enjoy talking about the old days."

Dr. Allen finally passed his dissertation defense against the use of bloodletting; it fulfilled the final requirements for his medical degree. His research was supported by Dr. Dudley, proving that bloodletting did not benefit lunatics. However, the dissertation was not accepted into the medical journals of the time, nor was it published by the *Transylvania Medical Journal*. Instead of trying to get his research accepted into other journals, Dr. Allen shifted his focus to the asylum and planned to organize it into the best medical care for lunatics.

By 1844, Transylvania Medical School had lost several members of the faculty, and Dr. Dudley had assumed two of those positions. That same year, Dr. James C. Cross was unceremoniously kicked off the Transylvania Medical School faculty after suggesting that Dr. Dudley give up one of his professorships at the medical school, showing the power that Dr. Dudley still had. Dr. Cross had been the first physician to work at the Kentucky Lunatic Asylum. Problems at the medical school continued.

*   *   *

While the asylum had kept up with the current building standards of Hunt's day, Dr. Allen wanted it to reflect a new age of medical care in insanity. The original building had one large center hallway on each floor, with individual rooms off of the hallways. The smokehouse and kitchen were on the right. Privies were well placed outside, and the airing yards were fenced. All were adequate facilities except for the back of the facility.

In the back of the original building was a building of box rooms for the sick. The box rooms were most disturbing to Dr. Allen as he saw them; they were too isolated, too far away from any medical care. Since the box rooms were not adequately heated, were poorly ventilated, and were only large enough for a bed, they were to be torn down. Dr. Allen had gained approval from the Kentucky legislature for the necessary money to build another building in the place of the box rooms over the next few years. He spent many hours at the asylum, watching and planning the best possible facilities.

Dr. Allen and Pindell, as chairman of the Board of Commissioners, were discussing the asylum plans and Kentucky politics. Pindell was still politically well connected in Kentucky state government and aware of political activities. They were sitting in Dr. Allen's office on the first floor of the original building.

"I guess you have heard that Henry Clay Sr. lost the presidential election; I am sorry to hear that," Pindell said. "Yet he is well respected in Kentucky."

"Yes, that is true. I also understand that Dr. B. W. Dudley had a dinner for Clay, following his defeat. I was invited but I am devoting all my time to this asylum," Dr. Allen said as he looked out into the main hallway. Everything was quiet since the last meal had been finished. All the lunatics had retreated to their rooms.

Dr. Allen had asked for Hunt's previous office, which was opposite from the dining room and had an outside door. He could view the airing yards to observe the more disturbed patients and seek better solutions to their care. His office was across from the steward and matron on the main floor. While he visited patients in their rooms, his office was large enough for the Board of Commissioners to meet. He was pleased with the arrangement.

"I understand that Senator James T. Morehead and Cassius Clay attended Dr. Dudley's dinner," stated Pindell.

"Also, I understand that Henry Clay Sr. blamed both men for his defeat, but mostly Cassius for his stand against slavery."

"That is unfortunate, but Henry Clay Sr. is known for defending his cousin's opinions against slavery, and the general public is afraid of Henry's position," responded Pindell.

"While I can understand Henry Clay's belief that all ideas should be heard and defended as the American ideal, his cousin Cassius shows extreme views and the American people are afraid of such extremes. I know I am," stated Dr. Allen.

"While I believe in the abolitionist ideas, it is the extremes that such individuals as Cassius have gone to and his other immoral behavior which leaves me to reject his ideals. I think that is true of many in Kentucky."

"Well, I'm more interested in taking care of the needs of the insane than debating such social issues with Cassius," added Dr. Allen.

"Yes, we agree. However, I am sorry for Henry Clay Sr. I think he had some good ideas and is tolerant of different ideas. I was surprised that Dr. B. W. Dudley was such a supporter of him.

"Actually, Dr. B. W. Dudley was more into supporting his son, William, and William's political interest," added Dr. Allen. "William is interested in government work in Washington, and Henry Clay Sr. is still the person to know from Kentucky."

Pindell laughed, "So that is why Dr. Dudley is into politics."

"I'm glad to be out of politics," laughed Dr. Allen. "My eight years in the Kentucky Senate was enough for me. I'm working on a book of rules and regulations for the keepers. They need to have some written standard for working at this asylum."

"I have never heard of such a thing. It certainly would be helpful. Remember, some of the employees cannot read," commented Pindell.

"Yes, I know, and the rules will be explained to them. I hope by establishing standards, the asylum will attract better educated keepers and officers. I hope that you as chairman of the board will approve this book."

"Yes, I will be most pleased to approve its publication, once I read it."

"There are those who will object to any standards, such as the politicians who want us to hire their supporters. However, we need to set standards. I had hoped you will support me as you usually do," said Dr. Allen.

"Yes, I will. Are you prepared to fire any officers or keepers if they do not follow certain standards?" asked Pindell.

"Yes, I am. Anyone seen abusing any inmate will be fired. I cannot tolerate such behavior," added Dr. Allen.

"Abuse, I can understand, but who will report the abuse? As you know, some officers and keepers don't like each other and will claim reports of abuse to get others fired," added Pindell.

"As superintendent, I will determine that. I expect to be around and observe for myself. I also want harmony within the asylum, and those officers or keepers who are always complaining about others need to be disciplined. I will establish ways to handle those types of problems."

"I'm sure you will," answered Pindell.

"Remember, I expect to be at the asylum every day so that I can observe the difficult employees. With these rules and regulations, I will have a way of firing those who create such problems," added Dr. Allen.

"Well, I will support your plan."

"We have a wonderful facility, but some of the officers or keepers have been allowed to do as they wish, without proper direction, and I must deal with them. I need the authority to fire them as I see best. Also, I plan to change the title of keeper to attendant," added Dr. Allen.

"Change it? Why?" asked Pindell.

"The title attendant is used for those who follow professional standards, whereas the title of keeper is just that, without any standards. This change is important for setting standards. Officers are the ones in charge; that will stay the same, but they must attend some training to become officers."

"Yes, I will support you on this," said Pindell. "However, you must remember that many employees were politically appointed, and if you fire them, you will have to answer to the politician who got them their jobs."

"Yes, we both know how politics works. That is why I will have a published standard that will show the expected behavior, and if those employed do not follow it, then I can fire them. As long as there are standards, our political friends cannot interfere. We must have the authority here; politicians should not have the control," added Dr. Allen. "At least, I expect so."

"I will support you. Just let me know what I need to do," Pindell said as he shook hands with Dr. Allen.

There were 100 rooms in the facility and 173 patients, too many for the limited facilities. Pindell's administrative and political connections were needed. He was excited that Dr. Allen was proposing the most progressive methods. While Pindell had observed the decline of the Transylvania Medical School, he did not wish the same upon this asylum. He was determined to do his part to keep it going.

At the end of 1845, Pindell wrote his second annual report to the governor. He stated that we "cannot present to you a favorable statement of the condition of the institution which is so much desired. The average number of patients increased since the last report from 177 to 212, and further financial support is needed. While there are thirty acres attached to the asylum, at least one hundred acres more are necessary for the health and comfort of the patients. While the Board of Commissioners has expressed their fullest satisfaction with the superintendent and general management of the asylum, cleanliness, neatness, and good order are everywhere visible. All our officers and attendants exhibit an anxious desire to promote the comfort and enjoyment of the patients. Their duties are now defined and they are required to faithful perform them. Every patient is examined daily by the medical officer with kindness and gentleness that marks the conduct of everyone in our employment."

Dr. Allen had enforced the rules and regulations for the asylum and was proud of his achievements with patient care and training of attendants. He found that better patient care came from hiring qualified attendants.

There had developed in America a group of asylum keepers who moved from state to state and asylum to asylum; they demonstrated poor care and no interest in the patients. Dr. Allen had established higher standards for his attendants and gained a habit of only hiring employees referred from people he knew and respected, not from politicians. He knew that politicians tended to recommend only those who contributed to their political interests, not based on any qualities.

On this day, Dr. Allen had an appointment with Dr. B. W. Dudley at his home on Second Street. While Dr. Dudley's home was often used for classes in the early days of Transylvania Medical School, medical students now attended a second Medical Hall near Dr. Dudley's home. Today, Dr. Allen observed that that Medical Hall had fewer students. Dr. Allen entered Dr. Dudley's front room after a maid allowed him entrance.

"Dr. Dudley," exclaimed Dr. Allen, "I am pleased to see you. I understand you wanted to see me, sir."

"Yes, I am hearing good things about you at the asylum," said the feeble and weakened Dr. Dudley. "And how are your wife and family doing?"

"My wife and daughter are fine. How may I help you?"

"I have a case that I want you to review," he said, directing Dr. Allen into his office. "This is the case of Dr. Abner Baker in Louisville, Kentucky.

He graduated from the Louisville School of Medicine, obviously a poor school to graduate a lunatic from. That school has no moral standards." He showed his obvious dislike for the school.

"Now, Dr. Dudley, I can understand your displeasure with that school," said Dr. Allen, "but what is the case about?"

Dr. Dudley continued, "After Dr. Baker's recent marriage, he killed his brother-in-law, Daniel Bates. A court acquitted Dr. Baker on the grounds of insanity, but the Bates family wants Dr. Baker executed. The Bates family has enough political pull to see that he is executed."

"Do you have the testimony of both the commonwealth and defendant?" asked Dr. Allen.

"Yes, I do. This case is important because Dr. Baker was recognized as insane prior to his killing of Daniel Bates, and it is being handled as a felonious intent case rather than a case of unsound mind. We of the medical community need to intervene for the insane. It is a sad, sad case, but Dr. Baker has been of unsound mind for years." Dr. Dudley sighed, showing his tired and weary manner.

"He needs our help, like any insane person does. I will do what I can. Such a misuse of the law is always unfair to the insane. I agree, we as physicians must voice our opinions. When should I report back my results?" asked Dr. Allen.

"The court needs your report by July. I will send one and M. C. Johnson will send one. Do you know him?" asked Dr. Dudley. "He is associated with the Northern Bank, but he has some legal interest in insanity."

"Yes, he and I have discussed some of the problems and legal issues with the insane," Dr. Allen said.

"Johnson married the sister of Cassius Clay, but she died the next year. While he has had many difficulties following her death, he still has an outstanding legal mind," stated Dr. Dudley.

"Yes, I have heard."

"M. C. Johnson has faced some bias against him. He was not allowed to march in his graduation because he was considered too ugly," continued Dr. Dudley.

"And I remember him being close friends with Mr. Hunt when he was chairman. I knew then that he had an interest in insanity issues," added Dr. Allen.

"I know that he is a brilliant man, but he has times of wavering interests. The loss of his wife, his difficulties with his brother-in-law, Cassius Clay, and personal bias has not always led to his staying with specific things," added Dr. Dudley. "However, with this issue, M. C. Johnson is strong."

"Well, you can depend upon me. I, also, wish to champion the importance of lunatics getting treatment in an asylum rather than just being punished," added Dr. Allen. "The law should not depend upon those who have political connections but upon what is right. All lunatics must have treatment and not punishment."

"I will await your decision on this case; we can discuss it further after you have familiarized yourself with the facts," Dr. Dudley said.

Dr. Allen excused himself and left Dr. Dudley's home. As he was leaving, he again noticed that the Medical Hall of the Transylvania Medical School was nearly empty. He had heard rumors of the school's declining enrollment.

*   *   *

On June 3, 1845, Cassius Clay published the *True American,* his antislavery newspaper. A mob attacked his offices and dismantled the press. The old sheriff, along with younger ones, was there to keep peace. He observed the split between families and friends again over the slavery issue.

Dr. Allen returned to see Dr. Dudley in early July. Dr. Dudley had submitted the following to the court:

The Undersigned has heard the evidence in the case of Dr. Baker, and conceives it a case of monomania as conclusively made out as can be found upon record. Dr. B.W. Dudley, MD.

Dr. Allen submitted his opinion as follows:

Kentucky Lunatic Asylum, July 24, 1845: I have examined fully the testimony, both on part of the Commonwealth, and the defendant, in the case of Dr. Abner Baker for the murder of Daniel Bates. After having seen a great number of insane persons, and after an uninterrupted intercourse with more than two hundred of them for twelve months, I feel no hesitancy in giving it as my opinion, Dr. Baker had been, and was at the time of the murder, affected with monomania, upon the subject of his wife's chastity, and ideas naturally connected with it: with symptoms indicating a strong tendency to degenerate into general derangement. That all cases of crime of violence, in which previous mental disease is proven, should have the whole benefit of the presumption that such disease may, in a moment, run into irresponsible mania, and the unhappy patient be judged fit for confinement and not for punishment. With the facts of the case before me, I should feel that I was omitting a duty to justice and humanity to withhold my earnest recommendation of Dr. Baker, as an object deserving, if not demanding, Executive clemency.

He signed it as Jno. R. Allen, Superintendent Kentucky Lunatic Asylum.

Dr. Allen asked Dr. Dudley, "What did M. C. Johnson say? Did he concur with us?"

"Yes," stated Dr. Dudley. "He gave his views as to the effect of monomania upon the criminality of acts committed under its influence. He had no doubt that a monomaniac, under the influence of an insane delusion, will kill or commit another act, and concludes it is not criminal. We have others who have also written an opinion on this case with the same conclusions."

"Well, I hope our opinions will carry some weight," Dr. Allen stated as he made plans to leave Dr. Dudley's home.

"I really appreciate your help with this case. It really was a case where scientific analysis was needed. Medically trained individuals need to be more involved in these cases rather than letting politics rule," added Dr. Dudley as he looked toward the Medical Hall.

Dr. Dudley continued, "I guess you have noticed that our Transylvania Medical Students have dropped off. There are fewer students at the Medical Hall."

"Yes, I have noticed; what will happen to the building—the second Medical Hall that we were so proud of?" asked Dr. Allen.

"Well, I hope to save the Transylvania Medical School," Dr. Dudley said, as he bade Dr. Allen farewell.

Dr. Allen had heard more rumors that the medical school would be closing. But he decided not to discuss that possibility with Dr. Dudley. Instead, he changed the subject. "I am busy preparing the asylum for a visitor, Dorothea Dix. She visits asylums and is responsible for the creation of some other state asylums. She also believes in the responsibility of state support for the lunatics and has been very successful in gaining more facilities. We have a lot of work to do to show her what a state asylum can do. She will be impressed, I hope."

"I am sure she will be," Dr. Dudley said as he and Dr. Allen shook hands.

Several weeks later, Dr. Allen received the October 1845 *American Journal of Phrenology* in his office. The articles still seemed to be theoretical and not applicable to his current asylum work. But it was the only available journal that dealt with common human problems.

Later that month, M. C. Johnson came to the asylum and asked the matron if he could see Dr. Allen. The matron showed him to Dr. Allen's office.

Johnson was visibly upset; his hands were shaking and he was unkempt in his clothes. Dr. Allen asked him to please take a seat in his office. He followed Dr. Allen into his office and said, "I just heard that Dr. Abner Baker was executed."

"What? I am shocked," stated Dr. Allen. "I thought Judge Buckner had been successful with a habeas corpus. The governor was supposed to respond and have an inquisition."

"Except that the governor did nothing, and the execution was carried out," Johnson said. "I just cannot believe that someone who should have been sent to an asylum was, instead, hung as a murderer. The Bates family had the political power while the medical professionals did not."

"Well, I am so upset over this injustice. Insanity is so misunderstood," contributed Dr. Allen.

"Yes, it certainly is. I see so many problems in my law practice; the law can only provide a standard, not a method of care. There are so many injustices in this world, even with the law. Well, I must go," Johnson said as he started to bid Dr. Allen good-bye.

"Yes, that is why I left the legal profession," added Dr. Allen.

"I wish I could. I really don't practice much. I am more involved in banking, where things can be more predictable. I still have trouble with the unfairness that I see," added Johnson. He appeared to be despondent, so Dr. Allen offered to show him around the facility, thinking that he would be encouraged over the progress at the asylum.

"Thank you, sir; however, I must hurry back to my bank. There is always something going on there," Johnson said. "Someday I might take you up on your offer. This is an interesting place." He started to leave. "You know, I had much respect for Chairman Hunt and often discussed legal issues and insanity with him. I still visit him at his home, although he is very frail." Then, he headed to the door of Dr. Allen's office.

Walking Johnson to the front door, Dr. Allen stated, "Yes, Chairman Hunt is missed by many, including me. He did so much for this institution and Transylvania."

*　　*　　*

Dorothea Dix had made a name for herself by visiting state asylums and recommending improvements with the appropriate state legislatures. She visited the Kentucky asylum in 1847 and praised the facility for the benefits that it provided to the lunatics. Dr. Allen had her meet some of the lunatics, including their most famous, Theodore Clay. He was sitting in his room, dressed in clean, matching clothing. This was unusual for a lunatic, but he had his own servant provided by the family, who saw that Theodore had the finest clothing that money could buy.

Mrs. Dix, with several years of experience with lunatics, asked, "You are Theodore Clay?" She sat next to him in his room.

"Yes, madam; I am also president of the United States," responded Theodore Clay.

"Sir, if you are president, why should you be here?" asked Mrs. Dix.

"My family does not recognize my powers; they have forced me to be here. They are jealous of me; see, my father lost when running for president, but I made it."

"Sir, are you happy here?" Mrs. Dix asked kindly.

"No, I have many things to do, and my horse and papers have been taken from me. I have no respect here," added Theodore Clay as he proudly displayed his exquisite coat. "I have difficulty getting decent clothing here."

"But, sir, I understand your family provides beautiful clothing. Your clothes are much nicer than the usual ones here." Mrs. Dix showed a profound interest in Theodore Clay. "Many here have much poorer clothing."

"But I have been unjustly confined here. I can never been happy here because I am prevented from doing important work," replied Theodore Clay.

Mrs. Dix dismissed herself from Theodore as he continued to talk about those in Lexington who have abused him. He especially disliked Dr. Dudley, who had advised his family about his care and restricted his use of the horse at the asylum.

Mrs. Dix spoke to Dr. Allen about Theodore Clay in his office. "I see that Theodore Clay is a very interesting person. However, he has no insight into how his own behavior got him into trouble."

"That is true. He had every opportunity as a child but never learned to accept responsibility," Dr. Allen said. "Earlier, he had an alcohol problem, which probably led to his difficulty with the law, but now, he does not see that he did anything. More recently, he became very threatening toward his family, and they have done everything for him. It is a real shame."

Mrs. Dix was amazed over Theodore Clay's excellent manners. "He is different from most pauper lunatics, not the typical asylum lunatic. Why is he not in a private facility?"

"The family has exhausted much of their money with his care. Earlier, they did pay for a private physician but they stopped that. Theodore Clay is often interviewed by medical students at this asylum because of his good verbal skills."

"Yes, I can see that," answered Mrs. Dix.

Dr. Allen continued, "There was a second son, John M. Clay, who recently had a similar problem. John does fine as long as he lives with his family and limits his alcohol usage."

"However, I understand that many here do not have families, like Sarah Norton, who had no home," added Mrs. Dix.

"Yes, you saw her also?" asked Dr. Allen.

"Yes, she is so sweet, but no one knows where her family is."

"True; she was admitted in 1845 at the age of twenty-seven. She had lived on the streets and was abused by many who would not pay her money after she worked for them. She was in poor health when she came. She never went to school, and no one knows of her family. She has thrived here, mostly on the attention that she gets. She is mentally slow but trainable. We have given her safety and a home," said Dr. Allen. "She has really become a good worker here at this asylum. We are proud of her."

"I can see lunatics like her benefiting from this institution. She would have died if this facility did not take her in," said Mrs. Dix.

"Yes, that is the purpose of this facility, to care for those who cannot care for themselves or whose families will not care for them," added Dr. Allen.

"Yes, I agree but I still question Theodore Clay being here. He is not a pauper who requires state support."

"Others like Theodore who are considered dangerous by the law must be restrained from hurting innocent citizens but not punished. They deserve treatment and to not be treated like criminals. Jail is not appropriate for them they need humane treatment in a lunatic asylum also."

"So I see," replied Mrs. Dix.

"Unfortunately, many of the insane still end up in jails. Jail is not a solution for the lunatics, they are in and out. A state asylum can provide better and necessary care for them," added Dr. Allen.

"I do have one concern: why have twenty-five patients, from a total of 271 patients, died in your asylum? That number of deaths appears to be higher at this asylum than at other facilities," Mrs. Dix said, as she compared the numbers with similar facilities. "I was shocked to see such figures."

"Yes, I am also concerned about that," stated Dr. Allen. "We have many difficult lunatics, and many were in poor physical health when admitted, such as Sarah Norton."

"But she has recovered. Have you called in for some expert opinions?" asked Mrs. Dix.

"Yes, and we have applied some of their advice. We are trying to discover the problem of why this facility has a worse death rate than others in the United States." Dr. Allen showed his embarrassment.

Dorothea Dix was very supportive of Dr. Allen, and she praised the asylum for its work, choosing to ignore the concerns over the high death rate. Instead, she went to the Kentucky legislature to request funds for a second state asylum, since the one in Lexington was full beyond its capacity. Dr. Allen had hoped that Dix's visit might help to provide pressure for his requests at this asylum while she was seeking funds for a second one.

In April 1847, Dr. Allen received the *Journal of Insanity*. He constantly read books related to care for the insane. In this issue was an article written by Dr. Buttolph, first assistant physician at the State Lunatic Asylum at Utica, New York, titled, "Modern asylums." Dr. Buttolph discussed the modern asylum, including:

Proper warming and ventilation of the buildings is necessary within the facility. Medical treatment should be in harmony with possibilities of relief and a more particular examination should be made of the bodily health and mental state of the patient. ... The insane person should be informed that they will receive the appropriate medical and other treatment, and when restored, will return home. They should be introduced to the Attendant in whose care they are placed, and if but partially insane, be informed more particularly of the regulations; being made to understand, that the enjoyment of certain privileges, will be connected with their ability for self-restraint, and that they will be withdrawn when abused or deemed injurious. Treatment should be divided into medical and moral, with the former, including the use of medicine, baths, regulation of diet, & the latter, all those means and influences brought to bear upon the person in his new situation; as association with others, employment, exercise and amusements, rising and retiring, habits of order and cleanliness, attendance on religious services, and the like. ... Next in importance to the medical, is the moral treatment of the insane, and indeed this is, in many cases, either superior to the former, or all that is required for the recovery of the patient.

Dr. Allen was encouraged by the similarity of his work at this asylum and the recommendations of Dr. Buttolph. Dr. Allen shared this article with members of the board, and they shared his enthusiasm.

An outbreak of cholera hit Lexington again in 1849, and 345 people died. Among the victims were the son of Dr. Allen and the beloved John W. Hunt. The asylum had lost a great leader. Dr. Allen especially felt both losses.

At the same time, the Kentucky Lunatic Asylum had sixty cases of cholera, and twenty-two died. Since most of the cholera cases came from the geographic area of north Lexington and the asylum was located in that area, twenty-two cases were not considered unusual. However, Dr. Allen suspected differently. The continued high death rate was becoming more visible.

In his 1850 report, Dr. Allen stated that he was concerned over the large mortality rate,

The throng of inmates which we have had to accommodate in a house without sufficient room might generate the disease. This disease is the most obstinate, even with the sane. With the insane, it becomes doubly formidable with their frequent resistance of remedies. Regarding this malady's mysteriousness in all phases, we have no theory to offer as to its origin. I can say with truth, that the condition of the asylum, as regards to its cleanliness and other hygienic precautions was, perhaps, better than ever with your direction, we have planned and built of brick, a stable and attached a corn crib and cow shed of suitable material with ample lofts for providers and straw. These very necessary out-buildings have been long wanted, but a hope that land might be purchased upon which they were to be erected, has postponed their building. The small parcel of land purchased by you during the year is commodious. In addition to the aids rendered in brick-making, we have made sixty five rods of turnpike road, leading from the front yard to the nearest point on the Georgetown road, giving us a turnpike to the city.

That year, Dr. Allen called in more experts to evaluate the medical problems at the asylum. The death rate continued to be very high. The cause of the high death rate continued to be elusive.

One group of experts recommended that all smoking and tobacco be banned from the facility. That recommendation was followed, but there was no improvement in the death rate. Another group of experts recommended that spittoons be removed from the living areas, but that did not reveal any decrease in the death rate. Dr. Allen was becoming very discouraged. He could not determine the cause.

Dr. Allen did get some financial help from the Kentucky legislature in 1851. A new building was completed, as he relayed in the following:

We are happy to be able to announce to you that the late addition to the building, which has been so long a desire, is now completed and will be soon occupied. Now, in the house about finished, we are gaining lodging for 10 males on each ward and each ward will have two day rooms, a large porch admitting at all times a current of fresh and pure air. From this porch is entered on each floor, a well arranged privy, bathing, and dressing-room. There is a large leaded cistern in the attic, holding about two hundred and fifty barrels of water, intended to supply the water-closets and to be used in case of fire. In the basement, we shall gain store-rooms, comfortable servants' lodgings, & apartments heretofore, very much needed. Above all other consideration, we have now afforded a complete classification of our inmates, the basis of curative treatment.

On the second floor, we have located a large hall, thirty-eight by thirty-one, which, in honor of the benevolent Mr. James Strode Megowan, who kindly made a donation to the asylum, we propose as "Megowan Hall," to be used on all occasions.

Rev. Chipley had become too feeble to continue on the Board of Commissioners, and he was replaced by Judge Buckner, father-in-law of Dr. Allen. Rev. Chipley's son, Dr. W. S. Chipley, had married Miss Elizabeth Fanning, who came from a long line of noble ancestors from Georgia. After establishing a large medical practice in Columbus, Georgia, Dr. Chipley and his family moved back to Lexington to care for his elderly parents around the 1850s. In 1854, Dr. Chipley became a professor of theory and practice of medicine in the declining Transylvania Medical College, hoping to salvage the school from ruin.

Dr. Chipley had met Dr. Allen at the Transylvania Medical School, where Dr. Allen had been chair of materia medica and medical botany since 1851. They both shared an interest in care for the insane, but by this time, Dr. Allen was less enthusiastic about his methods since he continued to feel personal blame for the asylum's high death rate.

Although Dr. Allen had an interested in phrenology, he was aware that Dr. Caldwell, the father of American phrenology, had disappointed many Lexington citizens, including Dr. Chipley. While Dr. Allen found solace in reading the most current phrenology journals of his time, he had no one in Lexington whom he could share his interest with. The two doctors appeared to have nothing in common.

In 1852, Rev. Chipley died, and his wife, Amelia T. Chipley, moved in with Dr. Chipley and his family in Lexington. Dr. Chipley had established himself with a large medical practice in Lexington by the time of his father's death.

*　　*　　*

Dr. Allen decided to have a serious discussion with Richard Pindell, chairman of the board, in the fall of 1852. He really felt defeated and could not see any solution; he told Pindell, "I just cannot determine why our death rate is so high. We were not so concerned when the death rate was high in '49, but the death rate continues to be high, now. I have done everything I can do, called in experts and tried their recommendations, but there is no improvement. The slow, continuous death rate makes me think that there is something within the facility that is adding to our problem, but I cannot determine what." Dr. Allen hit his fist on the table, showing his frustrations to his friend.

"I am so sorry. I have full confidence in you, and if you or the experts cannot determine the cause, I have no answers," added Pindell. "I just hope you will continue to do your best, which is all that we can ask of anyone."

"I'm having difficulty accepting such a failure," Dr. Allen stated. "I'm used to finding or working toward a solution; this is just beyond me and my training." He again slammed his hand against the chair. "I don't know anything else to do."

"Obviously, it is beyond the experts' ability, so maybe you expect too much. You are too hard on yourself," contributed Pindell. "Do you remember hearing about the early days here?"

"Yes, I heard so much from Chairman Hunt. I remember how he got so discouraged at times when no one seemed to support the asylum. Then, I had some answers; now, I have none," Dr. Allen said sadly.

"You have solved many problems here but the high death rate is different; no one seems to know. Outsiders assume that we have horrible things going on here because of the high death rate, but nothing could be further from the truth. What is causing it is not yet known. Mr. Hunt often felt discouraged but he kept going until you came along with your training, and now, you must continue the course until other solutions are found," added Pindell.

"Well, you have a point," replied Dr. Allen.

"Actually, there were about fifty original Lexington contributors, but

Mr. John W. Hunt was left alone with the responsibilities until you came along. You rescued the asylum. Your achievements have been dwarfed by the current problem."

"Yes, I hear what you are saying. I will think upon your words of wisdom." Changing the subject and hoping for a happier conversation, Dr. Allen asked, "By the way, what has happened to Mr. Hunt's home, Hopemount, since his death?"

"John Wesley's daughter, Henrietta Hunt Morgan, is living in the house. She returned to her childhood home after his death. Henrietta Morgan has seven children, with five being sons. She has an active family; therefore, the house is busy again as it had been in earlier days with John W. Hunt's twelve children." Pindell knew that his friend always enjoyed hearing about the local citizens.

"That sounds good, especially that the house is active with children," added Dr. Allen. "As you know, my wife and I have just lost our son. We still have one girl living. My wife is obviously upset, but she is still young and can have another son. I am sure her being upset and my not being able to find a solution to the death rate is all just too much for both of us at this time. I need time to think."

"I am so sorry! You have many disturbing concerns, and I'm sure this asylum is not helping. But I would hope you will continue with your services here," added Pindell. They continued talking about the Lexington people that they had known together, as Chairman Pindell knew that Dr. Allen tended to relax more when they shared such stories.

In 1853, Dr. Allen received word that Dr. Caldwell had died. Dr. Caldwell's death, even at the age of eighty years old, was an additional disappointment for Dr. Allen. Since Dr. Caldwell was still disliked in Lexington, he could not discuss this loss with anyone.

In 1853, Pindell's yearly report specified that a new building was needed. He supported Dr. Allen's recommendation for "a better mode of warming the buildings, suggesting that the whole facility needed to be improved with the use of steam and reducing the danger of open fireplaces." Also, for additional means of safety, Pindell "requested the use of gas for lights. Since the erection of gas works in the city of Lexington, it would require about $2,500 to connect with the city pipes, and furnish fixtures."

Dr. Allen reviewed his superintendency of the asylum at the end of 1853, looking at January 1, 1854, as the start of his tenth year to be superintendent. He stated the following in his yearly report:

My ambition has been to be instrumental in making the best of this institution which with its many defects and then to leave it to hands that are better qualified to develop its usefulness. There have been many difficulties I have met with, and many other obstacles, in the pathway of its greatest usefulness.

Pindell had reasons to be hopeful since his father, Thomas Hart Pindell, had become mayor of Lexington in 1854. Thomas Hart Pindell had used the second Medical School Building, which was then empty, as a city hall. They were keeping the building available as city hall and hoping to revive the Transylvania Medical School. Yet, new students were choosing other medical schools over the old Transylvania Medical School.

Dr. Allen continued to be discouraged over his inability to determine the cause of the growing high death rate at the asylum. And the declining Transylvania Medical School was also a blow to him. Dr. Allen had enjoyed teaching medical students as a diversion from the grind at the asylum, but that opportunity was ending. This was all too much for him.

At the end of 1854, Dr. Allen was offered a teaching position at the Jefferson Medical School in St. Louis, and he quickly accepted the offer, resigning from the Kentucky Lunatic Asylum. After Dr. Allen made the decision to leave Lexington, he felt better than he had in months.

Dr. Allen had worried most about his wife's reaction to leaving Lexington, but she surprised him. Elizabeth understood his reasons for leaving. She had recognized how depressed he had become since his son's death, his enthusiasm at the asylum was gone, and the medical school was closing, which all led her to see that something had to change. She saw that change coming with a new job offer.

Dr. Allen and his family left Lexington on a coach on the national road going west. Many of their personal items were to be shipped later. Elizabeth hoped that those items would never be sent, because she secretly hoped to return to Lexington in the future. Yet she knew her greatest responsibility was with her husband and their one remaining child.

Sources for Chapter 5

Allen, Dr. John R. *Rules and Regulations of the Kentucky Lunatic Asylum.* Lexington, Kentucky: James Virden, 1845.

Allen, Dr. John R. Yearly Report. *Kentucky Documents.* Frankfort, Kentucky: 1845.

Allen, Dr. John R. Yearly Report. *Kentucky Documents.* Frankfort, Kentucky: 1848.

Allen, Dr. John R. Yearly Report. *Kentucky Documents.* Frankfort, Kentucky: 1851.

Barkley, Dr. A. H. "Early Medical Lore Connected with the Bluegrass Region." *Lexington Leader.*

Buttolph, Dr. H. A. "Modern Asylums." *Journal of Insanity* VI (April 1847): 364–378.

Cotter, R. *Phrenology: An Annotated, Historical Biobibliography and Index.* Metuchen, New Jersey: Scarecrow Press, 1989.

Crozier, C. *Life and Trial of Dr. Abner Baker Jr* From Special Collections Lexington, Kentucky: University of Kentucky, 1846.

Deese, W. "Graduation data about Dr. John R. Allen and Dr. W. S. Chipley." Transylvania University Library from Special Collections Lexington, Kentucky: University of Kentucky, 2004.

Fowler, O. S. *The American Phrenological Journal* VII, 131, October 1845.

"Insanity in Kentucky" *Boston Medical and Surgical Journal* XXIV, 11, April 21, 1841.

"John Allen's Family History" *Kentucky Encyclopedia*. Lexington, Kentucky: University of Kentucky Press, 1992.

Kerr, B. and J. D. Wright. *Lexington: A Century in Photographs*. Lexington, Kentucky: Lexington-Fayette County Historic Commission, 1984.

Peter, Robert. *History of the Medical Department of Transylvania University*. Lexington, Kentucky: John P. Morton, 1905.

Pindell, Richard. "Report of the Managers of the Eastern Lunatic Asylum." *Kentucky Documents*. Frankfort, Kentucky: 1853.

Richardson, H. E. *Cassius Marcellus Clay: Firebrand of Freedom*. Lexington, Kentucky: University of Kentucky Press, 1976.

Wright, John D. *Transylvania: Tutor to the West*. Lexington, Kentucky: Transylvania University Press, 1975.

Photos

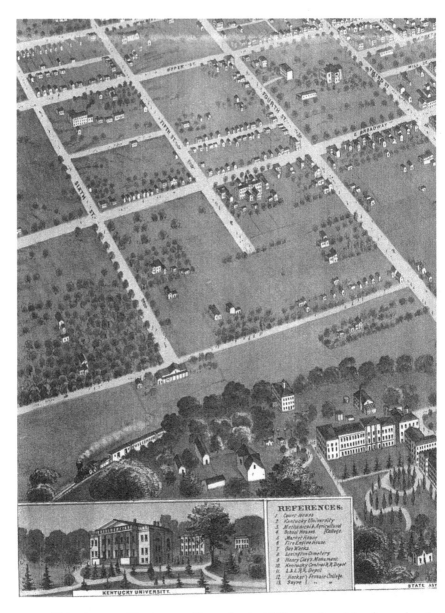

This picture of Lexington, Kentucky, in 1871, was found by the author in for the Insane, originally built in 1824.

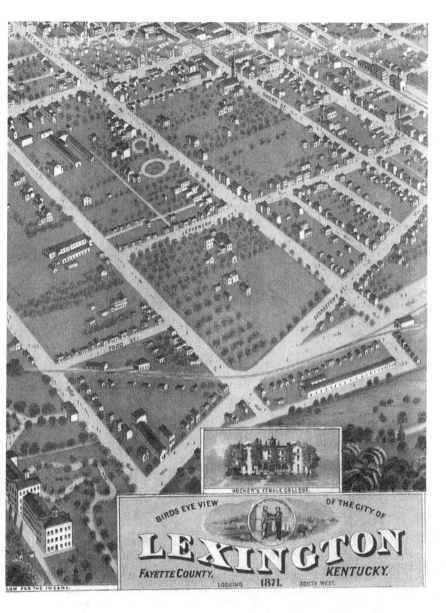

a Lexington antique shop. In the middle is a picture of the State Asylum

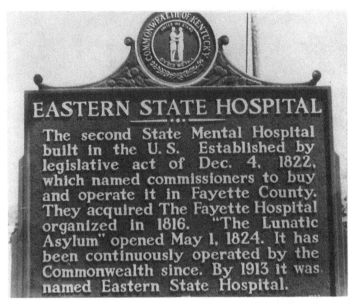

Official designation as continuously operating since 1824 and named Eastern State Hospital in 1913.

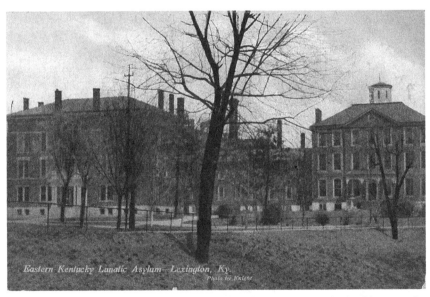

A postcard of Eastern Kentucky Lunatic Asylum dated 1911. The building on the far right was the first building. It is now called the Gragg Building. The building on the far left is the Administration Building, built in the early 1900s.

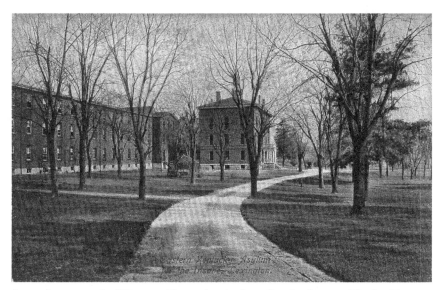

An early postcard of Eastern Kentucky Asylum for the Insane. The building in the middle is the Administration Building and on the left is the West Building, constructed in the 1860s. Notice the buildings were not connected.

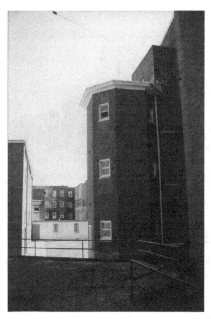

This is a current picture of one of two remaining octagonal-shaped bath closets from the 1860s. They allowed rainwater into the back of the West Building. It was considered the best institutional sanitization system at the time.

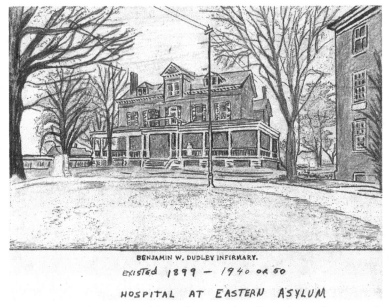

BENJAMIN W. DUDLEY INFIRMARY.
EXISTED 1899 — 1940 OR 50
HOSPITAL AT EASTERN ASYLUM

This picture is a machine copy of the Infirmary taken from the yearly report of 1899 and hand-colored by the author. The West Building is on the right, and they were later connected.

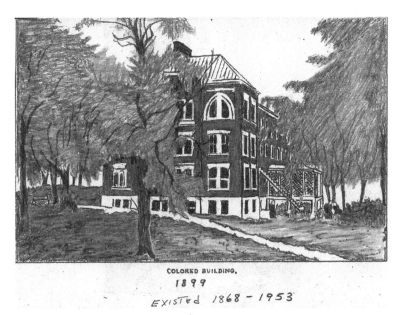

COLORED BUILDING.
1899
EXISTED 1868 — 1953

This picture called the "Colored Building" was machine copied from the yearly report of 1899 and hand-colored by the author.

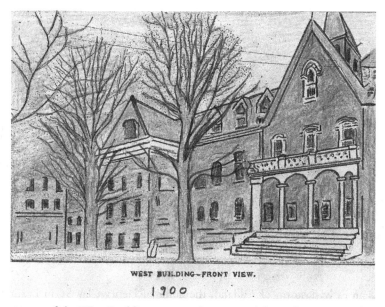

WEST BUILDING—FRONT VIEW.

1900

This picture of the West Building was machine copied from the 1900 yearly report and hand-colored by the author.

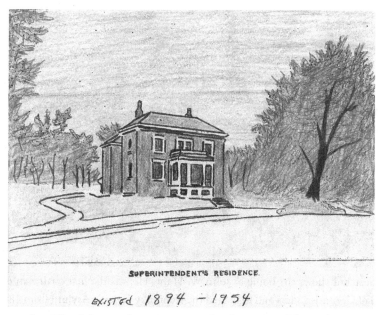

SUPERINTENDENT'S RESIDENCE.

EXISTED 1894 – 1954

The superintendent's home; this picture was machine copied from the 1900 yearly report and hand-colored by the author.

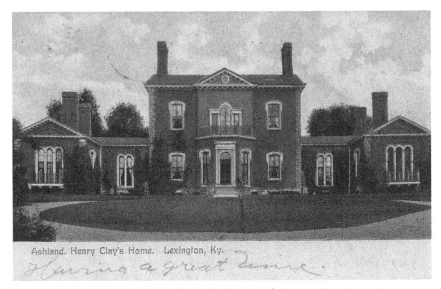

Ashland. Henry Clay's Home. Lexington, Ky.

This is an early postcard of Ashland, the home of Henry Clay Sr. in Lexington. Two of Clay's sons were admitted to the Kentucky asylum. The Clay family home is currently open for public tours.

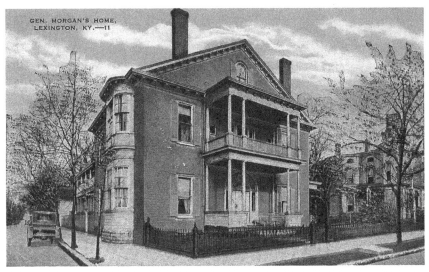

GEN. MORGAN'S HOME, LEXINGTON, KY.—11

This postcard shows the home of John W. Hunt. He was the first chairman of the Board of Commissioners and managed the Kentucky Lunatic Asylum from 1824 to 1844. His grandson, John Morgan, grew up in the house and achieved fame during the Civil War. This home is currently open for public tours.

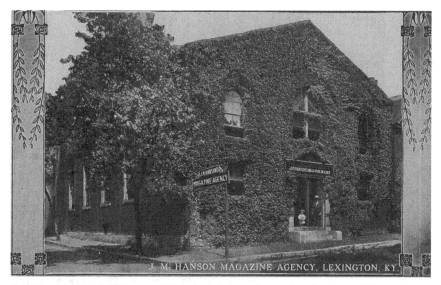

A 1913 postcard of the Hanson Magazine Agency, located in the original Transylvania Medical School building. The building was demolished in 1954.

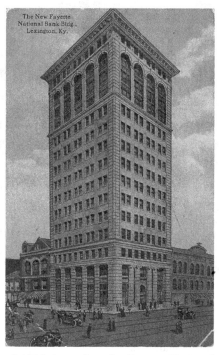

This postcard is dated 1914, just after the Fayette National Bank Building was completed; this was the second law office of Colonel John R. Allen.

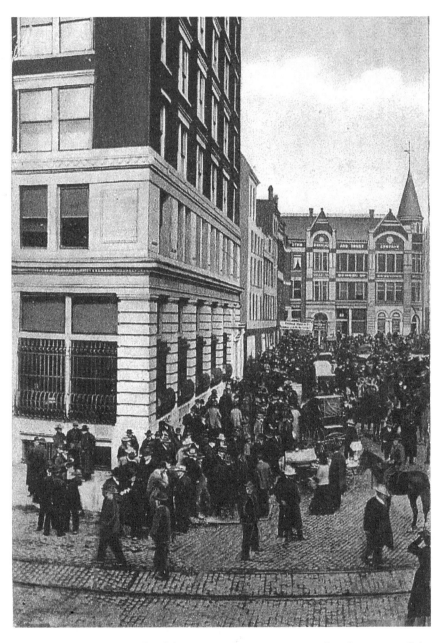

Two 1906 postcards of downtown Lexington, Kentucky, show part of the
the middle is a large three-story bank building where Colonel John R. Allen
attending a market day.

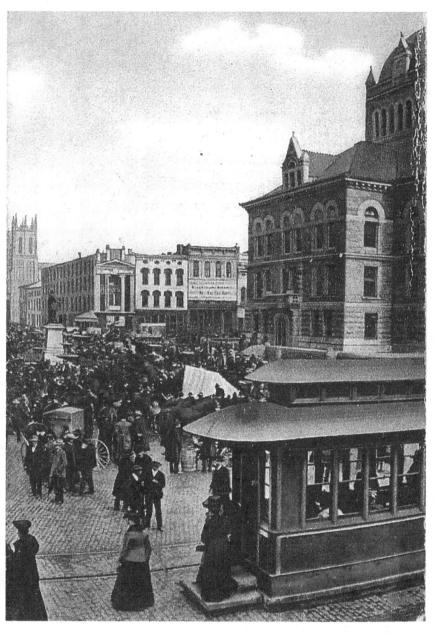

Fayette County Courthouse on the right side and a bank on the left side. In first practiced law with his uncle, Judge Buckner. The people were probably

Chapter Six

1855–1869

In April 1855, Dr. William S. Chipley was appointed the full-time superintendent of the Kentucky Lunatic Asylum. Dr. Chipley could not allow the asylum to be left without leadership, although he had observed Dr. Allen's frustrations with it. Because his father, Rev. Chipley, was an original contributor to the asylum and had been a member on the Board of Commissioners until his death, Dr. Chipley felt a duty to his family to assume the superintendent's role.

Richard Pindell, as chairman of the board, welcomed Dr. Chipley to the next meeting. Other members of the current board consisted of James A. Grinstead, James L. Allen, Richard A. Buckner Jr. (who had replaced his father, Richard A. Buckner Sr.), and Dr. S. M. Letcher. The board was divided between Pindell and Buckner, who had been supporters of Dr. Allen and defended his leaving the asylum. The other board members were critical of Dr. Allen's quick absence, his inability to reduce the death rate, and his purchase of warming devices they considered too expensive. Dr. Chipley had felt a duty not to take sides.

This meeting occurred in the room that Hunt and Dr. Allen had both occupied, the room that had always been used for board meetings. While the furnishings were the same, the room had draperies over the windows that showed the airing yard. This addition came when visitors became upset over observing the disturbed patients in the airing yard; Dr. Chipley also felt it was a distraction to him accomplishing his work.

Dr. Perrin, who had previously been a part-time assistant superintendent, was recognized by Pindell for accepting the temporary position as superintendent. Dr. Perrin had never wanted any full-time position since he could make more money in private practice. When Dr. Chipley took over as superintendent, the board had agreed to seek another assistant superintendent, since Dr. Perrin was ready to leave.

After the meeting was called to order, the chairman made the usual announcements and introduced everyone. "Sir," Dr. Chipley said, as he was recognized by Pindell, "I know of a local physician, Dr. T. P. Dudley, who is interested in insanity care. I would like to ask him to consider that position. He has helped me with my private practice here in Lexington, and I would appreciate his help in the position as assistant superintendent and physician."

"Yes, certainly, if you know of someone who might be interested, do seek his opinion so we can proceed further," answered Chairman Pindell. "Does everyone else agree?"

"Well, we need to know more about his training and experience," stated Dr. Letcher. "Is this Dr. T. P. Dudley from Lexington?"

"He is part of the Dudley family from north of Lexington. He has been trained elsewhere and has not been in Lexington long," stated Dr. Chipley.

"But is he related to Dr. B. W. Dudley?"

"I think Dr. B. W. Dudley is his uncle. As you know, all Dudleys around Lexington are related, but I'm not sure how he is related to Dr. B. W. Dudley," added Dr. Chipley. "If I remember, Dr. T. P. Dudley's father is Dr. B. W. Dudley's brother."

"Well, let us see if Dr. T. P. Dudley is interested in the position. The pay is low but opportunities for private practice will make the position more lucrative," contributed Dr. Letcher. "However, he might prefer private practice."

"I will talk to him, but money is not a major consideration for him," stated Dr. Chipley. "He is a very loyal person who believes in holding up one's duty and responsibility, and I appreciate that."

"As you know, that position pays only $250 a year," added Pindell. "I am requesting that the governor consider the amount of $500 for that position since that is the amount of similar facilities, but I have not gotten any answer."

"That is certainly nothing to interest another physician," added Dr. Letcher. "I would hope Dr. T. P. Dudley is adequately trained."

"Oh, yes, he is more interested in better care for anyone he is called upon to help," stated Dr. Chipley. "And he is loyal to me. I will talk to him."

"I have also asked that the governor allow a specific amount of $25,000 a year with which we can adequately run the asylum," stated the chairman. "With a specified amount, the facility can plan their yearly purchases."

"Yes, a specified amount each year would help," added Buckner. "We can make definite plans rather than running to the governor for each item."

"The problem is that the governor does not want to give the amount that we need; he wants us to accept less. Last year it was $20,000 and $15,000 the year before, so our debts only increase. We need the whole sum of $25,000, and I will use what political power I can to gain support for that amount," stated Chairman Pindell. "Any other issues we need to discuss?"

"Sir, may I have time to discuss the problems that I see at the asylum?" asked Dr. Chipley. "This board must decide some of those issues in the future, and I wish now for your consideration."

"Of course," stated Chairman Pindell. "Please, do!" He saw the enthusiasm that he had seen in the earlier days of Dr. Allen.

"As each of you know, I assumed this superintendent position last month after Dr. Allen left, but I understand that he had verbally contracted with Mr. Greenwood for the work and material to the much needed warming apparatus throughout the facility. The board approved the sum of $6,000 for completion of that work, but Dr. Allen realized that the completion would require more than $6,000 and stopped the agreement with Mr. Greenwood, leaving the institution still unheated. I believe we need to go ahead with that project," added Dr. Chipley.

"Well, I object," said Grinstead. "As a businessman, Dr. Allen was wrong to negotiate such a big contract without getting the specific total amount on paper. Then the contractor could not have increased the amount as he wished."

"Yes, maybe the business deal was poorly done," Dr. Chipley continued, "but we still need the warming device; the institution is without heat. We now need another opinion, and I would like to hire an engineer who can help us with this problem. Mr. E. C. Barrett is willing to serve in that capacity. I now request that the board approve his position."

"I agree," stated Pindell. "I'm not sure where the money will come from, but we cannot do without heat. We need some expert advice, and this engineer can provide that."

All board members agreed.

"As you know, the institution has many needs for adequate care for our lunatics, and I will be requesting funds from the board and the governor after I complete my report at the end of this year," Dr. Chipley said.

"Yes, sir, your report will be helpful," stated Pindell.

"Although the back building was recently completed, a building on the other side burned in '53, and this facility is again lacking in enough apartments to handle who we have. We have many needs to be addressed, but the most immediate problem is the high death rate. I will be evaluating the high death rate that has plagued this facility for years. I hope to have some solutions soon," resolved Dr. Chipley.

The board agreed to wait until Dr. Chipley could finish his evaluation of the asylum. They agreed to meet again the following month and then adjourned.

Dr. Chipley was able to hire Dr. T. P. Dudley as assistant superintendent. He had assigned Dr. Dudley to regularly check each person and determine if he or she were showing signs of illness in addition to his own regular medical duties.

Dr. Chipley was somewhat upset with Dr. Allen for leaving so abruptly, but he had come to expect such from others. Dr. Chipley had had tremendous respect for Dr. Caldwell during his early years as a medical student, and then Dr. Caldwell disappointed him. Dr. Allen was just another professional who had disappointed him.

Dr. Chipley took his responsibility seriously and demonstrated it when his elderly father and mother needed him. He left a lucrative medical practice in Georgia to move his own family back to Lexington to help his own mother and father. Now his sense of responsibility had led him to the asylum.

Dr. Chipley's wife, Elizabeth Fanning of Columbus, Georgia, had followed him to Lexington; when she met Elizabeth Buckner Allen there, they became fast friends and shared their love for family and home. Elizabeth Chipley understood how hard it was for Elizabeth Allen to leave her Lexington family and move, so she continued to write encouraging letters to her. Their friendship grew.

Elizabeth Chipley had also encouraged their children to visit the deep southern part of Georgia, not knowing that it would one day rip their family apart. The Allen children were too young to develop any preferences. Yet both women continued to write to each other as they shared family concerns.

$$* \quad * \quad *$$

The Old Buffalo Trail was part of the national road going through Kentucky, while the street was still called Mulberry in Lexington. Yet the Central Kentucky Railroad had come into town on the northeastern side of the Kentucky Lunatic Asylum. The asylum owned four and a half acres of land needed by the railroad, and the asylum was paid for that land, and gained another adjoining eleven acres on the other side, giving the asylum more usable land on the opposite side. Chairman Pindell had been pleased with this transaction and the final outcome.

As the Medical School of Transylvania University continued to decline in pupils in 1855, most of the professors had left. Those remaining were Dr. E. L. Dudley, who taught surgery; Dr. J. M. Bush, who taught anatomy; Dr. W. S. Chipley, who taught theory and practice; Dr. S. M. Letcher, who taught obstetrics; Dr. H. M. Skillman, who taught physiology and institutes of medicine; Dr. A. K. Marchall and Dr. B. P. Drake, who taught materia medica and botany; and Dr. Robert Peter, who taught chemistry and pharmacy. The opening session had only thirty-eight students, despite many advertisements in various newspapers.

In June 1855, Dr. T. P. Dudley, assistant superintendent of the asylum, observed an increase in sickness among the lunatics and summoned Dr. Chipley. "Sir, I have found three inmates with ice cold skin. One has a blue appearance. I am concerned." Dr. Dudley added, "I have tried to make them comfortable."

"We must check on them frequently, putting blankets and warming them up. Where are their rooms?" asked Dr. Chipley.

"Two are on the third floor Ward 4, male side, and another in the female side, first floor Ward 1. I have already summoned blankets and warm clothing. Two had limited clothing, so I have sent for additional clothing," added Dr. Dudley.

"Have you notified the matron and the steward?" asked Dr. Chipley.

"Yes, sir, both will be checking their clothing and changing the clothing as necessary. Mr. Rice will be purchasing more blankets since all our blankets are being used. Although this is June, many of our more frail patients are cold and have difficulty staying warm. I have authorized the purchase of more blankets."

Dr. Chipley checked on each of the three inmates and noticed that they improved with proper food and clothing. This routine continued as twenty more patients showed signs of cholera, similar to what had been reported in other parts of the city. Dr. Chipley noted that the laundry facilities of the asylum were slow and difficult when clean clothes were needed in a hurry. The sick patients required more watching and changing of clothing.

While the illness did subside, the attendants were exhausted. Dr. Chipley continued to seek ways to remove every cause that he thought to be capable of causing the malady. He searched every room of the facility, seeking any unusual source. He had all rooms cleaned with special care.

Then in the first of July 1855, even more patients became sick. Dr. Chipley noticed that some of the attendants were showing signs of the illness as well. While much of the early illness had been associated with the longer term and weaker residents, the attendants were usually healthy and previously not subject to illness in the asylum. Now, the attendants were also getting sick. He speculated over the events of the last few days.

By the middle of July 1855, most of the 202 asylum inmates had been attacked by the disease. Dr. Dudley was constantly checking each one and observing more of those who had shown the symptoms. He was growing weary and, like most attendants, was working without any rest. All employees were committed to their duty and refused to leave it.

Meanwhile, Dr. Chipley continued to look for a solution. He looked at the year of 1849, when cholera had killed fifty-five patients in May and June. Dr. Allen had meticulously recorded those who lost their lives and identified ones who died quickly from those who lingered. Inmates such as Matilda O'Bannon of Logan County, age sixty-nine, died as quickly as J. W. Settle of Barren County, age sixteen, while Mary Johnson of Louisville, age seventeen, and Alcy Richardson of Boone County, age sixty-two, lingered longer before their death.

What was the connection? Dr. Chipley wondered. It certainly was not age. He noticed one pattern: everyone who died of the disease was from some other county than Fayette County, the county of the facility. While Fayette County inmates did get the disease in the asylum, they were less likely to die from it. Why?

Could it be the water supply at the asylum? Dr. Chipley asked himself. Those from the Lexington area appeared to be more immune to the Lexington water. Also, while Lexington had had cholera several times, those from the north side of Lexington, where the asylum was located, were observed to have suffered less.

Dr. Chipley had one idea. He decided to observe the water supply that came from their unfailing water spring. Then, he would consult Dr. Letcher, who might have some knowledge of the Fayette County area water, since he refused to drink any other water except from his own artesian well.

Dr. Letcher, while a board member of the asylum, had been a physician in Lexington for many years. He responded to Dr. Chipley's special request by visiting the asylum.

Dr. Letcher was a quiet, small man; he entered the front door of the asylum building and was greeted by Rice, the steward. He asked to see Dr. Chipley. Rice directed him to Dr. Chipley's office. They greeted each other.

"Sir," started Dr. Chipley, "I admire your knowledge and dedication. As you know, cholera has been a difficult problem for years at this institution. Several have tried to find answers, but with no success."

"So how may I help you? I also have limited answers," replied Dr. Letcher.

"I would like your professional opinion," he said as he offered Dr. Letcher a chair in his office. "As you might not know, I have suspected our water supply because it is excellent for purging new patients. The new patients always react to our water supply, especially those from outside of the county. Can there be such as thing as too much purging, maybe resulting in a disease such as cholera? What are your observations?"

"I, too, have observed that patients from this area are more resistant to the purging effect of drinking water at this facility," stated Dr. Letcher. "I have had some of my own personal concerns about the water and will only drink from artesian wells. The past cholera in Lexington convinced me of that. Remember, Dr. B. W. Dudley said he realized that there was contaminated water in Lexington. He always boiled his water, and neither he nor any of his family got sick with the cholera. While we all have hoped that the asylum was different, maybe it's not."

"It is really bad here," Dr. Chipley said as he banged his hand on the desk.

"I have heard that almost everyone here is sick, including many employees," stated Dr. Letcher.

"Yes, I have been getting help from community physicians and volunteer nurses. The situation is growing more serious. As of today, thirty-five inmates have died, including seven employees and Dr. York, who had just finished his medical training. I will try anything to help," Dr. Chipley stated seriously.

"What other evidence do you have about the water supply?" asked Dr. Letcher. "It has long been a source of drinking water. In fact, I understand that this 'unfailing' spring was why the asylum was built at this location."

"Yes, the unfailing spring has been a source of pride for pure water since the beginning of the asylum," responded Dr. Chipley. "For me to point to it as the source of contamination, many will reject my conclusion."

"I would hope that you have some other evidence more than just speculation?" stated Dr. Letcher.

"I do; yesterday I had an attendant put some soap into our washhouse, and that same soap came up in our drinking spring twenty minutes later. I observed this occurrence several times. There must be some connection between the spring drinking water and our waste water, of which we have been unaware. How can we determine the problem without wasting a lot of money and time? Actually, I have little time, as my employees are sick and exhausted."

"This is very serious," added Dr. Letcher.

"Yes, it is, and I am doubtful as to how to proceed."

"I would suggest hauling in water from another part of city for the whole Asylum, and restrict all water usage to the hauled water and see what happens," suggested Dr. Letcher. "Then, if the disease is reduced, more permanent changes can be made, but for now, you must stop using the current water source. I agree with your conclusion."

"I will do that! We at least have a plan. I will request that all water for the asylum be hauled in from the other side of town. Then, we can see if the disease continues as usual," Dr. Chipley said, showing his first real enthusiasm to a longtime problem.

"If that proves to be the cause, then you would be justified in asking the governor for money toward having a well dug," added Dr. Letcher. "There is good water at 125 feet in most parts of this town, as I have found with my artesian well. There are other citizens in the northern part of Lexington who have had their own wells dug because they suspect the water supply."

Dr. Chipley was relieved to find that Dr. Letcher, who had a tremendous amount of experience, also suspected the water supply as a culprit. He began to tap the floor with his foot as his excitement increased, realizing that he might be close to eliminating the sickness that had been so rampant in this institution.

Dr. Chipley contacted the appropriate people to haul water into the asylum from other parts of town. Within one week, there were no new cases, and the cholera threat was over. Dr. Chipley was a hero to everyone associated with the asylum, including Dr. Dudley.

Chairman Pindell requested a sum of money from the governor to dig an artesian well for the asylum. It was immediately given, as Dr. Chipley's discovery had already preceded the request. The local citizens were pleased to see their asylum redeemed from the negative assumptions about it.

However, it took several months for everyone to completely recover, including Mr. and Mrs. Rice, the steward and matron. All attendants had been given the opportunity to leave the asylum to reduce their exposure to the disease, but all had stayed and did their duty. Mr. and Mrs. Rice were most symbolic of that dedication. They stayed and survived. Dr. Chipley was proud of all who stayed regardless of the danger to themselves. The attendants viewed Dr. Chipley as their idol.

*   *   *

Lexington was fast becoming a city. A large, three-story brick building, the Odd Fellows Hall, with an opera hall on the second floor, was completed. The building was to have a seating capacity of fifteen hundred people; it could hold important meetings, and the opera hall was to attract famous shows.

The Lexington Gas Company occupied the southeast corner of West Main and Patterson Streets. The manufacture of artificial gas for street illumination was completed by a New York firm, and Lexington was the first city west of the Allegheny Mountains to have illuminated lights. Downtown Lexington was becoming progressive, with a night lighting system and opera house.

In 1857, Elizabeth Chipley received a letter from Elizabeth Allen in Keokuk, Iowa. Elizabeth Allen wrote that her husband, Dr. Allen, had taken the professorship at the Jefferson Medical School for only a short time. The weather did not agree with Dr. Allen, and they moved on to Iowa, where he gained a lucrative practice through friends. Elizabeth Allen added that she was pregnant and hoped that this child would be the son that they wanted. Elizabeth Chipley had wanted to share the letter with her husband, Dr. Chipley, but he was too busy.

In 1858, another letter came from Elizabeth Allen, stating that she did have a son and had named him for his father, John R. Allen. They were still living in Keokuk, and Dr. John R. Allen had been persuaded by his friends to run for state senate, and he was elected. They would be visiting Lexington in the summer of 1859.

Dr. Allen, now a senator from Iowa, visited Lexington with his family in 1859. They arrived on the Kentucky Central Railroad and were met by Judge Buckner.

While Dr. Allen was proud of his achievements as an Iowa senator, he was uncertain about his previous friends and professional associates. He knew that some viewed him as a traitor for departing the asylum so hastily. While he had written to several of those friends and family, he was still unsure of their understanding.

The Buckner family had supported Dr. Allen's decision to move, especially after he later returned to politics and law. Judge Buckner viewed him as a political ally and eagerly awaited seeing his nephew, John Jr., and growing niece. Judge Buckner had assured Dr. Allen that everyone was so busy with the political issues of states' rights and slavery that other resentments were lost. His sudden departure was forgotten since Dr. Chipley had been so successful with the asylum. Dr. Allen was pleased to hear that the asylum was doing so well.

Dr. Allen was a rejuvenated person. His earlier enthusiasm and exuberance that had faded in his last years at the asylum were back. Elizabeth was equally happy and content with her new son, John Jr., and older daughter. After a few successful years in Iowa, they were a happy family returning to Lexington, following their despondent departure. Dr. Allen wanted to mend his broken relationships, while they would notice a significant change in Lexington.

Lexington was more of a divided town as neighbors took sides against each other. The Buckners were for the Union side, while the pro-Southerners had their supporters in the Hunt-Morgan family. Across the street from the Hunt-Morgan home was Dr. Peter's family, who were pro-Union. Cassius Clay was active in the new Republican political party, proposing that it adopt a strong antislavery platform, while his wife's family the Warfields, were pro-slavery.

The Transylvania Medical School was still in the process of closing in 1859. Dr. Robert Peter, dean of the medical school, was a giant in analytical chemistry and had served in that faculty since 1833. He continued to serve in the different universities that Transylvania had merged with. Dr. Peter became part of the history of Lexington and the Transylvania schools.

The Transylvania Medical Building that Dr. Allen had attended was conducting their last session with twenty-three students and six to graduate. Across from the medical school was Dr. B. W. Dudley's home, where Dr. Allen visited. They discussed the earlier days of the Transylvania Medical School and its closing.

Dr. Dudley asked Dr. Allen, "Did Dr. Peter teach you when you were at Transylvania Medical School?"

"Oh, yes, he did. He was an excellent teacher in chemistry. Remember, I was there in the late thirties and early forties. Dr. Peter came in 1833 to Transylvania Medical School. My main interest was not in chemistry, so I was not one of his most outstanding students."

"Well, Dr. Peter has sure fought hard to keep Transylvania Medical School, but now, there is just too much competition from other schools," stated Dr. Dudley. "The school just does not attract new students now."

"I am so sorry; it was such a good school for many years."

"Dr. Peter has calculated with this last session that Transylvania Medical School trained 6,456 students in its long history and sent out 1,881 doctors to mostly southern and western states," stated Dr. Dudley.

"Very impressive," said Dr. Allen. "The school has provided education and medical care to many isolated areas."

"Yes, it did, and I am proud to have been part of it. I made some mistakes, but teaching at Transylvania Medical School was not one of them," stated Dr. Dudley.

"The school served as a real educational beacon in the wilderness of Kentucky," added Dr. Allen.

"Well, I guess Dr. Caldwell was correct in 1837 when he said that Lexington was a 'mere western village, too small, too quiet, for a medical school,' so he left for Louisville. But there are 1,881 doctors who did not think so; not bad for nearly fifty years of existence. Will the Louisville

Medical School last fifty years? I don't expect to know, but this one did. Anyway, sir, why are you not practicing medicine full time?"

"It is just a matter of opportunity. My friends in Iowa wanted me to run for the Iowa Senate. I agreed to serve one term. My interest had been with lunacy care, but I was too frustrated with the Kentucky asylum. I left it because I did not seem to be getting anywhere. It was good for me to leave. I do have a small private practice in Keokuk," contributed Dr. Allen. "I prefer helping individual people rather than the political groups."

"Do you not plan to return to Kentucky, since you still have family here?" asked Dr. Dudley as he leaned back in his chair.

"No, my wife is now resigned to not being in Kentucky. I hear we will be at war soon, and Kentuckians will be divided against each other. I do not wish to see that."

"Yes, it is bad. One of my sons is thinking about moving to Mississippi, where at least everyone is pro-Southern. Here," Dr. Dudley sadly paused and then stated, "old friends will split and Kentucky will be a bad place to be during this time."

"Iowa is not that way; no one wants anything to do with war," added Dr. Allen. "Iowa hopes to stay out of war. I just have trouble seeing old friends split over this issue."

"Well, I'm an old man and don't expect to live through such an experience. However, it makes me sad. As a young man, I was willing to duel over my issues, but as an old man, I see the foolishness of such. But the young men of today are planning to go to war. I had my foolish days, so must the next generation, I guess," Dr. Dudley said sadly.

"As you know, my brother-in-law is a strong Union supporter, and he is ready to go to war. I have trouble with his quick action toward war without regard that such an action will be against Southerners and old friends. So many are on a path to war; all Americans will be hurt. While I really sympathize with the South, I have trouble with war. What about the asylum; is there any political conflict there?"

"Of course, I guess you have heard that your brother-in-law, Judge Buckner, has already left the board because of Richard Pindell's pro-Southern sympathies. Richard Pindell pushed for Captain John H. Morgan to be on the board, causing a great deal of anxiety. Captain John Hunt Morgan is an organizer for the Southern resistance army. Fortunately, James A. Grinstead and Charles S. Bodley have kept their personal preferences out and have remained on the board. Also, Dr. John R. Desha is on the board, trying to stay neutral," completed Dr. Dudley.

"How about Dr. W. S. Chipley's leanings. Is he on any side?"

"He is an interesting person. Dr. Chipley follows 'duty' and does as he feels will be his duty. I do not know his leanings yet, but I would suspect he will lean the way the state of Kentucky goes, since he feels his duty is to the state."

"I understand that he has several sons who will join the Southern cause. Does the Chipley family not realize that they might be fighting each other?" asked Dr. Allen.

"I'm afraid not too many people are considering those possibilities at this time, but Kentucky will feel the conflict worse because of its internal divisions. I just cannot believe it," puzzled Dr. Dudley.

"Are there several Transylvania Medical School graduates who will fight for the Southern cause?" asked Dr. Allen.

"Oh, yes, one is Dr. Luke Blackburn, who lives in Mississippi. My son might join him there. I just hope there will be no war."

"But we have some good memories," stated Dr. Allen as they continued to reminisce. "In 1845, they thought that our medical knowledge should influence the outcome of Dr. Abner Baker's death penalty. They sought all kinds of medical opinions about Dr. Baker's long-established insanity and found lawyers who supported our opinion that he needed to be institutionalized rather than given death. Instead, the governor did as his followers wanted. We believed that we could influence political outcomes with our medical knowledge." They both laughed over their naiveté.

"Yes, I remember our expectations, but we tried. The political forces were against us," added Dr. Dudley. They remembered about the sheriff getting bodies to study at the medical school. "Yes, that sheriff really helped me," added Dr. Dudley. "I think he is dead, now."

"Oh, I am so sorry to hear that; those sheriffs really helped the early settlements, but that one sheriff seemed to care more about the community. It was not just a job to him, it was his community."

"Yes," added Dr. Dudley, "he knew everybody in this town."

"Do you remember the attorney who was very upset over the death of Dr. Baker? He was associated with the Northern Bank," Dr. Allen said.

"Oh, that was M. C. Johnson. He is still around, but not in politics. He is now president of the Northern Bank."

"He was so upset about the Dr. Baker case and the misuse of politics," stated Dr. Allen. "I often wonder about him, he was such a caring person."

Both men continued to talk for a while until Dr. Dudley showed signs of being tired.

"Sir, I have talked to you beyond your endurance, please excuse my rudeness," stated Dr. Allen. "I must let you rest. I will visit you again, if you will allow me such an honor."

"Please do, I did enjoy this conversation. Return anytime. I am an old man, with nothing but the past."

Dr. Allen left the home of Dr. Dudley, looking over at the old Medical Hall and remembering how it was once a grand building.

The next day, Dr. Allen went to visit the Kentucky Lunatic Asylum. He did not wait for an invitation from Dr. Chipley since he was not sure he would get one. He went with his brother-in-law, Judge Buckner, who had recently resigned.

Dr. Allen knew that political ideals were more important to Judge Buckner. He was unhappy with how he saw the country going and wanted to participate at the national level of politics, while Dr. Allen was more interested in personal relationships. For now, they had agreed to visit the asylum. Their carriage turned from Broadway onto Fourth Street, proceeding west. Nice, large, imposing brick homes stood on each side of the street as their carriage wheels sounded against the bricked streets. The street had become very fashionable.

"Who took your place on the board?" Dr. Allen asked.

"Captain John H. Morgan," Judge Buckner said.

Morgan was the grandson of John W. Hunt and son of Henrietta Hunt Morgan, who lived in Hunt's home. He was captain of the Lexington Rifles, which was organized in 1857. The military company drilled every week.

"However," stated Judge Buckner, "they are all pro-Southern."

"Oh."

"These Southern sympathizers are adding to the lawlessness in the town." Judge Buckner showed some agitation by moving and rubbing his arms.

"The city does seem lawless. What happened to the old sheriff that knew everyone in town and knew how to smooth over things?" asked Dr. Allen.

"He was killed last year by William Barker, someone just passing through town. We have a lot of slave traders around town, trading wherever they can, while the anti-slave factions are also around. Each group is looking for trouble," added Judge Buckner. "The Southerners are the worse."

"Why can't the law handle the lawlessness?" asked the bothered Dr. Allen.

"Some of the old law officers are still here, but others just take the law into their own hands. This William Barker who killed the city sheriff was just asked some questions by him. He killed the sheriff while others grabbed Barker and put him into jail. The townspeople were so angry over the sheriff's death that they stormed the jail, dragged Barker from his cell, and hanged him from a large beam out the second-story window. Mr. Barker hung there for several hours in the hot July sun and was finally removed," explained Judge Buckner. He continued with the story, "Although Mr. Barker had killed a beloved citizen of the city, he did not have any trial. Such lawlessness ruled angry citizens who were already upset over the sheriff's killing. Such lawlessness cannot continue," stated the shaking and fidgety Judge Buckner. Such emotions were rarely expressed by him.

"It sure sounds awful," thoughtfully added Dr. Allen.

"Last year, Captain Ben C. Blimcoe was murdered at his front door by Alexander Warren from Madison County. The sheriff and Lexington Rifles prevented further mob action. Even Dr. E. L. Dudley, formerly of the Transylvania Medical School faculty, is organizing a Home Union Guard to protect the city. Yes, things are bad," stated Judge Buckner.

They continued talking as their carriage entered the grounds of the asylum. They stopped in front of the original building, which stood tall among the trees facing Fourth Street. The entrance road had been paved with bricks, while a new cast-iron fountain consisting of a statue of a female on a dolphin stood at the front of the building. They got out of the carriage.

Dr. Allen walked toward the fountain, looking amazed, and asked, "Sir, what is this?"

"That is the fountain that David Sayre presented to the asylum. It is rather nice, isn't it?" Judge Buckner approached the fountain.

"David Sayre had opened a school for girls called the Sayre Female Institute. He first established the school in 1855 on the northeast corner of Mill and Church Streets and moved it two years later to the mansion of Edward P. Johnson on North Limestone, opposite Second Street. Johnson had the first statewide carriage service before the trains. Johnson moved on to another city, and his mansion is up for sale."

"So David Sayre donated a fountain to the asylum. The water must be difficult to jet out," Dr. Allen said.

"The water comes from a rain-holding container within one of the buildings. The fountain is beautiful but the water supply is sparse at times. It is often a source of drinking water for the inmates who wander the grounds," added Judge Buckner. "As you can see, the grounds have been beautified, with a flower garden on the left." The flowers were in bloom and the aroma added peacefulness to the whole area.

"I see the kitchen is still on the right side," Dr. Allen said as he looked around.

"Yes, but the kitchen is connected with underground tunnels to the main building," answered Judge Buckner as both men stood looking around.

"I have heard that Dr. Chipley completed the steam heating apparatus so that there is steam in each area for warmth and heated water. He also found the impure water that contaminated the facility for years, and the facility has a new artisan well; is that all correct?" asked Dr. Allen.

"Yes, Dr. Chipley has done well with the facility. It is one of the best equipped facilities in the nation," added Judge Buckner. "It is a proud facility, and I may return to serve on the board sometime later."

They walked toward the original building and knocked on the front door of the asylum. The steward, Mr. Rice, opened the door and greeted them. Rice announced that Dr. E. L. Dudley was waiting to see Judge Buckner in the next room, while Dr. Allen was left to look around.

William and Jane Rice were hired by Dr. Allen in 1845 as steward and matron, so they were most happy to see him and demonstrated a pride in the asylum. They had heard that Dr. Allen was in town and wondered why Dr. Chipley had not invited him to the facility. They happily announced Dr. Allen's presence to Dr. Chipley, who had just returned from his early morning rounds. Dr. Chipley was still as neatly dressed as ever and did not show any aging.

"Sir, pleased to see you," Dr. Chipley said, noticing that Dr. Allen was much more relaxed than when he previously knew him.

"Yes, so am I. May I have some time with you? I would like to renew our past association," Dr. Allen said.

"Yes, however, I have no time today. I'm sure Mr. Rice can show you around and answer any questions you might have," stated Dr. Chipley as he left their presence.

Rice was disappointed in Dr. Chipley's response. He had assumed that Dr. Allen would be welcomed anytime. Rice quickly offered to show Dr. Allen around.

Dr. Allen, aware that he might face further rebuff, turned to Rice and said, "Sir, I would most like to know about some of the residents, such as Sarah Norton. She was admitted here when I was superintendent. Is she still here?"

"Yes, she is. She is doing well. When we had the epidemic in '56, all employees and several patients were sick on her ward. Dr. Chipley hired extra nurses to attend to the wards, but Sarah Norton knew what to do. She has been here so long that she is a real asset to the facility. She works hard here and enjoys it."

"I remember when she was admitted, she was poorly fed, dirty, and unable to care for herself. She never had anyone to care for her until she came here, then she found the care that she needed. I'm glad to hear of her doing so well," responded Dr. Allen.

"You remember Theodore Clay?" asked Rice.

"Yes, he was one of our best-known patients. I remember him telling me one day that this was one of the best boarding houses around, 'but it sure had some fools for residents,'" laughed Dr. Allen. "He was a real character."

"Yes, he has been, but this year, his condition has grown worse."

"Oh, I am so sorry," Dr. Allen stated sadly.

"Theodore Clay is now demented and a hopeless idiot, no longer the lunatic who entertained students with his claims of presidential powers and quickness of speech," stated Rice. "It is sad."

"Doesn't anyone from the Clay family visit him?"

"His brother, John M. Clay, visits some. As you know, Henry Clay is dead. His wife lives at their home, Ashland, with John. The family continues to be generous with the asylum; a relative, J. B. Clay donates a full-blooded calf each year, adding to our stock," Rice said proudly.

"I noticed that the train runs by the northern part and you seem to have more cultivated farm; does this mean that there is more land?"

"Yes, the farm is growing in size, and many of our inmates occupy themselves with work on the farm. Actually, those who work tend to be less subject to illnesses," added Rice. "The train does not cause much difficulty; most of our lunatics look forward to seeing it. I assume you have noticed the new furniture that is in the facility?"

"Yes, I did notice. Dr. Chipley has succeeded in gaining more financial support from the legislature?"

"Yes, he has. Dr. Chipley has really helped this facility. He discovered the cause of our high death rates and had artesian wells dug. He had the main sewer beneath the basement floor removed and replaced with large cast-iron pipes."

"That is great; so the basement gives you more rooms?" Dr. Allen was renewing his old excitement as he was able to witness some of the improvements.

"Some, but we have 228 inmates and have room for only 200; there are plans to build more buildings; however, if the war comes, I'm not sure when the new buildings will be built," added Rice.

"Do you think there will be war?" asked Dr. Allen.

"Yes, I am afraid so. I have two sons who have already gone south to be ready to join the forces when needed," Rice said quietly.

"What about Kentucky?"

"Kentucky is divided. My wife and I will stay and support the South from our positions," added Rice.

"I'm not sure you should be telling me that, since I understand Judge Buckner and Dr. E. L. Dudley are very much pro-Union. They were both on the board at one time and might see that you get fired over such statements," added Dr. Allen.

"Sir, I trust you. While you live in Iowa now, I know from your previous actions here you are pro-Southern. I would only tell you of my Southern preference since there are too many pro-Southerners around. Do you plan to return south if war breaks out?" asked Rice.

"I do not know yet. Iowa is so different. Many Iowans have moved away from the conflicting states and do not wish to be bothered with such talk of war," added Dr. Allen.

"But you are in the Iowa legislature; you might have to support the Union cause. Iowa cannot stay out of the conflict forever," stated Rice.

"I know that, and I will have to make a decision. At this point, I will wait and pray that war never comes," stated Dr. Allen. "May I see more of the grounds?"

Both men walked around the grounds of the asylum as Dr. Allen asked questions. "There is a new house on this side of the asylum grounds?

"Oh, that is the new superintendent's house."

"When was it built?" asked Dr. Allen.

"Last year, but Dr. Chipley has not moved there yet."

"Oh? Why hasn't he moved there?"

"As you know, he has been residing in his family home in Lexington, but a home was built on the asylum grounds for his comfort during war time. He will be expected to live on the grounds if there is a war," added Rice.

"So, even the state of Kentucky is planning for war! All other employees will live on the grounds, isn't that true?"

"Yes, we all will live in the basement or in rooms on specific wards while we are working. My wife and I also own a farm in the next county, which I leave in the hands of a sharecropper. We visit the residence on our days off; most of our possessions are at our residence, but we live at the asylum while working. If war comes, we might consider moving some of our possessions to the asylum. No one expects the asylum to be invaded," added Rice. "Asylums are usually protected during war."

They reached the original building again and returned to Rice's office on the northwest side. They both rested in new chairs. The old furniture had been replaced by additional state funds, and Rice was proud of them.

"Sir," nodded Dr. Allen, "I have really enjoyed seeing you again. I remember you being so helpful to me when I was here. I was so busy then, I never really had time to know my employees such as you." He continued to admire the furniture.

"You hired my wife and me," Rice said. "You were always fair with us. I will always appreciate the respect that you showed to us during your time."

Rice was expecting to see Dr. Chipley in the hallway as Dr. Allen had asked to see him.

Rice continued talking, "It was true, we were so busy previously there was just little time to know each other. But we had a mutual respect for each other and our work."

"Yes, I was so busy trying to solve all the problems that I faced, that I was not really someone to know," added Dr. Allen. "I just hope Dr. Chipley can understand why I left so much in a hurry; my own sanity was at stake. I had to leave."

"Dr. Chipley is a stickler for duty, and I'm sure he disapproved of what he saw as a neglect of duty by you. While Dr. Chipley is good in the position as superintendent, he is unchanging in what he considers as one's duty. However, many of us will be facing what we consider to be a duty with the coming war, and no one knows the outcome, which is scary," added Rice.

"Yes, I can imagine that," replied Dr. Allen.

"Remember, you did a lot of good for this asylum during your time.

You changed the workers from the morbid title of keeper to a quality standard of attendant."

"Well, I tried."

"You established rules and regulations for all who worked here. You provided a solid basis for the growth and development of this institution, so don't ignore that important part," stated Rice.

"Yes, you are correct. While Iowa does not yet have a state asylum, there is a growing awareness of that need, and I see so much to be done there," added Dr. Allen.

"And good workers are the key to good care."

"Yes, I certainly agree to that," nodded Dr. Allen.

"However, I shall like to keep in touch with you; may we write each other?"

"Yes, I shall be happy to keep in contact with you. I hope you and your family will survive the coming war," Dr. Allen said as he stood to shake hands.

Rice escorted him out of his office when they ran into Dr. T. P. Dudley, who was observing the dining room across from Dr. Chipley's office.

Rice introduced Dr. Allen to Dr. Dudley and then excused himself. Rice had some additional duties to complete and could not understand why Dr. Chipley had not returned.

"Sir, I understand you are the assistant physician?" asked Dr. Allen.

"Yes, sir, and you are Dr. Allen, the first superintendent here. May I help you?"

"I understand you are doing a wonderful job here, I hope you can continue in the service of this asylum." Dr. Allen was aware that he was stalling for time until Dr. Chipley would return.

"I will always serve under Dr. Chipley. He has done wonders for this asylum, and I will continue to do my duty here." Dr. Dudley stoutly stood.

Judge Buckner and Dr. E. L. Dudley entered from another room into the hallway. Judge Buckner introduced Dr. Allen to Dr. E. L. Dudley.

Both recognized each other as having been professors at the Transylvania Medical School. They exchanged conversations about students whom they both had taught. Then Dr. Chipley entered the hallway and asked Dr. Allen to follow him into his office. Dr. Allen excused himself.

Dr. Allen entered Dr. Chipley's office, the same office he had as superintendent. Dr. Chipley offered him a seat as Dr. Allen noticed the new furniture and draperies.

"I must ask you to pardon me for not seeing you earlier; I had other duties and had not planned on a visitor. I hope Mr. Rice was able to answer all your questions?"

"Yes, he did very admirably." Dr. Allen looked around. "I like your new furniture."

"Your brother-in-law insisted that I was rude to you, and for that, I am sorry; there is really no excuse for my rudeness," continued Dr. Chipley. "Your visit was unexpected, and I admire your spirit."

"Sir, my brother-in-law is a much more politically correct person than I. Although I have had my share of politics, I do not demand any indulgence. I understand your devotion to duty and admire your ability to stay devoted to duty as you have here at this institution, while I did not have that same endurance," stated Dr. Allen.

"Well, huh, huh, thank you, I didn't expect such a compliment. I did think that your departure was too soon for the good of the institution," stated Dr. Chipley.

"See, the longer I stayed after continuing to fail, the longer it would have taken for you to discover the solution to this facility's death rate. I am grateful to you for accepting that duty," added Dr. Allen.

"I really haven't seen it that way," stuttered Dr. Chipley with surprise. "You left so quickly."

"I'm for the best of this institution. I devoted ten years of my life, put sweat and energy into it, but at the end, I was unable to find an answer to the continuing high death rate. I had difficulty getting money from the governor, I had difficulty with purchasing a heating system, and the demise of Transylvania Medical School was just a final blow to me. Then I had personal losses with my children, and it was all too much at the time."

"Well, you did cast off your duty to this institution quickly."

"Yes, I did," Dr. Allen said as he stopped to take a breath, and then he continued, "But really, Dr. Chipley, I had lost my effectiveness. I had to let go, which was the only thing I knew to do. Now, I realize someone else had to find the solutions that I could not find. You did that, and I am grateful." Dr. Allen smiled.

"Well, I was angry at you for leaving."

"It has taken me a while to realize that I was not the person to help the asylum to reach the level you have achieved," Dr. Allen said.

"I never thought of it that way," stated Dr. Chipley.

"Dr. Chipley, as your father often preached, there is a time and place for everything, according to the Bible, and I believe that. It was not the time for me to make great changes, but it was time for you to do that. And I am grateful to have seen you again." Dr. Allen sat back confidently in the chair.

"Well, we did see each other as professors at Transylvania Medical School, but I never really knew you," added Dr. Chipley.

"I really did not understand myself, when I was here. I was so busy proving myself and was never able to resolve some of the basic problems of the asylum, such as the high death rate. Yet you did. Today, everything came more into focus as I visited this asylum. I wish to thank you for our conversation."

"Yes, I have enjoyed it. We must write to each other since we share a long history," stated Dr. Chipley. Then he added, "I understand you have a son?"

"Yes, I would like to bring him here to see the asylum when he is older and can understand what this place meant to me. He is too young to understand now, but we will be returning to visit relatives, and I will bring him to the asylum when he is old enough to understand." Dr. Allen looked around the office.

"I wish my sons were still too young and not planning to leave for war. I'm afraid that they are old enough to decide issues for themselves. They have often visited Georgia; they will fight for Georgia and the Southern cause."

"And you?" asked Dr. Allen. "Will you support the South?"

"As superintendent of a Kentucky state facility, I will see that the asylum follows the side that Kentucky follows."

"So you might be on opposite sides from your sons?"

"Yes, it might come down to that; I am sorry but I have a duty to this state-supported facility. So I have no choice but to go as Kentucky goes. I only hope Kentucky follows the South in this conflict, as my sons have already chosen."

"Such will be typical of many families. I hope you and your family the best, for all of you." Dr. Allen started to excuse himself.

Dr. Chipley rose from his chair and stated, "I understand my wife has been writing to yours over the past few years and expects to call upon your wife about a visit to our home. Will you and your wife visit one afternoon so we both can talk more?" Dr. Chipley was feeling much more comfortable with Dr. Allen.

Dr. Allen stood up; he was surprised that he felt so good about Dr. Chipley and stated, "Yes, I shall wait for your invitation. I must leave now to go back to the county to check on my family. My wife was visiting her parents' farm with our son."

"Where are you staying in Lexington?"

"We are staying in town at the Phoenix Hotel on the southeast corner of Main and Mulberry Streets. We have two comfortable rooms there. You may contact us there."

"My wife and I will find a time we can invite you, sir." Dr. Chipley stood up with Dr. Allen.

"Yes, thank you for a most satisfying visit." Dr. Allen left the room. He looked around inside the building where he had spent so many hours for ten years. He left the original building and found his brother-in-law waiting out front at the water fountain.

Judge Buckner asked Dr. Allen if he was ready to return to the family farm. Dr. Allen nodded his head, and they left the grounds.

Dr. Allen and his wife did visit the Chipleys several times. The Chipleys enjoyed seeing Dr. Allen's daughter and son, John Jr. They made plans to stay in touch.

Dr. Allen and his family needed to return to Iowa before winter set in. While the Allens had renewed old friendships and proudly displayed their children, two-year-old John and an older daughter, they planned to return more often since travel was easier by train. They were able to ride the train all the way to Keokuk.

Their train pulled out of Lexington on the Kentucky Central Railroad and passed by the asylum; Dr. Allen could only reflect upon his experiences of the last few weeks. Both he and Dr. Chipley had come to realize how much they had in common, while their wives spent time together. Both Drs. Allen and Chipley talked about patients in their various stages of improvement. The loving care demonstrated in each case was what the asylum was known for, and Dr. Allen was proud to have been a part of it. He missed that in Keokuk as a senator.

*   *   *

Early in April 1861, excited groups of citizens gathered on Cheapside, on Jordan's Row, in hotel lobbies and in the old courthouse to discuss the attack on Fort Sumter. Outside the telegraph office at Mill and Short Streets, anxious individuals were awaiting the outcome. Some rejoiced at the fall of Fort Sumter, while others received the news with regret. Nowhere were the sentiments more mixed than in Lexington, Kentucky.

Henry T. Duncan II, a Harvard University graduate, returned to Lexington to serve as a member of the Union Army. He was born in one of the most pretentious county estates, Duncannon, on the Old Buffalo Trail nearer Paris, Kentucky. He married the granddaughter of John Brand, Lillie Brand. It was a fine wedding of two old families from the Bluegrass area. Lillie was born in Elmwood, a house on Fourth Street and Walnut. Elmwood was built by her father, William Brand. Their wedding took place at her grandfather's home, Rosehill, on Fifth and Mulberry Streets.

Others were ready to join the Southern side, such as Captain John Hunt Morgan, who served on the board from 1860 until the war started. After Captain Morgan left, Dr. Letcher resumed as a board member of the asylum.

Richard Pindell had strong Southern ties that put him against other members on the board. He served as chairman on the Board of Commissioners until 1862; his tenure as chairman was eighteen years, only two years fewer than Chairman Hunt. Pindell continued to serve as a board member in poor health for eight more years until his death.

In 1862, David Sayer became the third chairman of the Board of Commissioners, while Cassius Clay and M. C. Johnson were appointed as board members. Clay served only one year, since he did not remain in Lexington due to the war. Johnson continued to serve as a board member for many years.

After Lincoln's inauguration, Cassius Clay expected to be appointed secretary of war, but Lincoln was committed to Simon Cameron. Instead, Clay accepted an appointment as minister to Russia. Before leaving for Russia, he had two assignments to complete, one for President Lincoln and the other personal.

His first duty was to visit Kentucky and see if Kentuckians would support a program of emancipation. He reported back to Lincoln that there was a loyal element in Kentucky that supported emancipation.

The second duty was to make arrangements to send his family and children, except for his son Green, who had volunteered as a Union soldier, on to Philadelphia. His relations with Mary Jane and her Warfield family were even more strained. His wife, Mary Jane, refused to leave Lexington. Clay's participation in Lincoln's official Emancipation Proclamation was his life's aspiration. He was disappointed to realize that his wife did not share his dream.

Union troops occupied Lexington and had minor clashes with Confederate sympathizers. They maintained order and control without much difficulty. Later in the fall of 1862, the Confederates under Kirby Smith moved into Lexington.

Dr. Chipley, as superintendent, wrote his yearly report on October 1, 1862. This is his description of that time at the Kentucky Lunatic Asylum:

Gentlemen: I am called upon to make the thirty-eighth annual report of this institution under peculiar circumstances. We are surrounded by the forces of the so-called Confederate Government ... claims to exercise the functions of the Executive of the State of Kentucky; the stars and bars, the emblem of disorganization and anarchy, have replaced the stars and stripes." ... On the second day of last month the forces under the command of Kirby Smith, entered this city, and placed it under the despotic sway of military rule. I allude to this fact because it was well calculated to affect the material interests of this Institution, and, if the occupation is to be permanent, we may not hope to escape the blasted fortunes of other similar institutions within the limits of the Confederacy, whose inmates have been driven from their comfortable abodes to suffer and to perish as those of their unfortunate class did before. ... The history of the unjustified and wicked rebellion which now curses our county warrants us in saying that the rebel forces act as if they considered it to be their special mission to ravage the county they traverse, to plunder its citizens, and to destroy all the evidences of civilization, and prosperity that may happen to fall in their way. Instructed by the history of these lawless forces, I endeavored, as far as possible to shield this Institution from these terrible results. ... As soon as I learned that the Federal forces had fallen back and left the country open to the depredations of the enemy, I directed the steward to purchase a supply of groceries, flour, clothing, shoes, etc., sufficient to cover the time beyond which I do not believe it possible for the invaders to hold this position. It was well we did so, although to accomplish the purpose, we were compelled to pay an advance on former prices. ... Our farmers were being plundered of their slaves, cattle, horses, and grain; our merchants compelled to open their doors at the point of the bayonet, and all are forced to adopt the absurd notion that Confederate script is money, and to receive it without question as to its value. The cost of articles of prime necessity has already advanced to famine prices. But for the provision made to supply the wants of the asylum, in anticipation of the arrival of the enemy, our expenses would have been enormously increased. ... Up to the present period no material direct assault has been made on the Institution. How long we are to be exempt, the future alone can tell. At this moment we are threatened with a rigid enforcement of the Southern conscript law, and if time permits this gross outrage, we may be deprived of the services of some of our most efficient and faithful employees.

In the midst of a struggle for national existence, it is believed to be eminently proper to exclude disloyalty from the public institutions of a loyal State. While we still regarded the ability and faithfulness of our employees, it is also important to know that they are not traitors. Hence, all the Officers and male employees in this Institution are required to take and subscribe the oath of allegiance to the Government of the United States, pledging to discountenance secession, and to give no aid or comfort to the so-called Confederate Government.

Mr. and Mrs. Rice, steward and matron at the asylum, refused to take the oath of allegiance and resigned. They had been employed since 1844.

In late fall of 1862, Dr. Robert Peter, previous professor at the Transylvania Medical School, received an appointment as acting-assistant surgeon in the US General Hospital in Lexington. That same time, thousands of wounded Union soldiers started pouring into Lexington from the bloody fields of Perryville. Since the second Medical School Hall was empty and used by the city of Lexington, the authorities gave Dr. Peter permission to use that hall for a hospital. The trustees of Transylvania surrendered all their buildings to the Union Army without opposition, as Union soldiers were everywhere by winter of 1862.

The John W. Hunt-Morgan family lived at Hopemount and all were pro-Southern. Even Aunt Betty, the old colored nurse from New Orleans who had raised all the Morgan boys, would hear about Southern troops on their way to Lexington. She would often fill the family silver pitcher with ice water and stand for hours on Main Street, waiting for one of her boys to visit.

John Hunt Morgan had entered the conflict as captain of the Kentucky Volunteers in the division of General Simon Bolivar Buckner. He was promoted to command a regiment of cavalry under Braxton Bragg, and later, as brigadier general, as he conducted famous raids in Kentucky, Ohio, and Indiana. The family kept silent about his activities but rejoiced in any of his Southern victories. They refused to speak to their pro-Union neighbors.

*   *   *

On the morning of May 22, 1863, the second Medical Hall was destroyed by fire. Flames destroyed the medical library and training apparatus that had not been removed when the Union Army converted the hall into a hospital. The structure had been filled with sick and wounded soldiers who were evacuated safely.

The destruction of this second Medical Hall seemed but another somber stroke in the death-knell of the once proud Transylvania Medical School. The first Medical Hall located at Church and Market Streets still remained. This first thirty-year-old Medical Hall had been purchased by the Hill Street Methodist Church in 1857 and it continued during the Civil War as Morris Chapel.

On September 4, 1864, Captain John W. Morgan was killed; his death was a heavy blow to the Confederacy and his family. Two of the boys, John and Tom Morgan, never came back, while four other grandsons of John W. Hunt lived to carry Aunt Betty's casket to the family plot years later.

General Lee's surrender at Appomattox Courthouse in Virginia was received in Lexington on April 9, 1865. Demonstrations followed far into the night with fireworks and gunfire. It was a day of rejoicing for many but of overwhelming sorrow for the friends of the South, who remained off the streets and in their homes. The Hunt-Morgan family stayed in their home, Hopemount, on Mill and Second Streets, while Dr. Peter's Union family rejoiced one block over on Second Street.

During the Civil War, Dr. Allen had moved his family to Memphis, Tennessee. He had served one term as senator from Iowa but became discontented. As a physician, he felt his skills were not being used. Elizabeth understood his need and accepted another move. His son, John Jr., was still a child but he respected his father's dedication as a physician.

Memphis had been occupied by Union forces as the Confederate naval forces were defeated in the Battle of Memphis. Memphis was designated by U. S. Grant to serve as the hospital and supply base in the attack on Vicksburg. Dr. Allen saw the hospital as an opportunity to serve as a physician, and he viewed Memphis with the potential of a growing town.

The Transylvania Law Department was very influential in Kentucky during the Civil War. Of the six governors of Kentucky from 1851 through 1867, all had studied at the Transylvania Law School, and three had graduated from there (Harrison. 1985).

*   *   *

After the war, the Memphis and Charleston Railroad linked the Atlantic Ocean with the Mississippi River traffic and made travel to Kentucky even easier. Dr. Allen stayed in touch with his family and friends in Lexington. Judge Buckner, his brother-in-law, continued to practice law at the Northern Bank Building on Short Street.

One of the letters from Dr. Chipley in 1867 glowingly described the appropriations that the State of Kentucky had set for the institution with the erection of a new modern three-story building. The capacity of that institution was to change from 250 to 500, expecting to accommodate all the Kentucky lunatics.

Dr. Chipley was so pleased with the changes occurring within the institution that he invited Dr. Allen to come see them when he visited Lexington. Dr. Allen was excited to be returning to Lexington.

In July of 1868, Dr. Allen and his family left on the train from Memphis to Lexington. They left Memphis around 7 a.m. and arrived in Louisville at 4:00 a.m. the next day on the Memphis and Louisville Railway. Then they caught the Louisville, Cincinnati, and Lexington Railroad, leaving at 6:00 a.m. out of Louisville, and arrived in Lexington five hours later. The Louisville, Cincinnati, and Lexington (later the L & N) Railroad used the three-story brick station of the Lexington & Ohio Railroad at the corner of Mill and Vine Streets. The old Kentucky Central Railroad tracks next to the asylum were still used by all trains.

The Allen family was thrilled over the improved railroads as they continued on with the last part of the train trip into Lexington. Dr. Allen read the *1868 Travelers Official Railway Guide* and noticed that it listed William A. Dudley of Lexington as president of the Louisville, Cincinnati, and Lexington Railroad. Dr. Allen excitedly stated to his son, "I knew Mr. William A. Dudley when he was in law school; he has done well for himself. His father, Dr. B. W. Dudley, is my friend."

Ten-year-old John Jr. responded but did not appear to understand the meaning from his father. He was more interested in seeing the passing landscapes, the horses, and the rock fences.

Dr. Allen continued, "William A. Dudley's father was my professor in the Transylvania Medical School. You will get to meet Dr. B. W. Dudley. See, son, Lexington has so many interesting people."

His son just answered, "Yes, sir."

Elizabeth Allen looked up from her handwork and said, "Dear! John Jr. doesn't understand the meaning those people have for you. He is too young."

"Oh, but he will. I want him to understand my interest in Lexington and even the asylum. I can hardly wait."

"We will be there soon," Elizabeth said as she looked at her watch. "Richard will be meeting us at the train station."

"John Jr., do you remember Uncle Richard Buckner?" asked Dr. Allen. "He has visited us several times."

"Yes, sir, I do. He bought me many books that I have read."

"Yes, he did." Dr. Allen smiled at his son as they prepared to arrive in Lexington. "You will learn to like Lexington as your mother and I do."

Several days later, Dr. Allen and his son went to visit the asylum upon the invitation of Dr. Chipley. Their carriage entered on Fourth Street, but the entrance was entirely different. There was a two-story entrance gate with one large room on each side. The doors opened upon request by an employee. A wooden fence now surrounded the Fourth Street part of the asylum.

Upon entering through the gate, Dr. Allen recognized the original building on the right, but on the left was a much larger building, three and four stories high. A middle entrance into the new building was four stories high with an impressive front. Dr. Allen stopped his carriage and gazed upon the site. Then he continued his carriage toward the original building.

Dr. Allen latched his carriage to the old post in front of the original building and led his son into the older building. Dr. Chipley's office was still in the same location, and Dr. Chipley recognized Dr. Allen as they came into the building.

"I am so pleased to see you, Dr. Allen, and this must be your young son?" Dr. Chipley said.

"Yes, and I am so captivated by the new building. We must see it."

"Yes, I will be happy to show it to you; however, now I have an emergency case, someone is sick on Ward 10. I shall ask my assistant, Dr. T. P. Dudley, to show you around. Then, he will bring you back here, and I shall be free to discuss what you saw. I hope you will not mind?"

"No, I know you are busy, and there are always unexpected emergencies." Dr. Allen continued to look around the original building for familiar parts. "We will be in Lexington for several weeks, and there will be plenty of opportunities for us to talk."

"This emergency is really something that cannot be left to my assistant; he will be most happy to show you around. His office is in the new building." The matron, Mrs. L. H. Vincent, showed them to his office.

They found Dr. Dudley in a beautiful new office as he greeted them and proceeded to tell them about the facility. His office was on the first floor of the new three-story building built after the Civil War. Dr. Dudley explained, "This institution is one of the most outstanding in the nation. We are leaders in the care of lunatics, and Dr. Chipley has achieved much national recognition."

"Yes, I understand that." Dr. Allen looked around as they walked throughout the new building. Dr. Dudley's loyalty to Dr. Chipley was commendable but a little much in Dr. Allen's thinking.

"Dr. Chipley has just returned from the Association of Hospital Superintendents in Boston, where he gained the most current information on caring for lunatics in this facility." Dr. Dudley continued to show the different parts of the new building. Everything was neat and clean.

"What are these back buildings?" asked Dr. Allen, pointing to octagonal-shaped buildings in the back.

"Those are the most current water closets. They are attached to the back porches; unpleasant odors do not enter the ward." Dr. Dudley walked over to the front of one such structure. "As you can see, rainwater is collected from a container in the roof and enters the octagonal building to clean the inside. It is most efficient and keeps the smell away from inside the apartments."

"Does that rainwater container provide water for other parts of the building?" asked Dr. Allen as he observed his son's reaction to passing lunatics. John was puzzled by the strange people but had enough manners not to say anything.

"Oh, yes, there is running water throughout the building."

"Oh, how interesting, the whole facility is beyond my wildest dreams," stated Dr. Allen as he held his son closer to him.

"The whole institution consists of three departments. This building is occupied by the white female patients and their attendants. The original building is for the white male patients and their attendants. A detached building near the railroad is the department for the Negro patients," added Dr. Dudley.

"So you have capacity for five hundred, I understand."

"Yes, we have two pleasure grounds, male and female with seats, flower gardens, and swings. From the annual income from the Megowan fund invested in a building in the city, we can provide for any diversion needed to relieve the tedium of hospital life."

Dr. Dudley was obviously proud of this institution and his association with Dr. Chipley. Dr. Allen enjoyed seeing the new buildings and the modern system of water closets. The smell was noticeably less on the wards.

The Allen family visited regularly at the home of Dr. Chipley. Dr. Chipley admitted to Dr. Allen that these last two years had been the most satisfying for him. "The State of Kentucky has finally recognized the importance of the asylum, and they are now providing financial support for it, as it should have in past years. I am beginning to see a real change in attitude toward insanity. This is what both of us have worked for when no one else cared." Dr. Chipley sat in his home chair.

Dr. Allen had never seen Dr. Chipley more relaxed and pleased. "Remember, John W. Hunt worked for this also. He worked under similar conditions as we," added Dr. Allen. "The time has come that insanity care is accepted, while in the past, we labored when it was unpopular."

"Can you believe that the Kentucky legislature is willing to build a whole different facility for the idiot cases?" asked Dr. Chipley. "A whole institution for the idiots from the lunatics is the more progressive way to go, and Kentucky is doing that."

"Well, I understand that you have had a lot to do with pushing for that and explaining the need for such a facility to the legislature," said Dr. Allen.

"I did petition for such a facility. It will be located in Frankfort, and all our idiot cases will be moved to that one place. The legislature is now willing to accept that our asylum is not for all unfortunate cases, but just for the insane."

"That sounds great. Iowa was planning a similar facility for their idiots when I left. They will be separated from the lunatic asylum, which opened in 1861," added Dr. Allen.

"It is really an exciting time in the care for the insane." Dr. Chipley looked out the window of his home. He could view some lunatics on the grounds as he was still living in the superintendent's home.

Both continued to sit and discuss the institution in the superintendent's house as the wives sat on the lawn, observing the lunatics roaming around. The grounds were beautifully cultivated around flower gardens. A full-time gardener was employed to cultivate the gardens and supervise the patient help.

The next day, Dr. Allen went to visit Dr. B. W. Dudley, who was now living with his son William. This successful son had bought the twenty-room Bodley House on Second and Market Streets, which had been built in 1812 by General Thomas Bodley, whose heirs sold it. During the Civil War when Lexington was occupied by Union troops, the house was used as federal headquarters. An American flag had been painted on the floor of the living room. It now provided plenty of room for Dudley's family and for the aging Dr. Dudley, who had sold his estate at the end of north Broadway.

Dr. Dudley was pleased to invite Dr. Allen into his son's home. Dr. Allen observed that the home had been furnished with the finest furniture and well matched with silk draperies and rugs.

"Please join me on this couch," Dr. Dudley said. "How was your trip?"

"Wonderful, we came to Louisville on the railroad, which is a great way to travel from Memphis. My family was most comfortable. When we lived in Iowa, the railroads were slower and more difficult. And how have you been?" asked Dr. Allen.

"Oh, as well as can be expected. As you can see, I have given up my own home. Good workers are hard to find, so I sold it. Of course, you heard that the medical school near my home burned during the war?"

"Yes, I had observed the empty lot the other day, and my brother-in-law told me what happened. Was that the final end of Transylvania Medical School?" asked Dr. Allen.

"Yes, I'm afraid so. Have you visited the asylum?"

"Yes, I did. The asylum is growing under Dr. Chipley's leadership. There are new buildings everywhere."

"Dr. Chipley has really been a leader in the care of lunatics. He has traveled extensively and educated the Kentucky legislature about the needs of the institution. I hope it continues," stated Dr. Dudley.

"Well, I see no problem. The institution has suffered from a lack of financial support by the legislature for years, and now that support has come. Dr. Chipley is the first one to fulfill the needs of the institution as we had wanted to do for years," Dr. Allen said enthusiastically. He kept eyeing the comfortable couch that they were sitting on. He had never seen one so elegant.

"Yes," responded Dr. Dudley, "the legislature has finally supported the first asylum adequately. If the legislature had supported the Transylvania Medical School instead of the one in Louisville, it would still be here. Unfortunately, the Kentucky legislature decided that Lexington could not provide an adequate medical school even though there were fifty years of proof. They supported the one in Louisville. The people of Lexington were dammed!" This elderly man showed some of his earlier spark that Dr. Allen had often witnessed.

"Yes, I know, since I was in both the Kentucky and Iowa legislatures. I always saw my job as doing what was best for the people, but some legislators put their power ahead of the people. So I'm back working as a physician; I'm much happier," commented Dr. Allen.

"You were always a people person, not one to seek power for your own purpose. You gave of yourself and have always done your best. Are you satisfied with living in Memphis?"

"Yes, my family and I are happy there. It has both Northern and Southern sympathy like Kentucky, and since my daughter is married, we will probably continue to live in Memphis. She married an attorney, and we hope to remain in that city."

"What about your son; how is he doing?"

"My son will probably attend a military academy soon. I enjoy my work and patients. What else can one ask for?" Dr. Allen asked.

"My other son, Dr. Charles Dudley, still lives in Mississippi. I miss him even though I am fortunate to still have William."

"Yes, I remember he went there before the war to support the Southern side."

"Well, he supported the Southern cause and has stayed there. He was a close friend of Dr. Luke Blackburn, who also practiced in Natchez, Mississippi. Dr. Blackburn graduated from Transylvania Medical School in 1835, and they were good friends. They both supported the Southern side. Dr. Blackburn was tried by the US military for his war efforts, but he escaped to Canada."

"Why was he tried?" asked Dr. Allen.

"It seems that Dr. Blackburn was accused of trying to send smallpox into the Northern troops. My son is still so bitter about what happened to Dr. Blackburn; he refuses to forgive and forget. Especially toward those of us who live in Kentucky—he is unforgiving toward us, his family."

"Oh, I'm so sorry over your loss of him," added Dr. Allen.

"Well, I had lost him long ago when Lexington was so divided and he left. He needed a mother and never had one."

"Your sons missed a lot," added Dr. Allen.

"I was not much of a father then, because I was always teaching. But he is still alive. He is just not willing to be a part of our family. However, there are families who have no hope of reconciling because of death. I still have some hope."

Dr. Allen saw the sadness in Dr. Dudley. He could only listen. They spent many hours together over the following few weeks.

Dr. Allen and his family returned to Memphis. This trip had been most satisfying since they saw some rebuilding of the city. Previously, there had been more discord. While the majority had reconciled with their friends and neighbors, a few families still appeared to hold onto their prewar beliefs.

The next year, Dr. Chipley was pleased with the effectiveness of his Asylum and with the Board of Commissioners. It was growing with 430 patients; they had capacity for 500. The asylum grounds were divided into the farm, buildings, and flower gardens.

*   *   *

On May 14, 1869, P. P. Johnson, an attorney for persons whose names were not given to the board, presented documents and affidavits in relation to the past management of the asylum. Upon examination by the board members, they decided to investigate the matter and requested the names of the accusers. On May 17, Johnson refused to disclose the names. Dr. Chipley, the superintendent, was notified and asked to reply to the accusations. He did, and the board members concluded that Dr. Chipley was free from all censure. Chairman David Sayre concluded that "seldom has the conduct of any public officer been subjected to such scrutiny."

Dr. D. L. Price, as chairman of the Democratic Committee, discredited Dr. Chipley for requiring all asylum employees to pledge an allegiance to the Union in 1862. The pro-Southern employees refused to make that pledge and were fired. While Dr. Chipley agreed to defend his professional reputation and personal integrity, he refused to justify his political stand in 1862. He was an ardent and sincere Union man with sons in the Confederate Army.

P. P. Johnson and Dr. Price represented the previous employees whom Dr. Chipley had fired. The fired employees felt that since Kentucky was neutral during the war, they should not have been fired. The pro-Southern employees of the asylum petitioned the Democratic political party to fire Dr. Chipley. Four of the board members viewed the political pressures from the Democratic political party to be unbeatable.

Dr. Price responded, "I did not write Dr. Chipley's gratuitous report of 1862, nor did I procure the testimony which P. P. Johnson has published."

Others viewed this as more of an attempt by politicians to gain control over the public institution rather than allowing a trained physician to control it. While the Kentucky legislature provided funding for the Kentucky Lunatic Asylum, the politicians were now demanding more control. Dr. Chipley would not allow such interference.

Sayre was chairman of the board, while M. C. Johnson, John R. Desha, James A. Grinstead, and Francis K. Hunt were board members. Sayer was the main supporter of Dr. Chipley but had to resign as chairman due to poor health; still, he stood by Dr. Chipley while others were calling for his resignation. He could not believe that four of the five board members were pressured by the Democratic Executive Committee of Fayette County to agree to Dr. Chipley's resignation. Sayre viewed Dr. Chipley's firing as coming from vengeful Kentuckians still fighting the Civil War without regard to any of Dr. Chipley's outstanding contributions as a physician and national leader in care for the insane.

However, there was another piece of evidence that could have damaged Dr. Chipley's reputation. In 1861, he wrote a book titled, *A Warning to Fathers, Teachers and Young Men: In relation to a fruitful cause of insanity and other serious Disorders of Youth*. It stated Dr. Chipley's belief that some insanity and physical illnesses were caused by masturbation, a belief that was not always supported by his medical profession.

His book, written to describe the dangers from masturbation, was possibly too taboo for the time. Kentucky society may not have been ready for Dr. Chipley's book, especially since it never gained any general or professional acceptance. While he quoted many other physicians and their observations on the subject, how strongly Dr. Chipley believed this idea is not known. The fact that he wrote the book and distributed it to the public could have contributed to his fall from the political arena of Kentucky.

In December, M. C. Johnson asked Dr. Chipley to resign "upon the request of a majority of the board." Sayre, the one board member who voted against Dr. Chipley's resignation, did not cave into the demands of the political party. Dr. Chipley first refused and then tendered his resignation on December 25, 1869.

Sources for Chapter 6

Chipley, W. S. Annual Reports of the Board of Managers and Medical Superintendent. *Kentucky Documents.* 1855, 1858, 1863, 1866, 1869.

Coleman, J. Winston. *The Squire's Sketches of Lexington.* Lexington, Kentucky: The Henry Clay Press, 1972.

Deese, W. "Keepers of the asylum." Lexington, Kentucky: 1990.

Deese, W. *The Medical Department from 1821 to 1859 of Students and Faculty.* Lexington, Kentucky: Transylvania University Library, 2004.

Harrison, L. H. *Kentucky's Governors 1792–1985.* Lexington, Kentucky: University of Kentucky Press, 1985.

Observer & Reporter. "Board of Managers of the asylum Met and Advised Dr. Chipley to Resign." December 1, 1869.

Observer & Reporter. "The Lunatic Asylum War." December 15, 1869.

Peter, Robert. *History of Fayette County, Kentucky.* Chicago: O. L. Baskin, 1882.

Peter, Robert. *History of the Medical Department of Transylvania University.* Louisville, Kentucky: John P. Morton, 1905.

Pusey, W. A. *Giants of Medicine in Pioneer Kentucky: A Study of Influences for Greatness.* New York: Froben Press, 1938.

Renck, G. W. *David Sayer, History of Lexington, Kentucky.* Cincinnati, Ohio: Clarke & Co., 1872.

Richardson, H. Edward. *Cassius Marcellus Clay: Firebrand of Freedom.* Lexington, Kentucky: University of Kentucky Press, 1976.

Simpson, Elizabeth M. *Bluegrass Houses and their Traditions.* Lexington, Kentucky: Transylvania University Press, 1932.

Chapter Seven

---◆·▸|◀·◆---

1870–1905

On January 1870, Dr. John W. Whitney accepted the position of superintendent of the Kentucky Eastern Lunatic Asylum. The employees were perplexed over what they had heard about Dr. W. S. Chipley's resignation. Dr. T. P. Dudley, first assistant physician, was a loyal supporter of Dr. Chipley and was devastated. The patients such as Sarah E. Norton, who had been in that asylum for around twenty-five years at this time, viewed Dr. Chipley as her loving father; she could not understand why he had left her. She cried for days. Other patients withdrew more into their own worlds and refused to socialize with anyone. The whole asylum was stifled and silent.

M. C. Johnson became the fourth chairman of the Board of Commissioners. He had been a member of the board since 1863 and knew how to avoid political division within all political parties. He had recommended that Dr. Chipley resign his position rather than face further investigations. He had also become a professor at the Transylvania Law School.

Francis K. Hunt, son of John W. Hunt, was still a member of the Board of Commissioners and was part of one of the major pro-Southern families in Lexington. He had been a local lawyer for years and usually was able to avoid political conflicts. All his sister's sons, including General John

H. and Calvin C. Morgan, had fought for the Southern cause. Although Hunt supported the demands of pro-Southern employees in the firing of Dr. Chipley, he claimed that his recommendation for Dr. Chipley to resign was based on his fear that the Kentucky Lunatic Asylum would be drawn into a long political fight between the Democratic political party and Dr. Chipley.

On January 1, 1870, Dr. Chipley moved his personal family effects to his mother's home at Rose and Maxwell, while he and his wife left town. Dr. Chipley made the decision to leave and never go back. Since the Chipley and Allen families were now long-term friends, the Chipley family decided to visit the Allens in Memphis. They notified Dr. Allen of their intentions. Dr. and Elizabeth Chipley rode the train to Memphis, watching the blurred landscape out their window. Dr. Chipley did a lot of thinking about the past as he was lulled by the rhythmic sounds of the train.

He had grown up in Lexington, and his father, Rev. Stephen Chipley, was the local minister and used herbal medicines. He often debated with his father about natural healing remedies over medical cares. He was influenced by Dr. Charles Caldwell and his theories on phrenology but was disappointed in Dr. Caldwell's early departure from Lexington. It was that final disloyalty to Lexington that hurt Dr. Chipley.

He had left Lexington after his graduation from medical school and established a medical practice in Georgia. While he and his father remained friends, he married a girl from Georgia and had a family. As his father's health started failing, he and his family returned to Lexington. Yet, his children remained loyal to Georgia and the South, dividing the family during the Civil War. He could understand his sons' loyalty to Georgia and respected their devotion to duty.

He had tried to rescue the medical school from closure. Yet it closed in the next few years in spite of all his efforts. He had enjoyed his employment at the Kentucky Lunatic Asylum and applied the newest knowledge of his profession. He had gained respect locally and nationally, stayed fifteen years, and loved his job with the people who worked with him and the lunatics within. Yet recently, he was being discredited by politicians who had no respect for the professional knowledge needed in caring for lunatics.

He saw the politicians as wanting to control his position, and he would not allow that. He had done the only thing he could: quit.

Dr. Chipley and his wife left Lexington at 7:20 p.m. on the train and arrived in Louisville at 2:30 the next day. He and his wife used the wait time to freshen up and eat some food, as their train for Memphis did not leave until 6:30 p.m. Dr. Chipley continued to think about the last fifteen years of his position at the Kentucky Lunatic Asylum. He was most disappointed over the way he had been treated after fifteen years of loyality.

His wife, Elizabeth, reached over to him on the seat. "Dear, you look worried. We must not distress our friends with our worries. Even your mother, before we left, assured you that you will prevail. I know you will. Your knowledge, experience, and financial resources will carry you through. Please, let us have a nice time in Memphis." She looked out the window.

Dr. Chipley admonished himself, *She is correct. I will rebound as usual.* He felt better. They slept that night on the train as they made their way to Memphis. However, he did not sleep well; it was a restless sleep as most had been lately.

Their train arrived into Memphis at 3:15 the next day, and Dr. Allen was there to meet them. John R. Allen Jr., at the age of thirteen, would have been with his father, but he was away, attending the Kentucky Military Institute.

Dr. Allen observed a difference in Dr. Chipley, but word of his resignation had not reached him. Their previous associations in 1868 occurred when Dr. Chipley had been in his prime. He was enthusiastic with the financial support of the Kentucky legislature and the new buildings. Today, he was not that same person. He was quiet, withdrawn, and perplexing to Dr. Allen.

Dr. Allen was four years younger than Dr. Chipley, yet both men had witnessed and shared a lot in their lifetimes. Both had been superintendents of the first Kentucky Lunatic Asylum. Dr. Allen left the asylum after ten years, moved to St. Louis to teach in the medical school, and then moved on to Keokuk, Iowa, where he was a physician and senator. After his term as senator, Dr. Allen moved to Memphis to help care for the wounded soldiers during the Civil War.

Dr. Allen did not want to be involved in the Civil War, but he was a physician who knew how to care for those who needed him. U. S. Grant had named Memphis as the hospital and supply base for the attack on Vicksburg. Dr. Allen showed that he could serve as a physician in a city that needed him. The Allen family stayed in Memphis and made it their home; their daughter married a local lawyer.

Now, both families were glad to see each other. Over the years, they had developed a bond that only two physicians of the time could understand. Their wives had grown together as sisters. They had maintained correspondence with each other.

While they visited social events of the city and the opera house, Dr. Chipley was most interested in Dr. Allen's medical practice in Memphis. Dr. Allen had an office on Main Street near the Mississippi River. Dr. Allen was pleased with his private practice in the city.

However, Dr. Allen's real pride and joy was his thirteen-year-old son. John Jr. had a quick intellect and love for books. He was succeeding in his course work at the military school in Kentucky. John Jr. had always wanted to return to Kentucky, and now he had his way as a student.

Dr. Allen's wife, Elizabeth, had always loved her husband but she had difficulty understanding his need for a challenge, which usually meant them moving. She had never wanted to leave Lexington but she had observed how depressed her husband had become and agreed to the change. She also realized how badly Kentucky families were torn apart during the Civil War and was grateful that they had escaped it. Now, Elizabeth Allen had adjusted to Memphis.

Dr. Allen's only living daughter was more like his wife; she had difficulty understanding her father. The daughter married John Greer, a Memphis lawyer who had aspirations of becoming a local judge. Dr. Allen was happy to help his son-in-law achieve that goal but his own political aspirations were gone.

Dr. Chipley finally decided to share information about his resignation with Dr. Allen. "I just had no choice but to resign," Dr. Chipley explained. "Can you believe how the politicians came after me? People I had assumed were my friends. I did what I thought was best in 1862, and that was war.

Obviously, it is now an unpopular one." He put his head into his hands, realizing how tired he was.

"Oh, I know!" responded Dr. Allen by laying his hands on Dr. Chipley's shoulders. "I know that politicians can be indomitable. I had hoped that things were still going well for you. The legislature was providing more than adequate funds for new buildings in 1868. You had been successful in so many ways. You must look at what you did achieve, not what you wanted to achieve." Dr. Allen continued to pat Dr. Chipley on the back.

"Yes, that was then. Now, the political climate has changed, and many pro-Southerners have gained power in Kentucky. Many are upset with my stand in 1862, but that was war. The asylum needs someone to care for the unfortunates, not to be a political football," he said, again sighing into his hands.

"Yes, many bad things happened during war. You did what you thought was best then. I am just so sorry for you, but you will survive." Dr. Allen continued to reaffirm his belief in him with pats on the back. They just sat together in silence.

Then, Dr. Chipley responded, "Yes, we will survive. I have made arrangements to rent the old Duncan home out past Mulberry Street on the Maysville–Lexington Road. It will be a private sanitarium." His demeanor changed into the old enthusiasm that Dr. Allen had known before.

"Oh, great, yes! Do I know the Duncans or their home?" Dr. Allen rested back into his chair, clapping his hands in response to knowing that Dr. Chipley had new plans.

"Yes, you know of them. The farm is still a major breeder of race horses. The home has been vacant since H. T. Duncan II settled into a Lexington home, called White Hall on Mulberry and Third Streets. Mr. H. T. Duncan II, although trained as a lawyer, has purchased a local newspaper, the *Lexington Press*. He married Lilly Brand, who was a granddaughter of John Brand. You remember John Brand?"

"Oh, yes, I remember the John Brand family and remember hearing of his early involvement with the asylum."

"Yes, H. T. Duncan II now has ten children; the youngest is two years old, Henry T. III. I have known the whole family for years."

"Well, you seem to have some good plans for a sanitarium. I understand sanitariums do well if you have the facilities to handle enough patients to make adequate money. I have not tried such a venture because it requires expensive facilities."

"I am just renting, and if the arrangements go well, then I might consider purchasing the home. However, I will not have to beg the state for money; the money will come from my own finances and income from patients."

"That sounds great," added Dr. Allen. "I'm so pleased for your plans."

"Unfortunately, I will not be able to admit those who cannot pay. I can only take patients who have their own income or families to pay, no state-paid lunatics. It will be very different."

"You will do well; I wish you the best of success," stated Dr. Allen as they continued to talk. Dr. Chipley was relaxing by the time they finished. Dr. Allen could understand the pressures of the past and it was comforting to have such a bond with someone who shared the same frustrations. They continued to share those experiences throughout the week.

Dr. Chipley and his wife left Memphis with a renewed interest in his future. Both families made plans to write more on a regular basis. They shared experiences that only they could know about.

Dr. Allen received his first letter from Dr. Chipley as he gave glowing details of his new sanitarium. He included an article about Theodore Clay from the *New York Times* dated May 19, 1870. Dr. Chipley asked Dr. Allen, "Do you remember him? You were there when his father died in 1852 and you had to notify Theodore of that event. I was there when a monument was dedicated to his father in 1861, but Theodore had no awareness of the event."

"Yes," Dr. Allen remembered but he was surprised to see the article in a New York paper. Then he remembered that Lexington papers never published negative articles about the Henry Clay family.

The article was titled "The son of Henry Clay: Thirty-eight years of hopeless insanity ended by death in an asylum." Dr. Allen eagerly read the article as it brought back old memories of Theodore Clay. The article read as follows:

Yesterday morning our special telegram announced the end of a weary life, in stating that Theodore, eldest son of Henry Clay, had died in the Lexington Lunatic Asylum after a long confinement. At thirty years of age Theodore Clay was a promising lawyer. He was the image and the hope of the statesman whose fame was on every tongue. It is true that there were whispers of wild living and of indifferent morals. It was hoped that ... the result of youth would be cast aside when circumstances called upon the mastered man to rescue himself and make his talent felt in the community. It was at this turning-point in his life that Theodore Clay began to pursue, with an unwearied perseverance, a young lady of Lexington, whom he had long loved hopelessly. The subject of his attachment was at the present time one of the brightest ornaments of Kentucky society, repulsed, firmly but kindly, every attention offered by the young man. He would not be refused and followed her in the streets by day, and wandered in the neighborhood of her home by night. Subsequently violent demonstrations tended to confirm the impression that the wretched truth could no longer be ignored and his confinement in the asylum became a necessity. That life, after thirty-eight years of imprisonment in what in the earlier days of this confinement he called, "a good boarding-house, but having some of the biggest fools he ever saw as boarders," has closed. For nearly thirty years he was one of the most noted of the inmates not only for his proud descent, but his graceful manners and flow of conversation rendered him an object of interest to all visitors. He labored under the hallucination that he was George Washington and was fond of assuming the traditional attitudes of the Father of his Country. At the occasional balls given to the inmates, he was always exquisitely dressed in the style of his day and was the beau par excellence. During all these long years, despite his general gentleness and cheerfulness of manner, he was restless and discontented, and required close watching. It was never having been considered prudent to allow him to go out into the grounds without attendants.

About the year 1860, his condition began to grow worse, and he soon after became demented, continuing in hopeless idiocy until a few days since, when Death, greater healer than time, placed him with the peers of his early manhood who had gone before him to the God that created him. And so ends the sad a story as the truth of history ever commanded to be written. Two sons of Henry Clay yet survive him, T. H Clay, ex-Minister to Honduras, now residing on his place, Mansfield, near Lexington and John M. Clay, the raiser of Kentucky horses, and one of the greatest turf-men living.

As Dr. Allen read the article, he could only reflect back when John M. Clay was showing similar symptoms as Theodore in the early 1840s. As a medical student, he was asked by Chairman Hunt for advice with this new patient. Dr. Allen came to believe that his advice may have helped to divert John M. Clay from the same fate as his brother.

While no one else knew that Hunt's advice came from an inexperienced medical student, that experience helped to encourage Allen to accept being the asylum's first superintendent. Now, years later, Dr. Allen was reading that John M. Clay was currently a great turf-man. Dr. Allen was proud of the part that he played in Clay's life but few knew it.

The next two letters from Dr. Chipley explained some of his patients at the sanitarium and his expectations for their cures. He had finally found a place where he could apply the most current treatment methods. Dr. Chipley was pleased, and so was Dr. Allen for his friend.

Dr. Chipley glowingly explained his methods used at the sanitarium. "Do you still take the *Journal of Phrenology*? Well, I have finally started an order and I enjoy the newer publications. Many of my more educated patients read the articles and find them helpful."

Dr. Chipley continued to praise the *Journal of Phrenology*. "Phrenology has advanced much more than what Dr. Caldwell had written about in his time. *Phrenology* has articles about people in 'The Life Illustrated' that is helpful to the general public. Another article, 'The effects of mind on the body,' in the October 1871 issue really applies to daily life and is unique for general understanding."

Dr. Chipley included the "Descriptive Chart for Giving a Delineation of Character" published in the 1869 *Phrenology* articles, which helped him to assess patients and to help them to help themselves. The descriptive chart gave an analysis of personality based on scientific knowledge and was a forerunner of psychological tests.

That letter also included an obituary of Dr. B. W. Dudley, dated June 20, 1870. While Dr. Allen had known that Dr. Dudley was elderly and living with his son, his death was still a surprise. Dr. Allen reviewed the following information about Dr. Dudley, realizing what a great leader he had studied with during his time at the Transylvania Medical School. The obituary stated the following:

In 1817 when a Medical School was added to the Transylvania University in Lexington, Dr. B. W. Dudley was elected to the Chairs of Anatomy and Surgery. Dr. B. W. Dudley condemned bloodletting while his skill with the knife soon gained him a national reputation with lithotomy as he was declared to be the lithotomist of the nineteenth century. Dr. B. W. Dudley had been reported to have operated on stones in the bladder 225 times and lost only six patients.

Dr. Allen felt that his hero had died. Dr. Chipley reminded Dr. Allen that he too had studied under Dr. Dudley; they both would miss him.

Another letter came from Dr. Chipley in September, stating that "David Sayre, the one board member who stood up for me, died on September 12. He had been in poor health but I remember him as a real supporter. He came to Lexington with nothing as a silver apprentice and made his fortune in banking after many years of hard work. Do you remember that David Sayre had purchased a two-story brick residence at the northeast corner of Short and Mill Streets to use as a bank?"

Dr. Allen responded in a later letter, "I had been aware of the Sayre & Company for several years but I did not remember a bank. I just remember that he was a very shrewd man."

Dr. Chipley added in the next letter, "David Sayre's nephew will continue the business at that same location. While the Sayre Bank will continue, I have lost a good friend."

Another letter from Dr. Chipley came later in 1870, relating another death important to Dr. Allen. Richard Pindell died in October after taking the "water cure" in Cleveland, Ohio. He was age fifty-eight and had been in ill health for several years.

Pindell had been chairman of the board at the Kentucky Lunatic Asylum from 1844 to 1861, as the second chairman, following John W. Hunt. He was an attorney and supported Dr. Allen during his ten years as superintendent.

In December 1871, Dr. Chipley's beloved sanitarium burned, and he described the details to Dr. Allen: "No one was hurt in the fire due to a strict enforcement of emergency evacuation knowledge of each patient and employee." However, he was again without a facility. While he had several offers of jobs, he accepted a position as superintendent of the College Hill Asylum near Cincinnati, Ohio.

That position was the best offer closest to Lexington, since his mother was still living there. He and his wife moved to an apartment at the Cincinnati asylum and regularly visited his mother's Lexington home at Rose and Maxwell Streets.

Dr. Chipley had rebounded into his new job by the next year. He was doing well and eagerly vested his energy into improving the Cincinnati asylum. He sent an article to Dr. Allen from the *Lexington Press* printed in August 1872, describing the Eastern Lunatic Asylum. Dr. Allen read with interest the article, which read:

One of the principal points of interest about our city is the Eastern Lunatic Asylum, located in the northern suburbs. Strangers who come to Lexington neglect to go through this institution, which deprives them of a visit that never fails to prove both instructive and interesting. Of all the great character of our State there is not one nobler than this asylum, reared and maintained as it is for the care and protection of the hundreds of poor unfortunates gathered there, God's best gift to the society they once adorned, the relatives and friends who loved and now mourn their mental death.

Oh! Insanity is a fearful misfortune, where the afflicted ones, now lying in intellectual darkness, will receive every comfort and be subject to all the influences necessary to promote their happiness. It gives us great pleasure to state that kindness now reigns supreme in the asylum, and that kindness is conducted throughout in all its departments with the spirit of the present enlightened age.

That gentle humanizing influences are brought to bear upon the poor unfortunate ones and that handcuffs, whips and all the other disgraceful implements of torture used in the past days through the fear or ignorance of those in power, are forever banished. And as an assurance to all who may have friends or relatives thus afflicted, we desire to say that under the humane and intelligent rule that now prevails under Dr. Whitney, and prevailed under Dr. Chipley, unkindness and harshness upon the part of a keeper is certain cause for dismissal.

It is known to those who have taken the trouble to investigate the subject, that from the days of the humane and enlightened Pinel, a complete evolution, accomplished successfully by the science, the humanity and perseverance of late years, Dr. J. W. Whitney who succeeded Dr. W. S. Chipley, as superintendent of the Institution, is as popular, as successful in his skill and experience as a physician. He is ably assisted by Dr. T. P. Dudley and we are quite satisfied that the health and comfort of all patients are carefully attended to.

Notable patients that the authors met in a recent visit were: First we saw "General Grant," the octogenarian, who stays in one of the upper wards, and insists on making his own hats and caps. He wore when we met him a queer combination of pasteboard, broom straws, carpet threads and odds and ends drawn from every quarter, bearing some resemblance to an old-fashioned skull cap.

General Grant informed one of the ladies, "It will only take me a few minute to make a prettier one for you lady," an offer that was not accepted.

Then, up in the female ward, we met Miss — with her prayer-book in hand who promptly replied to our remark that she had a pleasant place to live here.

She replied, "That depends, sir, altogether on what you have been accustomed to at home. Now, you may not have had anything better than this, but I—(there was a wonderful assertion of self-importance in the way she uttered the pronoun)—I was always accustomed to better accommodations. Why my room was as large again as this with three times as many windows and you may know this doesn't suit me, however, as much as you may like it."

The authors of the *Lexington Press* article were completely abashed, as they started to leave the room when Miss — called to say, "The State has done all it can for the inmates here, but it is so sad there are no religious privileges afforded."

The authors of this article ventured to remark that they thought religious services were held in the chapel every Sabbath afternoon.

She frowned negatively upon us and said that her "Minister, Mr. Shipman, came occasionally, but the poor patients couldn't understand him, and the swearing from the male inmates was so terrible she could not endure it or derive any comfort from Mr. Shipman whom she did so admire."

The authors wanted to leave the room but Miss — persistently followed them to let them know, "Mr. Shipman was her favorite, and that we needn't say anything at all to change her opinion of Mr. Shipman."

The authors of the *Lexington Press* article walked further and found their old friend, Fulkerson, associate of seventeen years in all the varied experiences of a newspaperman's life—as editor, reporter, correspondent and general writer—lying at full length of the dark shadows of a long hall as we passed by. However, it was not until the attendant told the authors who the old stooped man was, that they recognized him and called him by name.

Oh! There was a change, to find the old friend, the wit, the ready writer in every department, was indifferent, wandering. Once he was a man of indefinite wit, in the years gone by, the genius is dimmed, as poor old Fulkerson lies dozing and fretful in the ward of this insane asylum.

God bless our old friend and soon restore him to us with health and mental faculties refreshed and restored so that he may take up his life and continue it with more of hope and promise than he has ever had before.

The authors interviewed another patient who thought he owned the asylum, and they wrote of the kindness of the attendants. The article ended with praising the grounds of the Institution, the attractiveness of the lawn, the gardens and the whole surroundings and "interposed with flowers, shrubbery, swings, and other adornments to amuse and interest the unfortunate inmates."

Dr. Allen read the *Lexington Press* article with amusement, as he remembered the patients described in the article. He wrote to Dr. Chipley and stated that they would be visiting Lexington next year. His son, John Jr., would be exploring Lexington's law school.

An earlier local newspaper article reported on April 7, 1873, that Dr. Chipley had been selected as superintendent by the Eastern Kentucky Lunatic Asylum's Board of Commissioners from fourteen able and popular candidates. The board's selection was overridden by the governor twenty-one days later when a Dr. Bryant was appointed. There were more changes coming that year.

On April 28, 1873, Dr. George Syng Bryant became the new superintendent of the Eastern Kentucky Lunatic Asylum. The asylum's name was changed to reflect the presence of other Kentucky state asylums.

Another change was that the title, chairman of the board, was changed to president. Francis K. Hunt was that first president of the board. Interestingly, the first chairman of the board was Francis K. Hunt; his father was John W. Hunt. Now, the son, Francis, was the first president. In 1873, Francis Hunt was a successful lawyer; he taught at the Kentucky Law School and was the youngest of five remaining siblings.

Two other members of the board remained: Madison C. Johnson and Philip P. Johnston. While Johnson had been the fourth chairman of the board after David Sayre from 1869 to 1873, he avoided political entanglements by going along with the changes forced upon him. Johnston represented the new Democratic political power in Kentucky after the Civil War. He had helped to see that Dr. Chipley was fired. His brother, J. F. Johnston, was the secretary of the asylum board, which had become a full-time paid position.

Dr. Allen, in one of his letters back to Dr. Chipley in 1873, asked him if he remembered Dr. Luke Blackburn, who graduated from Transylvania Medical School in 1835. Dr. Allen remembered him as a young medical student from Versailles, Kentucky. He moved to Natchez, Mississippi, to practice medicine around 1846. He was pro-Southern and served as a civilian agent for the Confederate Army. He had won acclaim during the 1848 and 1854 yellow fever epidemics in the Mississippi Valley for effective quarantines. Anyway, Dr. Allen wrote, saying, "He came to Memphis, to give aid to the yellow fever epidemic, here. He recognized me and I recognized him after all these years."

Dr. Chipley responded in his next letter, "Yes, I have meet Dr. Luke Blackburn. He does have a good reputation with reducing epidemics, although I understand his actions during the war have been questioned. I understand he had to move to Canada after the war, to escape being put in jail for his activities during the war." They continued to discuss individuals that they knew.

*   *   *

The Kentucky Legislative Act of April 21, 1873, made three changes to all state asylums. The first required that the Board of Directors at the First Kentucky Lunatic Asylum carry out a "new system of effective and economical operations." The steward had the complete responsibility of purchasing all supplies, while the president of the board reviewed all purchases. The salary for the steward was to be doubled due to the increased responsibilities.

A second change among the three Kentucky state asylums was a major reorganization of all facilities. The Lexington asylum was to move all long-term cases to other facilities and accept the more recent ones. While differences in cases were often blurred, it created a hardship on local families visiting their loved ones. It was ceasing to be as a local facility.

A third major change involved the state reimbursement for each pauper patient, from $100 to $200 per year rather than a fixed administrative amount given to each facility. All changes were implemented because the first Kentucky asylum had become overcrowded with 550 patients, and the capacity was only 510. Reorganization appeared to be necessary for the Lexington facility.

Dr. Allen received a letter from Dr. Chipley in August 1873 asking if he remembered Dr. Dudley, who was the first assistant physician when he was there. Dr. Chipley wrote, "He continued to work at the asylum although upset over what he saw as 'radical changes.' I understand Dr. T. P. Dudley took a leave from his position and took a fatal dose of morphine. How sad, he was too devoted to the asylum. The asylum has lost another good friend. I wonder how many more it will lose?"

Dr. Allen could only shake his head. He sat down and stated to himself, "I cannot understand the politicians' lack of care and interest at the very place that should provide that care." Both observed that there was no mention of Dr. T. P. Dudley's death in the reports of the officers of the Kentucky Lunatic Asylum at the end of 1873. The reports specified that the first and second assistant physicians were Dr. William M. Layton and Dr. William H. Rogers. Dr. Dudley's death reduced the number of assistant physicians from three to two. If Dr. Dudley had still been there, one assistant physician would have had to leave due to cost-cutting measures. Yet no one seemed to care that a dedicated life to the institution had been lost in the process.

*   *   *

At the end of 1873, Dr. Allen and his family visited Dr. Chipley and his wife in Lexington for the holidays. John R. Allen Jr. was now fifteen years old and considering his future. He wanted to visit the Kentucky University Law Department in Lexington and his uncle, Judge R. A. Buckner. John Jr. wanted to follow in his uncle's educational steps but that was impossible. Judge Buckner had graduated from the Transylvania Law Department at Transylvania University, but the school changed after the Civil War.

Since Transylvania no longer had a medical school, it was no longer a university. By 1865, the Transylvania Board of Trustees, with M. C. Johnson as chairman, agreed to merge Transylvania and the Agricultural and Mechanical College into a Kentucky University in Lexington with four different colleges: the College of Bible, the College of Arts and Science, the College of Law, and the A. & M. College. The College of Arts and Science was a mixture of former Transylvania teachers, one of whom was Dr. Robert Peter, who was a senior member at age sixty. The law school continued to be part of the Kentucky University for years, although the classes were small.

During their visit in 1873, Dr. Allen and his family stayed at the Ashland House, a new hotel on Short Street between Broadway and Mill Streets. Judge Buckner lived at the Broadway Hotel, close to the Ashland House. The proximity of both hotels allowed for Judge Buckner and his nephew, John Jr., to spend more time together. Dr. Allen and his wife spent time at Dr. Chipley's mother's home on Rose and Maxwell Streets. Dr. Chipley and his wife would visit his mother at the same time, as they all enjoyed the time together.

John Jr. had talked to several professors at the Kentucky University Law School, including M. C. Johnson and Francis K. Hunt. He was pleased with what he saw and anticipated his last year in military school. He was enthusiastic to attend the Kentucky University Law School.

The Allen family returned to Memphis, where Dr. Allen went back to helping with yellow fever victims.

John R. Allen Jr. attended the Kentucky University Law Department from 1875 to 1877. Dormitory rooms were limited but he boarded in a nearby house as other students had done before him, as Jefferson Davis, president of the Confederate States, did when he attended Transylvania University in 1821–1824.

If a student such as John R. Allen Jr. was to arrive in Lexington to attend classes at Kentucky University, he would walk up the hill from Main Street, toward Church and Market Streets, where stood the old red brick building which once housed the first Transylvania Medical School of 1827–1849; by 1877, it was a church.

He could observe on the corner of Mill and Second Streets the handsome house of John W. Hunt, where his daughter, Henrietta Morgan, lived. A few blocks over stood a second Medical Building, with its fine colonnaded facade and cupola that once dominated Broadway. It was destroyed by fire in May 1863.

If John Jr. strolled north through the old college lot, he could see the General Bodley House, originally owned by Thomas Pindell and then sold to General Bodley. It was now in private ownership of William A. Dudley, the son of Dr. B. W. Dudley, the longtime professor at Transylvania Medical School.

Just northwest from the Bodley House was the previous location of the Old Transylvania Building, now a beautiful public park. The only building remaining on the old campus was the long, rectangular, single-storied kitchen and janitor's quarters, now used as a classroom for the academy.

Crossing Third Street would reveal the Old Morrison College building and the only remaining dormitory built in 1839; the others burned in 1861. Further back were ramshackled barracks built by the Union Army during its brief stay. The law school was crowded into the spacious halls of Old Morrison along with the Colleges of Art and Bible.

John R. Allen Jr. was taught by Madison C. Johnson, who had been on the Board of Commissioners of the Kentucky asylum since 1863 and served as the fourth and final chairman of the board. John Jr. was also taught by Francis K. Hunt, the first president of the board. Since both law professors had been extensively involved with the asylum, they were very knowledgeable in state and national legal issues related to insanity. They were both considered to be outstanding legal experts.

Johnson often talked about two local law cases of great interest. In the law case of Dr. Baker, Johnson often described how he had testified with Dr. Allen as superintendent of the asylum, resulting in the unfair execution of Dr. Baker in 1844. Dr. Baker had been declared a lunatic prior to killing his brother-in-law. This was an example of an innocent lunatic being killed and never gaining the care he needed, as Johnson often interpreted that case. Giving care and protection to lunatics was one purpose of a lunatic asylum, as M. C. Johnson believed.

The second case was a legal court commitment of a young lawyer to the asylum. Theodore Clay was court committed in 1833 to the Kentucky Lunatic Asylum for threatening John Brand's family. Johnson interpreted this early legal process as a protection from violence, which Theodore Clay would have committed if not put in the institution—a second purpose for asylums.

Although Theodore Clay spent the rest of his life in the institution, Johnson identified the legal process necessary in limiting insane persons to an institution and keeping the community safe. Johnson felt that lunatics should be institutionalized in state facilities rather than punished. He saw this legal process as a protection for innocent people and a way of getting proper care for the insane in our society.

Two other national cases related to insanity were discussed in the law school. The first case was Mrs. Packard, who in 1860 was committed to an asylum in Jacksonville, Illinois, by her husband and two doctors, who stated that she was insane when she tried to divorce her husband. By 1867, the law in Illinois had been repealed, and another bill required that a jury trial be completed before anyone could be committed to an insane asylum. This became a private war for Mrs. Packard, who continued to push for asylum law reforms.

The second case involved the well-known widow, Mrs. Mary Todd Lincoln, whose son, Robert, had concerns about her "irrational purchases" and financial incapacity. Since the conservatorship laws of Illinois depended on an insanity verdict, Mary Todd Lincoln was declared insane in the spring of 1875. Mary Todd Lincoln regained management of her own finances by proving that she had been restored to reason later that year. While the insanity laws were designed to provide care for the insane, in both of these cases the families were devastated by the process. The laws were changing to protect the rights of individuals who could prove that they had been unjustly determined to be insane instead of for the families.

Mary Todd Lincoln returned to visit her early childhood home in Lexington, Kentucky, after she had proven her sanity. She continued to have "buying manias" that required others to manage her finances, but not her son. Since the court process was so difficult to both, it was years before she was reunited with Robert. The legal process was so devastating to her son that he never intervened again. These cases were debated at the Kentucky University Law School.

M. C. Johnson was a lonely man who became a very outstanding lawyer in Lexington. He lived to see many more graduates of his law school influence state and federal governments.

Although Francis K. Hunt was the first president of the board at the Kentucky Lunatic Asylum, he was replaced by James A. Grinstead upon the governor's wish three years later. Hunt did not resist the changes. After Hunt left, each president of the board never stayed more than three years, and the institution suffered from the constant changing of presidents of the Board of Commissioners.

* * *

Early in 1877, Dr. Allen died in Memphis. He had remained on duty during another fatal outbreak of yellow fever. His son, John R. Allen Jr., had just finished law school and was studying for the Kentucky bar. He was devastated over his father's death and returned to Memphis to comfort his mother and sister.

His brother-in-law, James M. Greer, and his nephew, Allen J. Greer, took John Jr. to his mother's home. His mother was waiting for him in her usual chair, and John Jr. kissed her. She was still a very beautiful woman.

"I am so sorry, Mother, we will certainly miss Father."

"Yes," she responded. "You know he was so proud of you finishing law school as valedictorian. You are doing what you want to do, and your father died doing what he wanted to do, taking care of those who needed him."

"Yes, Father was always that way, he was known for his outstanding medical knowledge and his attention to his patients."

"He loved practicing medicine," replied Elizabeth Allen.

"Yes, he did here in Memphis. I remember other times when he had difficulty practicing medicine the way he felt best."

"There have always been other people, especially politicians, who tried to limit medical care, and your father would not stand for that. When he could not find a solution, he would move on, as we did in Kentucky, Missouri, Iowa, and finally to Memphis for better opportunities to serve."

"I only remember Memphis, since I was raised here."

"Your father was such a good man but he could not tolerate situations where there were no solutions, as he saw it. I had trouble understanding him," replied Elizabeth Allen.

"I could not study medicine because I observed the injustices toward those in the medical field. I viewed law as having more solutions."

"Well, I'm happy you have found law to your satisfaction. Obviously, we have many in our family who have," she said.

"Yes, I feel that through the application of law there is a greater chance of seeing injustices corrected. Of course, Father was able to practice both law and medicine, but in this modern time, such dual careers are not possible. Both law and medicine have more knowledge and require more study to master just one of them. I am satisfied with law," responded John Jr.

"Your father kept going back and forth from law to medicine, but when it came time to care for those who needed him, he was always the physician. I had difficulty with his changing and even leaving Lexington, since that was my home."

"I can understand that, Mother."

"But I soon adjusted to his ways. Your father was such an outstanding man, it was impossible for me to refuse to follow him anywhere he moved," added Elizabeth Allen. "I will miss him!" she cried.

The funeral was attended by many friends from Kentucky, Iowa, and Tennessee. John's sister, her husband, James M. Greer, and their two sons accepted Elizabeth Allen into their home, as she made plans to sell the family home. She decided not to permanently return to Lexington to live since John Jr. was still unmarried and roomed in a boarding house with his uncle, Judge Buckner. John Jr. returned to Lexington to finish his studies.

Dr. Chipley could not attend since he was away at the annual hospital superintendent's meeting. He and his wife sent messages to the Allen family expressing their distress over Dr. Allen's death. Dr. Chipley had lost his best friend, and the loss was deeply felt.

Dr. Chipley's position as superintendent at the College Hill Asylum near Cincinnati had succeeded beyond his wildest dreams; he and his wife now lived on the grounds of the asylum. His mother, Amelia Chipley, moved in with them, and they no longer needed her home on Rose and Maxwell Streets. The Chipley house was donated to the St. Joseph Sister's Hospital, and furniture from the residence was sold on April 7, 1877.

In 1878, John R. Allen Jr. was admitted to the Kentucky bar and became a law partner with his uncle, Judge R. A. Buckner.

When Cassius Clay acknowledged a baby born in Russia as his own son, the small society of Richmond, near Lexington, was horrified. The Warfield family was incensed and demanded that Mary Jane obtain a divorce on the grounds of abandonment. The *Cincinnati Enquirer* exploded in a heat of self-righteous outrage about the incident: "You see an early champion of freedom walking about boastfully with a bastard son, imported like an Arabian cross of horses, and swearing at her family (the Warfields)." Mary Jane did seek a divorce, which was granted in 1878.

That same year, the Kentucky legislature severed the Agricultural & Mechanical College of Kentucky from the Kentucky University. The city of Lexington provided its city park of fifty-two acres on South Limestone Street as a home for the A. & M. College. The Kentucky University continued to function independently, with a College of Bible and a law school.

Dr. Luke Blackburn, previously in Mississippi during the Civil War and a graduate of Transylvania Medical School, returned to Hickman, Kentucky, during the 1878 yellow fever epidemic. He provided medical care and became a hero to thousands of supporters. Dr. Blackburn announced his candidacy for governor of Kentucky that year; he easily won the Democratic nomination, and the "Hero of Hickman" became governor.

John Jr. attended the swearing-in ceremonies of the new governor; as a new attorney and registered Democrat, he wondered if the new governor remembered serving with his father in the yellow fever epidemic of Memphis five years earlier. At the reception line, John Jr. stood in line to shake hands with the new governor. When he reached the governor, he stated, "Sir, my father was Dr. John R. Allen. He was with you in the Memphis epidemic in 1873. Do you remember him, sir?"

The governor was surprised by the unexpected question and stood for a minute in silence. "Yes, I remember your father. We also went to Transylvania Medical School together. How is he?"

"I'm sorry to say he died in 1877 in the Memphis epidemic."

"Oh, I am so sorry to hear that," replied the governor. "Please give my secretary your address, as I wish to get back with you at some point; your father was a great man."

"Yes," answered John Jr. as he gave his card to the secretary. John Jr. had no interest in the politics of the situation, since most of those attending were seeking political favors. He had hoped to renew an acquaintance that his father had known. Since it appeared to be politics as usual, John Jr. left, knowing that his expectations were impossible. He would try later.

*   *   *

On February 11, 1880, Dr. W. S. Chipley died. He had spent his last nine years at the College Hill Asylum near Cincinnati. He completely redeemed that private asylum and instituted many reforms before his death.

His obituary stated that he was "warm and impulsive in his friendships, generous and courteous under all circumstances, he made friends rapidly and attached them firmly. As a medical practitioner, no man in the West has taken a higher position in treatment of diseases for which he had. He had achieved a very distinguished career."

Prior to his death, Dr. Chipley had never recovered from the personal loss of his best friend, Dr. Allen. Dr. Chipley had invited John Jr. to their home in Cincinnati, and he recognized the same quick intellect and wit of Dr. Allen in his son. Dr. Chipley's death three years later was another terrible loss that young John Jr. endured.

Dr. R. C. Chenault was the second superintendent to resign from the Kentucky Lunatic Asylum; he had been praised earlier for his work at the institution. In 1880, a law was passed in Kentucky authorizing the discharge of chronic inmates from asylums. Dr. Chenault disagreed with the law. He believed that chronic inmates should not be discharged since there were usually no families to care for them. Dr. Chenault viewed the law as the Kentucky legislature absolving its responsibility to chronic patients and putting them out of an asylum with no place to go. He resigned in 1880 over that issue.

Dr. Bartlett was appointed as superintendent of the Kentucky Lunatic Asylum and lasted for one year. Dr. Bartlett reported difficulty with the asylum's Board of Commissioners.

The board consisted of M. C. Johnson and Judge R. A. Buckner, the best legal authorities in the state. The other board members were R. A. Thorton, a respected lawyer; Major P. P. Johnston, a state senator; Major R. S. Bullock, sheriff of Fayette County; Mr. Thomas Mitchell, cashier of the First National Bank of the city; and Major B. G. Thomas, sheriff.

Two physicians on the board were Dr. Atkins and Dr. Price; both were respected in the city. John T. Shelby, secretary, and J. F. Johnston, treasurer, were also lawyers in Fayette County.

Dr. Waller O. Bullock was appointed superintendent in 1881. He was praised in 1882 by the *Lexington Transcript* of June 7 for impressing upon the board the effects of pure air in curative treatment. Verandahs were built in the rear of all wards so that the inmates could be exposed to more fresh air. Dr. Bullock served in the Confederate Army during the Civil War. He returned after the war to study medicine at the Louisville Medical School and practiced medicine in Lexington.

Dr. Bullock was also a critic of restraint methods and required that all use of restraints at the Kentucky asylum be available for his review. By introducing more physical activities for each patient, Dr. Bullock reduced the use of restraints from seven hundred hours under Dr. Chenault to Dr. Bullock's seventy hours. Dr. Bullock viewed exercise and diversions as the way to reduce the need for physical restraints, even for more disturbed patients.

Dr. Chenault claimed that Dr. Bullock's reduction in restraints was unhelpful to the institution and insisted that the governor reappoint him as superintendent. The governor did in 1883. Dr. Chenault considered restraints necessary for an orderly asylum. By reappointing Dr. Chenault, the politicians decided an issue that should have been a medical decision.

By 1882, the Agricultural & Mechanical College of Kentucky moved to its new fifty-two-acre campus on South Limestone. The three early buildings consisted of a three-story brick Administration Building, two-story brick residence for President James K. Patterson, and a four-story brick dormitory for boys.

Captain Charlton H. Morgan served as the steward at the Kentucky Lunatic Asylum from 1880 to 1883. He was the younger brother of General John Hunt Morgan and grandson of John W. Hunt, the first chairman of the Board of Commissioners of the asylum.

Captain Morgan had been a successful man. He had served with the US Consul in Messina, Sicily, until 1861, when he served under his brother in the Confederate Army. He was captured twice by the Union Army. He returned to Lexington in 1865 and was employed by the US Revenue Cutter Service for many years until he retired.

After retirement, he gained the position as a steward at the asylum in 1880. He was appointed by Dr. Blackburn, the pro-Southern governor. His employment was uneventful until Dr. Chenault was reappointed in 1883 by a different governor.

The *Lexington Transcript* (February 12, 1883) reported rumors about Captain Morgan's "morals." He was criticized for purchasing supplies without the Board of Commissioners' consent. The December 7, 1883, *Lexington Transcript* stated that Captain Morgan bought supplies upon

Dr. Chenault's request. The Board of Commissioners became upset over Captain Morgan's disregard for them. On December 8, the *Lexington Transcript* reported that Captain Morgan was to be replaced by Governor Knott.

While Governor Knott had promised Captain Morgan that he would not be replaced, his firing was a surprise to many in Lexington. The Morgan family was well respected in Lexington, so friends were indignant over his removal. Colonel T. Logan Hocker replaced Captain Morgan as steward.

After Governor Knott reappointed Dr. Chenault in 1883, problems at the asylum continued. On December 2, Dr. Chenault tried to remove the receiver, Mr. Reardon, from his position and replace him with John Marrs. Reardon refused to leave, and Governor Knott supported Dr. Chenault.

The Board of Commissioners disagreed with Dr. Chenault and the governor. Although the *Lexington Transcript* praised Dr. Chenault for improvements made within the institution on October 22, 1884, by the next year, the newspaper was printing complaints about the superintendent written by employees.

In a *Lexington Transcript* article titled "The Lexington Imbroglio," on October 20, 1885, two female employees made claims against Dr. Chenault, while other employees supported him. On October 1, 1886, another article described problems between Dr. Chenault and the steward, Colonel T. Logan Hocker; this article was called "The asylum Racket." While Dr. Chenault insisted upon hiring and firing all employees at the asylum, Colonel Hocker wanted to select employees under his supervision. Other employees took sides against Dr. Chenault, showing the conditions at that time.

Bessie Parkins, an employee who had worked at the asylum for eight years, reported, "I came out in the hall and saw Dr. Chenault sitting in the hall on a chair. I saw a girl patient, affected with mymphomania, sitting on his lap. She had both arms around Dr. Chenault's neck, kissing him. He came in frequently afterward, as often as six to seven times a day and called for her. He would be lying on a couch in the parlor and she rubbing his head."

Mrs. Perkins continued as a witness of "another girl, who is deaf and dumb and seemed to be fond of men's company, sitting in his lap, hugging up to him. I told her if she did not stop sitting in men's laps, I would put her in the strong room. I told her by signs."

The reports continued against Dr. Chenault, with another witness stating, "In one case a patient was crying, Dr. R. C. Chenault called her a bully and told us to throw her out."

Mrs. Perkins continued, "On another occasion, Dr. R. C. Chenault came to my door about half-past eight and shoved the door open while I was giving a dose to a patient. The patient had nothing on but a chemise. He stood and smiled at her, seeming to enjoy seeing her in this condition. She was ashamed and hid."

Mrs. Perkins continued, "He continued to be on a ward more than once when the patients were undressing. He knew the time they went to bed. I did not tell these things because I thought Dr. R. C. Chenault would influence the Board and I would be discharged and lose my place. I was a poor woman with three little children to support."

After all the witnesses, Governor Knott requested Dr. Chenault's resignation, but the Board of Commissioner disagreed with the governor. Regardless, Dr. Chenault was fired, but he continued to practice medicine in Lexington until his death.

The Kentucky Lunatic Asylum continued to be negatively referred to in the *Lexington Press* as "The asylum muddle reviewed." Local citizens were no longer proud of an institution that for generations had been important to their city.

*   *   *

In 1884, at the age of twenty-eight, John R. Allen Jr. retired as Colonel from the Lexington Guards and Second Kentucky Regiment. Members presented him with a gold-mounted sword, which became one of his most prized possessions.

On February 3, 1885, Colonel John R. Allen Jr. married Miss Eliza McCalister Duncan, daughter of Colonel Henry T. Duncan II and Mrs.

Lilly Brand Duncan of Lexington. The *Lexington Transcript* reported that the "wedding was elegant and in the presence of a large assembly of our best people. Promptly at 8 o'clock, the bridal party entered Christ Church on the arm of her father while the groom and his uncle, Judge Buckner, faced the altar. The bridal party was invited to the residence of Mr. H. T. Duncan II, on North Limestone. Later in the evening, Colonel John R. Allen took his bride to their home on North Limestone, known as the Ridgley property. The house was charmingly furnished and the bride was the recipient of many elegant and costly presents."

The only positive news about the asylum for several years was reported on December 2, 1886, in the *Lexington Transcript.*

The Board of Commissioners of the Eastern Lunatic Asylum had purchased a three story brick building on the corner of Limestone and Water Streets with funds from the Megowan Family and the resulting money will be used for providing patients with recreation opportunities.

This Megowan Fund was created by the family of Captain Stewart Megowan, an old soldier of the War of 1812 who was born, lived, and died in Lexington. He was a bachelor and made a bequest in a sum of money, the interest was to be used in furnishing amusements to the inmates of the Lunatic Asylum. For twenty-five or thirty years when David A. Sayre, M. C. Johnson, and F. K. Hunt served as Chairman of the Board of Commissioners, they set aside this fund for the purpose of adding pleasures and amusements to the patients.

On December 8, 1886, M. C. Johnson died in his home at Madison Avenue and West High Street. Colonel Allen, along with many of Johnson's students, would often visit Johnson's home and listened to his stories. Johnson often told stories about the old Transylvania University and the Law Department. He detailed the early Transylvania Medical School, the professors, and how the school had lost students by the early 1860s.

Johnson loved to tell how the law school remained as a part of the

Kentucky University and how the medical school was lost to the city of Louisville. He often told how after the Civil War, Transylvania University was merged with another college to create Kentucky University, upon his recommendation as trustee. Then, he would tell how Transylvania separated from the new Kentucky State College and how the old Transylvania professors faded out.

Johnson recalled the early Asylum with Dr. Allen as superintendent and Dr. Chipley following. He recalled the problems with Dr. Chipley and how he had advised him to resign, hoping to reduce future conflicts within the asylum. He often admitted that such did not happen within the asylum, since political interventions continued to erode the institution.

While Johnson remained on the board, he finally agreed to resign from his position on the Board of Commissioners in 1883, having served for twenty years. While the asylum had followed one political controversy with another since Dr. Chipley, Johnson had always been there to observe and make legal interpretations for his students.

Colonel Allen had always been fascinated with the old histories of Lexington. After Johnson's death, Colonel Allen missed his old law professor.

*   *   *

Problems with the asylum continued in the local newspaper. The *Lexington Transcript* reported on February 24, 1888, that the current superintendent of the Kentucky Lunatic Asylum, Dr. Clark, had criticized the steward, Colonel Hocker, for not obtaining competitive bids on products for the asylum. Dr. Clark also criticized Colonel Hocker for hiring a kitchen employee and florist, which Dr. Clark considered at waste of money.

On March 30, 1888, the *Lexington Transcript* claimed that Colonel Hocker was vindicated following an investigation into his department. Yet the Board of Commissioners recommended that competitive bidding would improve purchasing items for the asylum. The steward and receiver were to award bids together, while the superintendent would do the hiring. These disputes between superintendent, steward, receiver, employees, and

Board of Commissioners continued for many years, while the facility continued to grow in patients beyond its capacity.

Since the superintendent was often the only professionally trained employee, superintendents felt themselves to be the only ones qualified to run such a facility. Yet the politicians had financial control and considered themselves more qualified, while employees considered themselves more qualified to run their own departments. All this continued to cause various disputes between individuals associated within most American lunatic asylums, and those in Kentucky were no different. Patient care was affected by constant changes in employees and political policies.

In October 1889, the nephew of David Sayre died, leaving the bank his uncle had created to be liquidated. The Security Trust Company became the successor to David Sayre's bank, located at the same location of Short and Mill Streets.

On September 6, 1891, Henrietta Hunt Morgan, the only living child of John W. Hunt, died. She had lived her elder life in the home of her parents and had outlived her eleven brothers and sisters. She died at the age of eighty-five and had had ten children. She did not live to see the monument for her son, General John H. Hunt, built in downtown Lexington. He was considered one of the greatest and most gallant cavalry leaders of the Confederacy.

The Law Department at Kentucky University, which had operated from 1865 until around 1880, attempted unsuccessfully to reopen in 1889 and 1892. It was permanently closed in 1895.

Henry T. Duncan II, father of Colonel Allen's wife, was mayor of Lexington in 1894 and 1895. He had graduated from Harvard University prior to the Civil War and returned to Lexington to serve as a member of the State Guard during the Civil War. He had married Lilly Vertner Brand, granddaughter of John Brand, who had been an early board member at the asylum. They had ten children. Duncan established the *Lexington Press* in 1870 and continued to express his opinions and questions about Kentucky state government.

Another local newspaper, the *Kentucky Leader*, reported on February 3, 1894, that "the Eastern Kentucky Lunatic Asylum is to be discontinued, the ground sold off into town lots and the institution merged into that one at Anchorage, near Louisville. This startling information came from Frankfort." The current superintendent, Dr. Clark, was quoted as saying "that he did not think it would be advisable to extend the asylum buildings. The city was rapidly growing around the asylum and the water supply was inadequate. The old Board of Commissioners were divided at their last meeting on the question of asking for money for needed repairs at the Lexington Asylum." The board decided "to ask for no appropriations." No appropriations meant that the asylum was to be merged with the third Kentucky state asylum in Anchorage, Kentucky, near Louisville.

A statewide Joint Committee on Charitable Institutions was created to review the needs of the state. The committee recommended that "all three of the lunatic Asylums of Kentucky are overcrowded and it is absolutely necessary that provisions be made for the enlargement of each of them, if they remain," but they were uncertain about the Lexington asylum.

In reaction to the article about merging the Lexington asylum with the Louisville one, a Lexington newspaper responded with the following:

Is Lexington to be robbed of another of its Institutions? A Deep Laid Scheme to wipe out the Lexington Lunatic Asylum, then, Louisville will be enriched at the expenses of her sister City, and Colonel Hodges made an appeal for Lexington, but it fell on unwilling ears. Louisville parties were requesting that the asylum be merged with the one at Anchorage with new and elaborate buildings. The State would sell off the Lexington grounds.

For reimbursement of wrecking Lexington's "Great Institution," the oldest one of its kind in the West, the Louisville gangsters generously proposed a reform school or a penitentiary here. Was ever such generosity known, and in Louisville, too? The old Transylvania Medical School in the late 1860s was absorbed by the new Medical School in Louisville. Now, the asylum was being considered for merger to Louisville in 1894.

How the issue was resolved is not recorded, but Dr. Clark continued as superintendent until 1896, and money was appropriated for new buildings. Another residence was to be constructed for the superintendent closer to the front with an Administration Building and Infirmary. These last two buildings were to move the business offices and apartments for the employees from the main buildings to create more rooms in the female department. The Administration Building was to have a large hall for amusements for all the patients.

In 1896, Dr. W. F. Scott was named superintendent but lasted for only one year. His Republican brother-in-law, W. O. Bradley, had been elected governor in 1895 and appointed him superintendent. During that year, there were 236 new admissions with a total of 817 patients in a facility built for half that capacity. The asylum discharged 210 patients but still had 376 white men and 318 white females; 63 colored males and 60 colored females. The facility continued to be overcrowded for at least eighty more years.

The main conclusion in the "Seventy-second Annual Report of the Eastern Kentucky Asylum for the Insane" was "too much politics." The Board of Commissioners unanimously urged the amendment of a law regulating the officers and taking control away from the hands of the governor. The Board of Commissioners lost control when the governor interfered, so it was a matter of who had control of the scandalized asylum.

On July 28, 1897, the *Kentucky Leader* reported that the grand jury was considering "a recent report on the Management of Dr. W. F. Scott. He appeared before the Grand Jury on charges against him and he was the worst witness for himself." On July 29, another newspaper, the *Lexington Herald*, reported that Dr. Scott "was an honest gentleman, but utterly without the executive ability to manage the affairs of an institution as important as this."

On July 30, 1897, the Board of Commissioners demanded Dr. Scott's removal or all of the members of the Board of Commissioners would resign. The charges against Dr. Scott included that he was replacing experienced employees at the asylum with friends from his own home county, Pulaski.

After Dr. Scott had replaced the long-term employees, the National Guard had to be called in to control angry ex-employees. The inexperienced employees could not handle the more difficult patients, and other patients were upset over the changing of so many employees. The whole situation was chaotic.

The Board of Commissioners reacted to Dr. Scott by cutting the salaries of his appointed employees. The situation continued to be very tense, and bloodshed was feared. On July 30, the *Herald Leader* reported, "There was more bad blood among the sane than among the inmates of the Eastern Kentucky Lunatic Asylum." The article denied that Dr. Scott's removal was politically motivated since there were two Republican board members, R. P. Stoll and H. McDowell, who were against Dr. Scott's mismanagement and favored his removal.

Dr. Scott was removed by the governor and replaced by Dr. Edward W. Wiley, according to the *Kentucky Leader*, August 1 and August 10, 1897. Dr. Wiley had hopes of improving the facilities and conditions at the aging and overcrowded Kentucky Lunatic Asylum.

On September 11, 1897, Mrs. Elizabeth Buckner Allen died at the age of seventy-eight. Colonel Allen and his wife, Eliza M. Allen, attended the funeral in Memphis. They had often visited Elizabeth in the home of Judge and Mrs. Greer, sister of Colonel Allen. Judge Buckner, brother of Elizabeth Buckner Allen, went with them to the funeral.

* * *

The idea of another medical school in Lexington never completely died down. In the 1890s, the idea of attaching a medical department to the Kentucky University was established. The action came from the Kentucky School of Medicine in Louisville, which had thirty-six faculty members and well-equipped buildings. A contract with the Lexington university was approved on November 4, 1897.

The requirements for an MD in 1897 were not too different from those a half-century before at Transylvania Medical School. Instead of two years in the medical school, the requirement was now four years. Beginning in

1898, the Kentucky University of Lexington had a functioning medical department in Louisville. Apparently this arrangement did not work out, for in May 1898, the Kentucky University Medical School was abolished.

By 1898, an infirmary was established in the asylum in Lexington and called the Dr. B. W. Dudley Infirmary, in memory of one of the greatest physicians in Lexington. The superintendent, Dr. Wiley, reported other improvements at the old institution. Plans were being drawn for a complete system of heating and ventilating for the main Asylum buildings. A new cold storage plant was to be erected, and a trench for the new sewer was being dug with pipes laid. The walks and driveways were improved with a nine-foot iron fence that ran the entire length of Fourth Street, replacing a wooden one. The iron fence stopped at the handsome brick entrance gate that was built in 1869 under Dr. Chipley's direction.

On July 3, 1898, the *Kentucky Leader* reported a new electric light plant at the asylum. The buildings and grounds of the asylum were brilliantly lighted at night at about two-thirds the expense of the previous gas plant.

While the Eastern Kentucky Lunatic Asylum had survived threats to remove it, Dr. Wiley had plans to redeem the facility by the end of 1899, but his tenure as superintendent only lasted two years.

The asylum continued to face problems with changing superintendents as the employees changed with each different superintendent, and patient care was inconsistent or inadequate. Yet the number of patients continued to increase and the facilities became more inadequate. While the asylum had survived into the twentieth century, it was far from stable.

The city of Lexington was growing out while the downtown was starting to grow up. In 1899, a five-story building, the McClelland Building, was built on the corner of Short and Upper Streets. More floors were added to that building, starting a trend toward taller buildings in the city.

Lexington's growing out started with the introduction of streetcars. By 1890, a large brick powerhouse was constructed on the south side of Loudon Avenue between North Broadway and North Limestone Streets. The plant soon increased in size to provide electricity for general use. On the opposite side of Loudon Avenue was the Streetcar Barn. The streetcars provided transportation from downtown Lexington to surrounding areas as the twentieth century arrived.

For central Kentucky, including the Lexington area, the 1900s started with tearing down the last tollgate house on the Maysville–Lexington Road, having been built by private owners in 1830 on the original Old Buffalo Trail. After the trail merged with other roadways to become part of a national road, the tollgates ceased to be privately owned. That last tollgate house in Lexington stood on Harrodsburg Road in the vicinity of Waller Avenue; it was known as the Lexington, Harrodsburg, and Perryville Turnpike.

Mulberry Street had been the earlier name for Limestone Street, owing to its association with the Old Buffalo Trail. The name was changed to Limestone Street in 1902, when a new street numbering system was developed. Streetcars became common for everyday use as Lexington continued to grow outward.

*   *   *

Discord followed Dr. Scott, who had been superintendent at the asylum from 1896 to 1897; on January 17, 1900, his son, Lieutenant Ethelbert Dudley Scott, was killed by a former congressman, David G. Colson, in Frankfort, the capital of Kentucky. Ethelbert Scott was a thirty-year-old attorney who had been a first lieutenant in the Fourth Kentucky Volunteers, while Colson was a colonel in that regiment. A personal dislike developed between both men, resulting in Scott being dismissed from the service by a court of inquiry. Scott appealed to Washington DC and was reinstated by the War Department. On February 11, 1899, Lieutenant Scott returned to his regiment and seriously wounded Colonel Colson. Lieutenant Scott was arrested but the charges were dismissed because Colson did not appear at the trial.

According to the *Morning Herald* of January 17, 1900, about forty people were eating dinner in the Capitol Hotel in Frankfort when many shots were fired. The shooting threw diners into panic. Lieutenant Scott was shot six times and died instantly. Two innocent bystanders were killed.

Captain B. B. Golden, commonwealth attorney of the 27th District, was shot. While Colonel Colson was shot twice, he claimed self-defense and was acquitted of all charges on April 22, 1900. All this conflict occurred at the same time William Goebel, a Democrat, was killed as he took the governor's office. Kentucky was once again facing serious internal discord.

Phrenology in America was the pop psychology, along with the health-reform movements of the nineteenth century. Its publication, the *Journal of Phrenology*, had one of the longest histories of any nineteenth-century magazine. Phrenology was considered the science of the mind and implied that reform was possible through self-knowledge. However, newer sciences were beginning to refute some of the principles and teachings of phrenology by the early 1900s.

One such example, Dr. G. F. Stout published *A Manual of Psychology* (1899), which listed his criticisms of phrenology. He wrote, "The reading of character by the feeling of bumps on the head is not accurate, nor does it correspond to the development of the brain. Instead," he continued, "whenever we do a thing to a person, to see how he will take it, we are performing a psychological experiment. The experiment secures accuracy of observations and the connection of every result with its own condition while it enables observers in all parts of the world to work together upon one and the same psychological problem." The science of psychology was developing.

On February 18, 1900, Judge Richard Buckner, uncle of Colonel Allen, died in Lexington. He was considered one of the most prominent citizens of central Kentucky. He had studied law at the Transylvania University Law Department, graduating in 1837. In 1839, he was appointed commonwealth's attorney, continuing until he was appointed circuit judge in 1842.

Politically, he was a Whig and supported Henry Clay Sr. for the presidency. During the Civil War, he supported the Union. He was an honored and eminent member of the Lexington bar but had withdrawn from practice several years earlier after Colonel Allen took over his law practice. Judge Buckner had served on the Board of Commissioners of the

Eastern Kentucky Lunatic Asylum starting in the 1860s and continued in that capacity for many years. His father had served on the Board of Commissioners starting in 1844 when his son-in-law, Dr. Allen, was superintendent.

By the 1900s, the Eastern Kentucky Lunatic Asylum was constantly mentioned in the local newspapers; such as on January 4, 1900, an article in the *Leader*, "The asylum Report had issued a pamphlet as an interesting contribution to the Official State Report," reflected the perplexity that permeated the facility. In the *Lexington Leader* on June 1, 1900, other changes were reported: Dr. J. S. Redwine was appointed to be superintendent along with a list of other new officers. Another article on July 5 proclaimed, "Fourth at the asylum, where there many matters of importance at the asylum considered but no definite action was taken."

The Eastern Kentucky Lunatic Asylum for the Insane, as it was titled at this time, had completed an Infirmary, named for Dr. Dudley. It consisted of four private bathrooms, an operating room, diet kitchen, and ten private rooms with hot-air blast heating. By 1901, another article referred to it as the New Infirmary, without Dr. Dudley's name.

In 1901, Mrs. Short, a relative of Dr. Dudley, received a bequest for an operation he had performed in 1827. While the son's father could not pay Dr. Dudley for the operation, after that boy became a man and died, he had left a sum in his will to pay for his operation. Mrs. Short donated the money to the Good Samaritan Hospital in Lexington and was reported in the local newspaper.

On August 25, 1901, the *Lexington Herald* included a "Sketch of the Eastern Kentucky Lunatic Asylum" that gives a rare glimpse of that facility at that time. The article praised the facility for their work with the unfortunates:

There have been 3,450 persons admitted in its long history. Currently there are 450 white males, 350 white females, 70 colored males and 60 colored females. There are 144 employees on 18 wards. Sarah Norton who had been admitted in 1845 at the age of 27 years was still there. Dr. Redwine had three assistants, Dr.

L. H. Mulligan, Dr. R. H. Alexander, Dr. Minnie C. Dunlap, and three consultants, Dr. David H. Barrow, consulting Surgeon, Dr. F. H. Clark, Consulting Neurologist and Dr. Claude W. Trapp, Consulting Oculist and Laryngologist. Other employees include James H. Reed, Steward, Mrs. Betty Ruth, Matron, T. A. McLaughlin, Receiver, Miss Harriet Cleek, Superintendent of the Infirmary and Miss Mary Elder was Supervisor of Female Ward and Thos. Adams, Supervisor of Male Wards.

After 1903, the first and only remaining building of the Transylvania Medical School, erected in 1827, now housed the Jennie Hanson Magazine Agency. It had been used by the Hill Street Methodist Church from 1857 to 1866, and then it became the city library. A new library was opened on Second Street between Mill and Market, and the original Medical School Building was taken over by the Hanson Magazine Agency in 1903. It was demolished in 1954 to make way for a parking lot opposite Christ Church.

A law department was opened in 1905 at the Kentucky University while the university was created months after the Civil War ended. There were nine men on the faculty and the course was to run for two years. There were twenty-five students enrolled. While the University Law Library had moved earlier to the county courthouse as part of the Lexington Law Library, it was available to the law students. Applicants were advised (but not required) to attend courses in the College of Liberal Arts (the undergraduate school). The Law Department was established to provide lecture and textbooks; apprenticeships were considered to be inadequate for legal training by this time period.

For the year of 1905, the patient population at the Kentucky Lunatic Asylum had continued to grow to a total of 1,232. There had been 974 admitted before 1900 and 258 admitted after, as demands upon the institution continued to exceed its resources. There were around 135 employees, including many who had been hired as a political payback. The employee-to-patient ratio was one employee to every eleven patients, showing a severe lack of employees.

Dr. Redwine stated in a report, "We have been compelled to refuse admission to over a hundred patients during the past year. The facilities are so crowded, dangerous, unpleasant, unsanitary, and harmful. I cannot emphasize this hurtful state of affairs too much. The effect of overcrowding into the institution is so detrimental to any type of treatment, and the only solution is to build more buildings." As the overcrowded facility tried to cope, deplorable conditions continued and compounded.

At the end of 1905, the old administrative system of a Board of Commissioners was discontinued, and a new Board of Control was established the next year. The old Board of Commissioners, who had volunteered their time and expertise to the asylum for eighty-two years, had been local citizens. Now the Board of Control became paid employees with statewide control of two other state asylums.

That same year, Sarah Norton died at the age of eighty-eight. She had been at the facility for sixty-one years. She was a part of the old facility and its history. She symbolized the institution's dedication in caring for those who had no one to care for them due to their unfortunate circumstances.

Sources for Chapter 7

Bullock, Dr. W. O. "Dr. Benjamin Winslow Dudley." *Annals of Medical History* 7, no. 3 (1934): 201–213.

Deese, W. *Lexington, Kentucky: Changes in the Early Twentieth Century.* Charleston, South Carolina: Arcadia Publishing, 1998.

Gaillard, E. S. Annual Report of the First Kentucky Lunatic Asylum. *Richmond and Louisville Medical Journal* 17, no. 1 (January 1874): 128–129.

Grinstead, James A. and Dr. R. C. Chenault. Fifty-Third Annual Summary, *Legislative Document*, no. 7 (September 1877). Frankfort, Kentucky: Kentucky Yeoman Office.

Grinstead, James A. and Dr. R. C. Chenault. Fifty-Fourth Annual Summary, *Legislative Document*, no. 7 (September 30, 1878). Frankfort, Kentucky: Kentucky Yeoman Office.

Harrison, L. H., ed. *Kentucky's Governors, 1795-1985.* Lexington, Kentucky: University of Kentucky Press, 1985.

Hunt, F. K. and Dr. Syng Bryant. Yearly Report. *Kentucky State Archives.* November 1873.

Hunt, F. K. and Dr. R. C. Chenault. Yearly Report. *Kentucky State Archives.* October 1875.

Johnson, M. C. and Dr. John W. Whitney. Report of Officers of Kentucky Eastern Lunatic Asylum. *Kentucky State Government* 9 (October 1, 1872): 1–5.

Kerr, Bettie, and John Wright. *Lexington: A Century in Photographs.* Lexington, Kentucky: Lexington-Fayette County Historic Commission, 1984.

Kerr, Judge C. et al. *History of Kentucky.* Chicago and New York: The American Historical Society, 1922.

Lancaster, C. *Vestiges of the Venerable City: A Chronicle of Lexington, Kentucky.* Lexington-Fayette County Historic Commission. Cincinnati, Ohio: C. J. Krehbiel, 1978.

Levin, R., ed. "Richard A. Buckner Jr.," in *Lawyers and Lawmakers of Kentucky.* Chicago: Lewis Publishing Co., reprinted by Southern Historical Press, 1897.

Lexington Herald. "Dr. J. S. Redwine of Breathitt Co. Appointed Superintendent of EKLA, Replacing Dr. E. M. Wiley." May 27, 1900.

Lexington Herald. "950 Patients at EKLA and Entrances for New Patients Denied." March 29, 1902.

Lexington Herald. "Sketch of Eastern Kentucky Lunatic Asylum." August 25, 1901.

Lexington Herald. "Tribute to Judge R. A. Buckner." February 20, 1900.

Lexington Leader. "Asylum." January 24, 1897.

Lexington Leader. "Dr. Scott." August 10, 1897.

Lexington Press. "Asylum Improvements." June 7, 1882.

Lexington Press. "Conditions at EKLA." April 21, 1875.

Lexington Press. "Dr. Allen Died." December 4, 1877.

Lexington Press. "Dr. R. C. Chenault of Richmond Appointed Superintendent of EKLA." June 30, 1875.

Lexington Press. "Eastern Lunatic Asylum." October 21, 1877.

Lexington Press. "The Lunatic Asylum War." August 8, 1873.

Lexington Press. "A Visit to Eastern Lunatic Asylum and an Interview with Patients." August 8, 1872.

Lexington Transcript. "Asylum Board Members and Sketches of Their Careers." December 18, 1883.

Lexington Transcript. "The asylum Muddle Reviewed." December 18, 1883.

Lexington Transcript. "The asylum Racket." October 17, 1885.

Lexington Transcript. "Col. John R. Allen Weds Miss Eliza M. Duncan at Christ Church." February 4, 1885.

Lexington Transcript. "Death of Dr. W. S. Chipley." February 12, 1880.

Lexington Transcript. "Madison C. Johnson Dead." December 6, 1886.

Lexington Transcript. "Two Story Building at Limestone & Water Being Erected by Megowan Fund of EKLA." December 2, 1886.

Memphis-Shelby County Public Library *History and Facts about Memphis & Shelby County,* 2003.

New York Times. "The Son of Henry Clay." May 19, 1870.

Observer & Reporter. "Board of Managers of the asylum Met and Advised Dr. Chipley to Resign." December 1, 1869.

Observer & Reporter. "Dr. Chipley Resigns and Is Replaced by Dr. Whitney." December 25, 1869.

Observer & Reporter. "The Lunatic Asylum: Another Bulletin from the Battlefield." December 18, 1869.

Observer & Reporter. "The Lunatic Asylum, Latest from the Battlefield." December 15, 1869.

Observer & Reporter. "Richard Pindell Dies." October 8, 1870.

Observer & Reporter. "War Still Going on at EKLA." December 15, 1869.

Phrenological Journal. "Life Illustrated." April 1871.

Phrenological Journal. "Life Illustrated." August 1866.

Phrenological Journal. "Life Illustrated." December 1871.

Phrenological Journal. "Life Illustrated." February 1871.

Phrenological Journal. "Life Illustrated." March 1865.

Phrenological Journal. "Life Illustrated." November 1871.

Phrenological Journal. "Life Illustrated." September 1871.

Phrenological Journal. "Life Illustrated and Testimonials in Favor of Phrenology." October 1865.

Redwine, Dr. J. S. Reports to the Board of Commissioners. November 1, 1901, and September 30, 1903.

Richardson, H. Edward. *Cassius Marcellus Clay, Firebrand of Freedom.* Lexington, Kentucky: University of Kentucky Press, 1976.

Sapinsley, B. *The Private War of Mrs. Packard* New York: Paragon House, 1991.

Seventieth Annual Report of the Eastern Kentucky Asylum for the Insane. Frankfort, Kentucky: Capital Printing Co, September 30, 1894.

Seventy-Third Annual Report of the Eastern Kentucky Asylum for the Insane. Frankfort, Kentucky: Capital Printing Co. September 30, 1897.

Sixty-Fifth Annual Report of the Eastern Kentucky Lunatic Asylum. *Legislative Documents.* September 30, 1889.

Sixty-Second Annual Report of the Eastern Kentucky Lunatic Asylum. *Legislative Document* no. 6, September 30, 1886.

Sixty-Third Annual Report of the Eastern Kentucky Lunatic Asylum. *Legislative Document* no. 29, September 30, 1887.

Vernon, Edward *Travelers' Official Railway Guide for the United States and Canada, Containing Railway Time Schedules.* New York: J. W. Pratt, 1868.

Wells, S. R. *Phrenological Journal and Life Illustrated.* December 1871.

Wells, S. R. *Phrenological Journal and Life Illustrated.* October 1871.

Wells, S. R. *Wells' New Descriptive Chart for Giving a Delineation of Character According to Phrenology and Physiognomy for the Use of Practical Phrenologists.* New York: Fowler & Wells, 1869.

Chapter Eight

——◆◆◆◆——

1907–1969

A lthough members of the new Board of Control at the asylum were full-time paid employees, they had no special training (other than being appointed by the governor). The first chairman of the Board of Control was a well-known Lexington politician, Percy Haley. The board members had offices in Frankfort, where all of Kentucky's state offices congregated.

The First Kentucky Lunatic Asylum was renamed the Eastern Kentucky Lunatic Asylum as it was one of three asylums in the state, with a fourth state hospital created after World War II. The change to a Board of Control reflects a shift in more answerable state employees and statewide political control. While the process gained accountability, it lost the support of families from the local community of Lexington. The hiring of employees became controlled by statewide politicians.

By 1907, Dr. Redwine, as superintendent of EKLA, was sued by the Ketterer estate for the wrongful death of Fred Ketterer, but the case was dismissed since he had already been removed as superintendent. Dr. Robert L. Willis became the new superintendent in 1908 as the cycle of ever-changing superintendents and employees continued.

James H. Reed changed that cycle by staying at the hospital for nearly fifty years, until 1950. He may be the last known descendant of John W.

Hunt's to work at the asylum. J. H. Reed stayed with the Kentucky Lunatic Asylum as the name was changed to Eastern State Hospital.

* * *

On February 19, 1907, the dean of the medical school in Louisville cancelled their contract with the Kentucky University and ceased to use the Kentucky University for medical teaching. While there had been two additional medical schools in Louisville, the College of Medicine (1875–1907) and School of Medicine (1851–1907), all merged into one school. This was the last attempt to establish a medical school in Lexington for many years.

By 1907, the Good Samaritan Hospital moved to South Limestone Street. It was established in 1889 on the north side of East Short Street. Some of Dr. B. W. Dudley's estate contributed to its early development. That same hospital provided internships for many future physicians, including Dr. Logan Gragg, who became a future leader of Eastern State Hospital.

In 1908, the state college in south Lexington established its own law school with a three-year program. Although the Kentucky University Law Department continued for several more years, the State College Law School gained a reputation for having a better program.

In 1909, Henry T. Duncan III, law partner of Colonel Allen, followed in the footsteps of his crusading father and became a leader of reformers in the city of Lexington. He charged Louis DesCognets, president of the Lexington Street Railway Company, with providing funds for Thomas Combs's mayoral campaign. After Combs became mayor, Duncan claimed that expenditures for the Lexington road repairs were given without competitive bidding to his favored contractors. He accused Combs of buying votes. Believing that Lexington was under the control of Combs and political leader Billy Klair (see Bolin, 2000), Duncan ran for mayor in 1909, calling Klair and Combs "the Siamese Twins of Lexington politics." He lost the mayor's race by only 132 votes to Klair, but he believed that he had eroded Klair's power.

Klair became boss of Lexington in the first two decades of the twentieth century and was the "undisputed czar of Lexington politics by 1930" (Bolin. 2000). He was not only powerful within Lexington, his power had grown to statewide proportions. This included a group of power brokers in Lexington dubbed the Big Six of Kentucky politics. Besides Klair, the group included Ben Johnson of Nelson County, Michael J. Brennan of Louisville, Albert Yount of Morehead, and Frankfort's Percy Haley (all Democrats) and Maurice Galvin (a Republican from northern Kentucky). All six individuals built substantial power bases in Kentucky and controlled power throughout the commonwealth. Percy Haley was the president of the Board of Control for the Kentucky Lunatic Asylum during that time.

The Kentucky Lunatic Asylum continued to be a major resource for the local politicians to provide jobs for their supporters. With no job standards established, the local politicians offered regular paying jobs at the asylum. Patients continued to increase in numbers as the old facilities were becoming more overcrowed.

*   *   *

By 1912, the Kentucky University Law Department had only six or seven law students; most law students were attending the State College Law School. The Kentucky University Law Department was soon discontinued.

On June 4, 1912, Henry T. Duncan II died. He was twice elected mayor, with his last time being in 1900–1903. He was a defender against the "spoils system" and often protested the illegal use of public funds. His earlier services had done much to keep Lexington politics clean. But when his son tried to challenge the leaders of Lexington politics, he lost.

In 1912, Dr. Waller O. Bullock purchased the Bodley House on the northeast corner of Market and Second Streets; it stayed in the Bullock family for many years. Earlier, that same house had been the federal headquarters in 1862 and 1863, and later it was owned by William A. Dudley, president of the old L & N Railroad. William Dudley had brought his father, Dr. B. W. Dudley, an early leader at the Transylvania Medical School, there to live his final years.

On October 11, 1912, the last grandson of John W. Hunt and the last grandson to be employed at the asylum, Captain Charlton Hunt Morgan, died. He was the son of Henrietta Hunt Morgan. In 1861, he enlisted in the Confederate Army with his brother, General John Hunt Morgan. Captain Morgan married Miss Ellen Key Howard and worked in the Revenue Service for fifteen years. He returned to Lexington and was employed as a steward at the asylum from 1880 until 1883.

Captain Morgan lived his last four months at the High Oaks Sanitarium until his death at age seventy-four. That same High Oaks Sanitarium had been purchased earlier by Dr. R. C. Chenault after he left the asylum in 1885. After Dr. Chenault died in 1890, Drs. Silas Evans and George Sprague operated it for Mrs. Chenault until 1912, when Dr. Sprague purchased it with eight-three more acres. That facility continued to function at that location until 1945, when it became the new St. Joseph Hospital.

* * *

In 1912, the Kentucky Lunatic Asylum was renamed Eastern State Hospital. Since 1873, the name had been changed three times, using some variation of "Asylum." Now, it was striving to be a hospital, like most American asylums, and "Hospital" was included in the name, instead.

The asylum was originally developed in 1817 as Fayette Hospital. The hospital was not completed, and the original building was taken over by the state in 1824. That same facility had gone from the Fayette Hospital to the State Lunatic Asylum and now back to a hospital. This cyclic process of changing names was part of a national trend, but it was also symbolic of seeking better quality of care.

Since Transylvania University no longer had any graduate or professional programs, it became a liberal arts college and was renamed Transylvania College in 1915. That name has remained.

The Fayette National Bank, a fifteen-story building, was finished in 1915 at the northeast corner of Main and Upper Streets. That same year, Henry T. Duncan III, law partner of Colonel Allen, married Carolyn Goff.

The *City Directory* in 1919 listed Henry T. Duncan III and Colonel

John R. Allen's law office on the 15th floor of the Fayette National Bank Building, with a telephone number of 755. Their partnership started in 1901 when Colonel Allen dissolved a previous partnership of Broston & Allen. He had assumed that partnership, previously described as one of the oldest, strongest, and most successful law firms in Lexington, from his uncle, Judge Buckner. Duncan was considered one of the most brilliant young men to be admitted to practice. Their office in the Fayette National Bank Building was a crowning achievement for any law office.

The Board of Control of Eastern State Hospital continued to function with different leaders until 1920, when a new state organization was created. Eastern State Hospital was again reorganized under a statewide Board of Charities and Corrections. Grand juries continued to visit Eastern State Hospital with scathing negative reports. Urgent action was always requested, even promised, but the neglect continued, and the patient population continued to be over the facility's capacity. Local newspapers continued to report negatively about the institution.

*　　*　　*

In the early 1900s, a second Logan Gragg was born in Fayette County, Kentucky. His father, the first Dr. Logan Gragg, was a Fayette County physician who was identified as the attending physician for several members of the Rankin family in north Fayette County between 1930 and 1940, after he had graduated from the Ohio Medical School. That first Dr. Logan Gragg died on July 27, 1945. His father, W. O. Gragg, graduated from the old Louisville Medical School in 1854–1855 and practiced in Lexington in the late 1800s. The Gragg family practiced medicine in that same area of North Lexington for three generations.

The second Dr. Logan Gragg went on to become one of the outstanding leaders at Eastern State Hospital in the middle 1900s. As a local Lexington boy, he who had been told as a child, "If you don't mind your p's and q's, you will end up at the asylum on Fourth Street." He returned years later as a trained physician at that same facility where he had heard so much negativism in his youth, hoping to change things.

Two other employees who worked there and recorded their memories at a later time included Mrs. Anna Rogers, who was hired in 1922 as a nineteen-year-old single female. In 1968, she remembered, "I was immediately put to work on Ward I. Dr. Larue was superintendent and he claimed that there were twenty-three hundred patients. This would include those in the hospital and those on Convalescent Leave.

"I just knew it was very crowded," she continued. "Politics controlled everyone who worked there. We all just accepted that fact. I knew a political boss in my town, and he arranged for me to get the job. But the good employees cared about their jobs and viewed politics as the way in. We were determined to prove that politics did not control us."

Another employee who recorded her memories in 1968 was Mrs. Lucy Gamble, who was hired at Eastern State Hospital in 1923 as an aide. "Yes, knowing someone politically was the way to get a job. Everyone (including employees) either lived on a ward or in rooms next to their wards. For example, I worked on Wards I, II, and III. Living on the wards made it convenient to work," added Mrs. Gamble.

Mrs. Rogers explained, "We had two shifts, everyone worked twelve-hour shifts, and each ward had one or two employees at all times. We had one Sunday off monthly and one afternoon off each week."

"We had to have permission to leave the grounds, even on the days off," added Mrs. Gamble. "But it was fun because we were all there with the patients."

"Everyone lived on the grounds, and we all married each other. We all socialized together as employees and patients," Mrs. Rogers recalled. "Then a building was built in 1927, which the married employees moved into. This was what was later called Nurses' Building. The single ones continued to live on wards."

Mrs. Gamble remembered, "Patients attended plays in the old ballroom that they performed in. They also had dancing classes where the patients were encouraged to attend. The male and female patients were not allowed to mix except at socials in the ballroom."

Mrs. Rogers worked on the wards for one and half years and then took a position in the Occupational Therapy Department for the rest of her employment time. While she got the beginning job through politics, she advanced by having supervisors recommend her. She started working with patients as an attendant and later found a job opening as an occupational aide. She learned the job under the direction of a supervisor.

"I remember there was Occupational Therapy on each ward and the patients did displays for the Kentucky State Fairs. They often won blue ribbons for their entries," stated Mrs. Rogers.

Mrs. Gamble worked on the wards and on the telephone switchboard. When the supply officer left, she took over that job. She continued in some form of administrative job the rest of her employment time. "However, I was always filling in with different jobs as someone was needed."

Mrs. Rogers described the early facility: "There were no RNs in the twenties or thirties. Women worked only on the female wards and men worked on the male wards. We learned by watching the other employees. When we did get a nurse, her name was a Miss Rogers (and no relationship to me), and she started a training program for the aides."

There are photographs from the 1940s with Miss Rogers identified as superintendent nurse; Dr. Foley was the superintendent, and a Miss Cohran was the social director. Two other registered nurses identified in the 1940 pictures were Edith Chumley and Bessie McCord.

Mrs. Gamble stated, "All patients were transported here by train. There were aides who went up (to their homes) to get the patients, many times in sad, horrible conditions and would bring them back." She continued, "Often, a patient had to be brought out on a cot, and they were put in the train baggage car with an aide. It was often hard to bring them out of the mountains of Kentucky."

"Yes, the aides often told us how the local sheriff would meet them at the train station, and they would hike into some distant remote area to bring out a filthy, disturbed person who would often fight the aide," added Mrs. Rogers.

"Those patients were often difficult to get here, but they were well kept," added Mrs. Gamble.

"They had several dining rooms throughout the hospital. The women's dining room was part of Ward 10 and the men's was on Ward 16. They had china and white tablecloths that were changed twice a week. The patients took pride in their dining rooms and did much of the work. They were clean," Mrs. Gamble added proudly.

"And the doctors were well liked," added Mrs. Rogers. "Oh, there was always one that was not as well liked, but mostly all were liked, and they took care of the employees, too." Both Mrs. Rogers and Mrs. Gamble were proud of achievements that they observed during their employment.

In 1931, Miss Lilly Duncan died. She was the aunt of Elizabeth Duncan Allen and daughter of Henry Timberlake Duncan I. She was born in one of the most well-known Bluegrass estates in 1848, Duncannon. She also developed her own reputation in Lexington's society.

In 1870, Miss Lilly and her beautiful sister, Mrs. Mary Gibson, pooled their patrimonies and bought Ingleside, a mansion built in 1852. There Miss Lilly resided for the following fifty years and made it a show place. She had many parties and maintained political connections.

Upon Mrs. Gibson's death in 1910, Miss Lilly lived at Ingleside alone. Her memorial in the April 12 edition of the *Lexington Leader* stated, "Her recollection of Lexington which she saw grow from a pathetic little village to the current city, is not recorded. But she did a much better, higher thing. She bequeathed to the many that loved her, the enchanting perfume of a perfect life." She symbolized life of the wealthy in early Lexington.

On November 13, 1934, John H. Brand died at the age of ninety-three. He was the grandson of John Brand, a notable and outstanding figure in the early history of Lexington. They were survived by a granddaughter, Mrs. John R. Allen, and a grandson, Henry T. Duncan III, who was a law partner to Colonel Allen.

Colonel Allen died on March 22, 1937. He lived to the age of eighty and left no children. He was survived by his wife and two nephews, Colonel Allen J. Greer, of Buffalo, New York, and Rowan A. Greer, of Dayton, Ohio. His legacy was using political power for good, honesty, and upholding law and order over a long period of years in Lexington.

Politically he was a Democrat, but Colonel Allen was called to leadership in his party while "he was known as no party person at the bar of justice." As a result of this, he was time and again elected by Republican circuit judges as well as Democratic circuit judges.

Colonel Allen served as city attorney for Lexington, was county attorney for three terms, spent twelve years as master commissioner of Fayette Circuit Court, and served as the commonwealth's attorney for more than twenty years. His career was remarkable due to the local factionalism and bossism that controlled politics in Lexington and the state during his time.

Although both Henry T. Duncan II and III openly opposed the political powers and Colonel Allen was closely associated with them, he still survived in Lexington politics. Four of the six political bosses of Lexington were Catholics, and they controlled most of the political offices, Colonel Allen, a Protestant, still had an outstanding career; he refused to participate in the misuse and plunder of politics.

All this was described in Colonel Allen's obituary on March 22, 1937, in the *Lexington Leader.*

*　　*　　*

Overcrowding continued at Eastern State Hospital until it peaked in 1944 with 1,996 in-house patients. Mrs. Rogers remembered "the crowded conditions at the hospital."

Mrs. Gamble stated, "We were just pleased that there was finally a decrease in patients. More money for renovating the old buildings became available. While we were pleased, some of the older employees didn't see any need for changes. However, at the dedication of the renovation of the original building [in 1944], we had many visitors from Frankfort. We worked hard to show off while some employees wanted things to stay the same."

"Yes, the old wooden porches were fixed with concrete and the old buildings were fireproofed," added Mrs. Rogers. "The old employees finally approved of the improvements but they had been mostly baby sitters. I had difficulty getting employees to see the need for occupational therapy that gave the patients a challenge, not just something to occupy their time."

Mrs. Gamble stated that "when patients died who had no relatives, they would be buried on the grounds. In the early forties a social worker was concerned that there was no funeral service. So she created a chapel and saw that each dead patient had a funeral service. Then, later in the forties, patients' bodies were returned by train to their last known community."

"I remember that the aides used cars in the late forties to pick up patients and to return them to their homes," added Mrs. Rogers. "Things were better by then, and newer employees were more educated. There were several opportunities for more training."

This decline in population after 1944 was attributed to many factors in Kentucky: the creation of a fourth state mental hospital, medical developments, a "parole system" of community follow-up, and a hospital clinic, all similar to national trends in psychiatric care. Eastern State Hospital followed those trends.

The two-hundred-acre farm of Eastern State Hospital, which provided occupation for patients during the early years, was gradually being discontinued. James H. Reed, farm manager for fifty years, realized the changes were coming and retired in 1950. He had been educated at Transylvania University. His grandfather was Dr. Reed, an able physician in Clark County, Kentucky. His father was J. Henry Reed, who had enlisted and served under General Morgan's command during the Civil War. J. H. Reed was from an old and well-connected Lexington family.

J. H. Reed had described with delight how he would encourage withdrawn patients to work on the farm. While often criticized for making the lunatics work, he remembered how those who worked on the farm more often improved.

In 1950, Eastern State Hospital hired its first full-time master's-degreed psychologist, Jessie Irvine, who stayed many years. She was an advocate for patients' rights long before it became a popular term in psychiatric care. Other psychologists hired during the early 1950s were PhDs but did not stay long.

At the beginning of her employment at Eastern State Hospital, Irvine was both a psychologist and personnel officer. She agreed to be personnel officer until someone trained and experienced was hired. While Jessie preferred seeing individual patients, she had witnessed poor personnel officers who answered to their political bosses rather than to those at the hospital. Since she understood the need for a good personnel officer, Jessie kept both positions for two years.

The most current psychology theories were being applied in a city where the early theories of phrenology had been taught by Dr. Caldwell at Transylvania Medical School. Now, it was replaced by newer trained and qualified psychologists.

In 1952, Eastern State Hospital was once again reorganized into a Department of Mental Health. This change was expected to give the state hospitals more importance. Employees were being trained or hired according to national standards.

Local politicians controlled the hiring of all employees until a merit system was established in Kentucky by the middle 1950s. This change required that employees be hired and protected for their merit to do the job rather than based on one's politics or political connections. Those changes were slow and often irregular, as the old ways were hard to change.

Kentucky tried to follow national requirements toward what was called "professionalism." By 1955, thirteen out of the first sixteen state mental hospitals in America had at least one professionally trained psychologist, including Eastern State Hospital (Deese. 1991). While the Kentucky asylum was established for "curative purposes" in 1824, Eastern State Hospital was following the newer therapeutic methods by the middle 1900s. It followed the American trends in psychiatric care as it continued toward what was believed to be an acceptable state hospital, to include the most current treatment methods.

Mrs. Rogers recalled, "By 1953 all employees were working forty hours and five days a week. Conditions at the hospital were much improved for employees and patients."

Mrs. Gamble said, "All employees were being encouraged to live off of the hospital grounds as salaries improved. Employees had money to buy their own homes."

Since farm work was no longer available, industrial therapy was created to occupy and train patients for work throughout the facility, including the laundry and workshops established by vocational rehabilitation workers.

Mrs. Berta Oliver, laundry manager at Eastern State Hospital, said that she had been there since 1933, when the conditions were worse. She explained how "the laundry evolved into a therapy center in the forties and fifties. Although several patients had been trained for and later obtained specific jobs in local laundries, the primary purpose of industrial therapy in our laundry was to teach the patients to be responsible for any job they might obtain." Mrs. Oliver explained, "The laundry stimulated them to develop good work habits, self-confidence, and acceptable social behavior, all important in any job situation" (Oliver. 1961).

Dr. Logan Gragg first became the clinical director of Eastern State Hospital in 1953; he prescribed newly developed medications that created results that Drs. Allen and Chipley could have only dreamed about. The new medications were able to subdue the most difficult patients, who were often able to return back to their community; Dr. Gragg was able to witness a truly therapeutic hospital.

Dr. Gragg attended Transylvania University and the medical school in Louisville; he later served in the 29th Field Hospital during World War II and interned at Good Samaritan Hospital in Lexington; he had the unique qualities of a local physician that Chairman John W. Hunt had wished for back in 1840. Dr. Gragg changed that old asylum into an acceptable mental hospital, according to the expectations of the American Psychiatric Association.

The 1950s and 1960s were significant times for both Dr. Gragg and Irvine, as they witnessed changes in patients from the new medications and with changing treatment programs. Both Dr. Gragg and Irvine enjoyed telling this author about those times.

Irvine lived in Paris, Kentucky, in the same home where she and her sister, Katie, were raised. As a child, Irvine had not been expected to live. She often said that her will to live exceeded everyone's expectations. That experience set her up for a lifetime of determination by her own self-description. She claimed that determination proved to be valuable in her work at Eastern State Hospital. She often insisted upon each patient getting his or her specific needs met at a time when many were forgotten on the crowded wards. As always, when Jessie wanted something done, it was done, and it was always for a patient's benefit.

Jessie drove to Lexington from Paris each day. She would turn off of North Broadway onto Fourth Street, where old brick homes lined the street on one side and Transylvania College was on the other side. She observed how the houses became smaller and shabbier. On the right were tobacco warehouses and supply offices, which had replaced the earlier stockyards approaching the railroad crossing. After crossing the L. & N. Railroad tracks, she would see the imposing buildings of Eastern State Hospital on the right, behind an iron black fence.

At this time in the 1950s, the old two-story front gate house was gone, but the same road to the original building from Fourth Street continued. Jessie would turn left at the front of the Administration Building and park her car. All outside doors required a long brass key to open them, and Jessie had that key with her. She would walk up to a locked door in the middle section behind the Administration Building next to the female wards on the left and unlock the door to enter. She would walk toward the telephone switchboard in the back of the Administration Building and enter her office. She smoked as she went. Patients often followed her into her office, hoping she would give them a cigarette.

Her psychology office, which was across from the Personnel Office, had been a seclusion room. The Personnel Office was closed as long as she was expected to do both jobs. Her psychology office was simple, with a file cabinet for testing equipment. A simple table was available for administering the often used Rorschach test. Other tests included the Wechsler Adult Intelligence Scale and personality tests. Jessie fearlessly defended her use of psychology tests.

Eastern State Hospital consisted of several buildings, including the original and a three-story addition on the left built while Dr. Chipley was superintendent; another Administration Building had been added in the front and later attached to the older buildings. There was a dining and kitchen building added to the back of the three-story buildings, and two small octagonal buildings remained. On the right side of the original building was a new building that replaced the old "Negro" buildings, named for Dr. Wendell, a black physician. At the back of the facility were various small buildings that had been part of the old farm and a laundry building.

Because of earlier overcrowded conditions, some small farm buildings in the back were used for housing; they now remained empty. The whole hospital was heated by coal with an extension from the railroad track that went into the back of the kitchen area to store each delivery of coal. In the 1950s, the facility was still overcrowded and old. Smaller buildings such as the superintendent's home, a nurses' building, and a male employees' dormitory were still available but falling into disrepair.

Irvine first met Dr. Gragg upon his initial employment interview and instantly liked his quiet but competent manner. She orientated Dr. Gragg to the hospital as the personnel officer, but he was familiar with it already, having lived in the northern part of Fayette County.

They were instant friends. He also agreed with Jessie about the poor conditions of the institution; something had to be done. Dr. Gragg also recognized, along with Jessie, that electroshock treatment and electric coma treatment (ECT) were being overused at Eastern State Hospital. As clinical director, Dr. Gragg wanted to develop better ways to occupy the patients, who often lay on the hallway floors and hid in the old tunnels. Many others sat idle and withdrawn into their own worlds.

Jessie explained to Dr. Gragg her difficulty in hiring and keeping professionally trained employees. Many new employees witnessed distasteful experiences at the facility. She gave one example of Dr. Edgar Allen Moles, who was hired in 1951 as a psychologist. Dr. Moles left his employment a year later, due to "electro shock being the primary form of treatment with no therapy or psychology models in use." He refused to stay at Eastern State Hospital, but he did become a state official in the administration of the state hospitals in Frankfort.

Dr. Moles often told how "he observed the staff being so fearful of patients that they used ECT punitively as a means of control. No tranquilizers were used then, and broken bones often occurred. Patients were daily lined up in the halls for ECT. It was a horrible place to work." Dr. Gragg recognized that problem and started looking for competent employees who were willing to work in that state mental hospital regardless of the poor working conditions and inadequate care methods.

Electricity was first used for seizure induction in state hospitals in 1940 (Abrams. 1994) and spread throughout public hospitals with large populations of mentally ill patients. Eastern State Hospital used electroshock as early as 1946, according to the yearly reports. The 1947 Report of the Department of Welfare of the Commonwealth of Kentucky stated that a total of 130 patients were given ECT. The use continued to grow and dominated the attitude of staff. Newly qualified employees were horrified, and Dr. Gragg was determined to change that image.

He described in his handwritten notes of 1954 the forms of treatment used at Eastern State that year: electric coma treatment, insulin coma, and electro-narcosis. All this was too much, according to Dr. Gragg's observation.

Dr. Gragg was willing to try any new approach. He introduced the new drugs, Thorazine and Serpasil; Eastern State was the first state hospital to use these drugs in Kentucky. He later explained that "such drugs were not in the hospital budget so I had to get special approval from the governor to purchase them. The state was willing to try anything and I immediately was given permission."

As soon as Dr. Gragg noticed positive results from the new drugs, the other state mental hospitals followed his approach. This was the beginning of using new antipsychotic medications, leading to the future discharge of patients and the development of community care.

This process of discovering and testing newer medications continued for many more years in American state hospitals. For Kentucky, it started with Dr. Gragg at Eastern State Hospital in Lexington.

Irvine pushed for better trained employees. She did not hire someone who had a questionable personal history. Fearing that a new employee might be abusive toward a patient, she initiated the use of standard psychology personality tests to evaluate potential employees. She continued to administer personality tests for employee selection throughout her employment even after the psychology tests were determined to be discriminatory.

Jessie later became director of psychology full time and directed all her energy into developing individual and group therapy programs for all patients. She was well respected among the employees and patients.

Dr. Gragg described to this author his best example of a long-term patient who was dramatically changed by the new medications. He had observed a woman who had been locked in the basement of the facility and was given food through a hole in the door. She had a long history of violence during her years at Eastern State Hospital. She was so strong that it often took several attendants to restrain her. Restraining her enough to administer one of the new medications was a challenge for even the strongest attendant, knowing her reputation for hurting employees. Dr. Gragg suggested that they entice the patient by letting her reach through the hole in her door to get a favorite food.

When she did that, they were able to give her a first and second shot of the medication. Within a few days, she showed calmness that they had never seen in her. Later, the attendants and Dr. Gragg were able to open her door and give her more medication. The employees were amazed and cheered with Dr. Gragg. After a period of time, she continued to improve and verbalized an interest in herself. She showed rational behavior, while all the employees were thrilled over witnessing such a change in her. Later, as that same patient took an interest in her own appearance, she noticed that her left ear had been partly bitten off in one of her past fights. No one knew when or where the fight had occurred; she had been one of those forgotten ones. Since her appearance had improved so much after taking the new medication, the ear was even more unattractive.

She came to Dr. Gragg's office one day and asked if something could be done with her ragged left ear. Dr. Gragg made arrangements for the state to pay for plastic surgery on that ear. She continued to improve and was placed in a community home. She never returned to the institution.

Dr. Gragg often told this story as an example of the dramatic changes that were accomplished at that time. He claimed that the late 1950s were the most exciting times; he witnessed changes from the new medications with often-forgotten patients. It was "electrifying" to Dr. Gragg and his employees as they developed more innovative methods.

Mrs. Rogers developed more occupational therapy programs as the patients responded and needed more activities. The employees were excited to be part of such reformations in patients.

Yet, at the same time, politics within the Kentucky Mental Health Department reared its ugly head. In 1954, the head of that department, Dr. Gaines, resigned after the new governor would not allow him to run the Mental Health Department without political interference. Dr. Gaines told Dr. Gragg that he "was expected to fire employees from previous administrations and hire replacements approved by the new governor regardless of qualifications." Dr. Gaines left that position, which was viewed as a blow against professionalism in the Kentucky state mental hospitals.

In 1956, the two hundred acres of land that had been the farm land of Eastern State Hospital and owned by the state of Kentucky was sold to IBM Corporation. A typewriter manufacturing plant was dedicated that year and became a major source of jobs in Lexington, adding to the growth of the city. However, patients were no longer given opportunities to work on the farm. Dr. Gragg explained that most of the current patients were no longer from farming backgrounds, and farming was no longer a desirable job for patients. The hospital needed to get out of the farming business and concentrate on better care.

In 1956, Dr. Logan Gragg became superintendent (rather the clinical director) of Eastern State Hospital. He had proved his willingness to use any method to help patients, and the employees loved him for his concern for the unfortunates of society. His changes at Eastern State Hospital were recognized at both the local and national levels.

At the end of the 1950s, Eastern State Hospital was highlighted on a National Educational Television program as a "typical quality state mental hospital." The American Psychiatric Association credited Dr. Gragg with improving this old institution. Dr. Gragg and his employees achieved the status of a quality state mental hospital.

Dr. Gragg was interested in not only the present circumstances of the facility but also its past; he collected and preserved data from the early days of the asylum. His historical collections are preserved today by this author, who kept them from being thrown away in the trash.

In 1957, Dr. Gragg displayed some of that early history of the asylum in an open house. He was proud of the history of Eastern State Hospital;

a new building was named for Dr. John R. Allen, the first superintendent. Unfortunately, this tribute to Dr. Allen took place after his son, Colonel Allen, had died.

The Allen Building was created to combine the most current intensive treatment methods with short-term care techniques. Instead of placing a new patient among seventeen hundred others in the old buildings, the Allen Building provided specialized care in smaller groups.

Irvine was able to claim three psychology offices in the southeast side of the Allen Building. These three psychology offices were proof to her and others that psychology had finally become a modern and useful treatment modality. Psychology was no longer relegated to the abandoned seclusion rooms, as she often recalled. She continued as head of the Psychology Department until her retirement.

Also in 1957, a new medical school was started in Lexington. Groundbreaking ceremonies were held for the Albert B. Chandler Medical Center on Rose Street. The current leaders resurrected a medical school as the need became obvious. That facility was dedicated in September 1960 and named for the governor who initiated it.

This second medical center was dedicated 144 years after the Transylvania Medical School conferred its first Doctor of Medicine degree in 1816 and one hundred years after the last session was taught in 1860. The influence of the Medical Department of Transylvania University can scarcely be calculated, since it produced so many early physicians; the need for another one had been recognized.

As a final tribute to the early families associated with the asylum, Henry T. Duncan III, law partner of Colonel Allen, died in 1960. His son, John Allen Duncan, who was named for Colonel Allen, had followed the family tradition of attending what had become the law school at the University of Kentucky. While the Allen family in Lexington died out, the Duncan family continued.

So what does all this show for a small town in central Kentucky with one of the earliest asylums, as well as medical schools and law schools? Any one facility would have been remarkable for a small settlement, but there were three.

All three facilities have long histories. While the Transylvania Medical School failed before the Civil War, the other two facilities merged into different facilities into the next century. The asylum became a hospital, while the law department moved with the changing universities. After the new medical school was created, all three now exist in some form.

It shows a long-term commitment of families who contributed their time and money for developing these community facilities. The original members of the Chipley, Buckner, Duncan, Johnson, Hunt, Dudley, and Allen families have all gone, of course. But their names remain on buildings and streets in Lexington. They were part of concerned citizens who wanted to improve their world through education and with institutional care for the unfortunates of society. They contributed their time and expertise as the keepers and gatekeepers of the time.

*   *   *

And the story goes on for Eastern State Hospital. Dr. Gragg was so thrilled with the changes he observed at the hospital that he made sure that the local newspapers published stories about the place and proudly gave names to describe the events. He kept copies of those articles and later gave them to this author. Those articles give a glimpse inside that facility at a time when such publicity was encouraged and as therapeutic changes were being made. Although this author was there during some of the time, Dr. Gragg's articles are much better sources of information, and a chosen few will be described next.

On August 8, 1957, the *Lexington Leader* described an outing at Eastern State, where fifteen hundred patients attended the annual picnic. They participated in relay races and were entertained by a band. The food included forty-five hundred hot dogs, one thousand pounds of potatoes, and ice cream, pies, and other treats donated by individuals, clubs, and businesses. Patients who were unable to attend were served on the ward. A picture shows a large group of patients enjoying the picnic.

Another article that was undated from the *Herald-Leader* showed a photo of the new "resocialization and rehabilitation" unit at Eastern

State Hospital. It was a home-like atmosphere and was for the purpose of restoring patients to the community. The unit was called Uphill; seven women and twelve men were responsible for taking care of the unit, cooking their own food, washing their own clothes, and planning their own activities to live independently from hospital routine as possible. Patients would go to the hospital outpatient clinic to see their doctor and were responsible for taking their own medication. They had access to hospital personnel but acquired self-confidence in daily living with a near normal life. Another picture showed a bedroom of the Uphill Unit with Mrs. Jean Wood, nurse supervisor, and Mrs. Mary Washington, aide supervisor, assisting a resident.

An article on July 11, 1958, showed William Swann, a sixty-six-year-old patient at Eastern State Hospital who transformed a trash area into a beautiful flower garden. Swann was proudly pictured with his garden, and the article discussed how he created it.

Another picture on February 28, 1959, showed occupational therapy with men and women in the geriatrics admission unit weaving and making potholders. The men were "carding wool that came from sheep on the old hospital farm," while others were making "a pillow from ribbons saved from corsages and baskets of flowers." Employees that were pictured included head nurse of the unit, Mrs. Nancy Whitehead, and Mrs. Ann Rogers, occupational therapy aide. (This is the same Ann Rogers discussed in chapter 9.)

On March 16, 1959, an article discussed the Council of Patients at Eastern State Hospital; patients appointed representatives from each ward to take their concern about the institution to weekly council meetings. Most of the problems concerned food, clothing, recreation, or things that need fixing. Patients were encouraged to take part in their own environment and express their interest. The council was composed of two representatives from each of the twenty-three wards.

On March 18, 1959, a small article announced a dance for patients at Eastern State Hospital. Jock Godhelff and his orchestra played for a patients' dance at 7:30. The musicians for the occasion were provided through a grant from the Recording Industries Fund obtained in co-operation with Local 554, American Federation of Musicians.

On December 22, 1960, the *Lexington Leader* showed two pictures of Eastern State Hospital preparing for the holidays. There were about thirty sixteen-pound fruit cakes made for Christmas Day. The cooks proudly displayed them as their names were listed in this article. Turkeys with all the fixings were made to go with the cakes for approximately fifteen hundred patients. Table decorations included candles and greenery. Gifts sent in by thirty-eight community groups in eastern and central Kentucky would be handed out on Christmas Eve. One picture showed Mrs. Majel Moore, volunteer coordinator, handing a package to a patient who helped carry thousands of gifts from the receptionist's desk to the Santa Claus room in the basement.

On March 25, 1961, a picture showed Donald Shropshire, Eastern State Hospital administrator, and Mrs. Grace Turner, psychiatric aide instructor, honoring the twenty-five graduates of the aide program. The aides completed six months of training with three months of class work and three months of practical work under the supervision of registered psychiatric nurses. Eight current psychiatric aides received special certificates and pins for training in special areas of remotivation and resocialization. All these qualified psychiatric aides were expected to be employed at Eastern State Hospital.

Another undated picture in the newspaper showed carnival time at Eastern State Hospital. Patients in the wheelchair parade were pictured at the seventh annual patients' picnic-carnival. About twenty wheelchair patients were proudly lined up in front of the Administration Building.

On June 18, 1961, an article with pictures showed Dr. Evaline Plucknett, head of the outpatient clinic program at Eastern State Hospital, and other members of her staff, including Mrs. Catherine Joslin, secretary; Morton McAnally, psychiatric social worker; and Jessie Irvine, clinical psychologist. They were visited by Dr. Gragg, hospital superintendent. This article described the outpatient clinic team members who served for several years in four field clinics in the hospital's thirty-nine-county area. The clinics make it possible for many patients to remain at home who otherwise would have to be readmitted to the hospital.

June 29, 1961, the *Lexington Leader* had a picture of patients attending a picnic. There were eighteen booths at the picnic carnival at Eastern State Hospital. Approximately eleven hundred patients were entertained, with about one hundred volunteers and three hundred employees helping out. Relay races and other games were played. Hayrides were available with a picnic supper. The Pace Setters played for the group while the Buckskin Dancers performed.

In August 1961, an article in *Mental Hospitals*, titled "A Laundry Evolves into a Therapy Center," was written by Mrs. Berta Oliver, laundry manager at Eastern State Hospital. She described the process of how the laundry became part of the Industrial Therapy Department in 1955. Since the program started, an average of sixty-seven patients had worked in the laundry each day. Of those, 50 percent had adjusted to community life. The laundry stimulated patients to develop good work habits, self-confidence, and acceptable social behavior, important to any job situation. They took pride in returning all patient clothing in cleaned and pressed condition as the working patients improved in well-being and personal appearance.

On February 21, 1962, the *Lexington Herald* printed pictures and an article about honoring employees, a practice that Dr. Gragg encouraged. This one included Dr. Harold McPheeters, commissioner of the Department of Mental Health, who presented employee awards to 143 employees in a ceremony. The picture showed Mrs. Ann Rogers receiving a forty-year pin; Russell Kennedy received a thirty-year pin; and Mrs. Lucy Gamble was awarded a thirty-five-year pin. Other employees received pins for five, ten, fifteen, twenty, and twenty-five years of service.

On March 9, 1962, Dr. Gragg spoke at a Kiwanis Club meeting, stating that the hospital handled fourteen hundred patients a year on a budget of $4.50 per patient per day (a comparable figure for a private institution was $25 to $30). He stated that the purpose of the institution was to prevent needless hospitalization, treat inmates with respect and dignity, and rehabilitate them through consultation and therapy.

An article dated May 20, 1962, in the *Sunday Herald-Leader* stated that Eastern State Hospital had a new admission and outpatient clinic. The long article stated that it was located in the remodeled quarters of the basement of the Administration Building to handle the admission work once divided between two buildings. Dr. Stuart Brest was in charge of admissions with a specialized team that allowed more time devoted to each new patient. Previously, patients were admitted to different parts of the hospital by physicians who had many other routine chores to perform. Now, from 160 to 250 patients were seen each month, and about two-thirds of the patients released by the hospital became outpatients. Included with the article was a picture of admissions personnel: Dr. Brest was shown interviewing a patient, Mrs. Marian Gulley, secretary, Glenn Cole, a psychiatric aide supervisor; and Mrs. Pauline Iago, registered nurse, were also shown. Also included were Miss Sarah Toncray, admission psychiatric social worker, and Mrs. Marie Reynolds, admission clerk.

On June 28, 1962, in the *Lexington Leader,* a picture showed another patients' picnic at Eastern State Hospital. A hat booth became a favorite stop for the one thousand patients on the front lawn. Patients played games, visited booths, received a box picnic supper, and danced to music of the Blue Grass Hoppers. Smoke Richardson's Band played while a hundred volunteers helped.

On June 27, 1963, a picture in the *Lexington Leader* showed patients on another picnic at Eastern State Hospital. Women patients crowded around the hat booth as they selected hats to wear for the rest of the day. Approximately one thousand patients attended, played games, and visited the nineteen booths. Picnic suppers were served later.

On July 25, 1963, a photo was taken of Miss Mary Abbett serving a cup of punch to Dr. Logan Gragg during an Open House at Up-Hill. Others were Mrs. A. Moore, Miss M. Sprague, and Mrs. J. Dansby, volunteers, and Mrs. D. Johnson, hostess with Miss Abbett. The Open House was held in observance of Uphill's second anniversary. Eight women were living in the unit in preparation for leaving the hospital.

On September 10, 1964, a picture and article were published in a Lexington paper: "Mental Health Clinic Serves 200 per Month in Pikeville." The picture included visitors from Pike County who were being orientated at Eastern State Hospital. They were Miss Dolly Curry and Mrs. Margaret Stratton, public health nurses, with Hart Ransdall, psychiatric social worker in charge of the clinic, Mrs. Teressa Roche, psychiatric nurse at the clinic, and Mrs. Avanell Hunt, secretary. The clinic obtained social and medical data on patients before they were admitted to the hospital and worked with the families of patients, helping them understand the effects of mental illness and ways of coping with it.

Another undated picture in the *Leader* was titled "Volunteers Honored at Eastern State Hospital." Red Cross volunteers were honored for serving at the hospital as volunteers for the past ten years. Dr. Gragg, as superintendent, presented certificates to each volunteer, and their names were listed in the article.

On October 11, 1964, an article and picture were published by the *Herald-Leader* titled, "Some Patients at Eastern State Hospital Earn Token Pay." A program at the four state mental hospitals was launched in July to pay three to fifteen cents a day to patients (who had never been paid before). The state did not supply the money; it came from raising and selling vegetables to hospital employees; the article explained that "prices were not to give unfair competition to outside vegetable growers." Money also came from ironing shirts and washing cars for staffers. Eugene Lee, director of Industrial Therapy, stated there were 365 patients receiving pay in the five grades of earnings. Two patients were at the top grade of earning fifteen cents per day, while twelve patients were making ten cents a day. "Someday, we hope to be able to pay as much as a quarter an hour," Lee stated. "Patients do most of the manual labor at the hospital. While we would like for the hospital to be in such shape that patients would not be asked to do work that is not therapeutic, the boiler room, one example, could not operate without patient help." It was through this program that many working patients, who had no money at all, now had at least a little to spend as they wished. "This can be a good beginning," Lee said.

On July 7, 1965, a Lexington paper published before-and-after pictures of the cafeteria of Eastern State Hospital. The article, "Cafeteria for Patients at Eastern State Hospital Is Remodeled, Newly Equipped," said that the $100,000 project had started the previous November. The newly renovated and newly equipped cafeteria had Dr. Gragg as hospital superintendent and other hospital officials dishing up the food for the first patients at the noon meal. A total of 720 patients were served at each meal with forty employees and twelve cooks in the hospital's Dietary Department.

Another undated article published in the Lexington paper was titled, "New Program at Eastern State Meets Approval of Officials." Eastern State Hospital officials announced a new program for older men and women patients over fifty years of age to be housed in the Geriatrics Admissions Unit. This unit, a first in hospitals of the Kentucky State Department of Mental Health, created a healthy atmosphere of daily mixing and mingling among the patients. The new ward had fewer than a hundred patients and was under the full-time care of Dr. W. E. Rich. This article included several examples of improved patients on that ward.

On July 23, 1965, Eastern State Hospital launched a new project for Fayette County patients at a luncheon. The program was aimed at preventing unnecessary hospitalizations and shortening hospitalizations. Principals at the luncheon included Dr. Gragg, hospital superintendent; W. Van Meter Alfor, president of the Mental Health Association; Theodore Fasso, psychiatric social work consultant for Region 3 of the Department of Mental Health, Education and Welfare; and Dr. Cleta Elequin, psychiatrist and director of the Fayette County project.

In the *Lexington Leader* on August 12, 1966, there was an article and picture of a Honduran social worker studying at Eastern State Hospital. She was one of two social workers employed at the Hospital Neuro-Psiquiatrico in Honduras. The article talked about the hospital in Honduras and how she would apply her learning from Eastern State Hospital to her hospital.

On October 5, 1966, two pictures in the *Lexington Herald* showed hospital awards given by Dr. Gragg to Mrs. Lucy Gamble for forty years, Thurman Judd for twenty-five years, Mrs. Sue Wilson for fifteen years, Mrs. Mary Washington for ten years, and Dr. German Gutierrez for five years. Another picture showed Eastern State Hospital honoring six employees who were retiring in 1966. Dr. Gragg presented gifts to Mrs. Mason Williams for ten years in nursing education, Martha Lindsey for eight and a half years in social service, and Marvin Robert for fifteen years in maintenance.

Then on June 7, 1967, there was an article in the *Lexington Leader* titled, "Eastern State Hospital Gets Historical Marker: The Second Oldest in the U.S." A picture showed the dedication of a historical marker at Eastern State Hospital. Present were W. A. Wentworth, chairman of the Kentucky Historical Markers program; Dr. Dale Farabee, commissioner of the State Department of Mental Health; Mrs. Elmer Deiss, chairman of the Fayette County Markers Program; Dr. Joseph Parker, chairman of the Department of Psychiatry at the University of Kentucky Medical Center; and Dr. Gragg, hospital superintendent. The article gave a general history of Eastern State Hospital. The current administration included approximately 510 employees, including eighteen physicians. The treatment programs utilized the team approach with motivating more community interest. Patients were referred to a clinic in their area when they left.

On June 18, 1967, another article about hospital employees being honored was published. There were fifty-five employees honored for a total of 575 years of service. Mrs. Ann Rogers of the Occupational Therapy Department received a pin for the longest time of service, forty-five years, while Dr. Rich, staff physician, had fifteen years, Mrs. George Embry in the Nursing Department had twenty years, Mrs. Lester Baker, Occupation Therapy, had twenty-five years, and Mrs. Hugh Edwards, Nursing Department, had thirty-five years. Dr. Gregg presented the pins.

In July 1967, an article written by Earl E. Staton, executive director of the Kentucky Mental Health Manpower Commission, and published in the *Journal of Hospital & Community Psychiatry*, discussed the opening of a day care center for children of employees at Eastern State Hospital. For a small fee, the center provided a well-supervised program of education, guidance, training, and care for children from three to six years old. The center proved to be a valuable asset in recruiting and retaining hospital staff and continued for many years.

On July 27, 1967, the following article was published: "Eastern State Hospital Patient Load Drops below 1,000." The patient load had dropped for the first time in fifty-nine years. Dr. Gragg attributed the decline mainly to reorganization in the hospital's treatment programs, which had started a year ago. "Instead of one total program and one clinical director," he said, "we have five treatment services and five clinical directors." Patients in the hospital at the close of the year in 1958 totaled 1,690; in 1965, there were 1,218.

One picture printed in the *Lexington Leader*, April 17, 1968, showed a dedication ceremony for the new day care center at Eastern State Hospital. Pictured were Fayette County's Judge Joe Johnson, Mayor Charles Wylie, and Mrs. Norma Jean Levitch, future staff member of the center. The Jaycees solicited supplies for the Mental Health Service and renovated the building. Another picture included the opening of the day care center, with Dr. Gragg, superintendent of Eastern State Hospital, and Pete Perlman, president of the local Jaycees. On hand for the ceremonies were many city and state officials. The day care center was a joint program of the hospital and the Comprehensive Care Center of the Central Kentucky Regional Mental Health-Retardation Board. It was staffed by personnel from both agencies and provided psychiatric treatment for people who did not need full-time hospitalization.

That same year, awards were given to employees: J. T. Fraley, personnel officer of the Kentucky Department of Mental Health, presented service pins to Mrs. Iva Frazier, secretary to the superintendent, for thirty years, Mrs. Beulah Brown, Nursing Service, for twenty-five years, Miss Ann Benckhart, laboratory technician, for twenty years, and Dr. Gragg, hospital superintendent, for fifteen years of service.

On May 27, 1969, this article was printed: "Eastern State Working for a Program Called Open Hospital." Under the current program, only potentially dangerous patients would be locked in their wards. Others would have daytime freedom of the grounds and hospital. About half of the approximately sixteen hundred patients were already on open wards but more planned activities were needed. Open wards were not the objective, rather planned activities to occupy everyone were the objective.

Proudly displayed in the *Lexington Leader* on May 27, 1969, was this announcement: "Accreditation after 145 Years." That important article will be completely quoted:

Eastern State Hospital in Lexington, America's second oldest state hospital has made remarkable improvements within recent years and for the first time has been granted full three-year accreditation from the Joint Commission on Accreditation of Hospitals. Such accreditation is far from routine, ever for newer hospitals. High standards of patient care must be met and it is quite an achievement when an institution whose history goes back some four decades before the Civil War can meet those high standards.

Dr. Logan Gragg, who resigned as Superintendent of Eastern State Hospital around the time the accreditation inspection was being made, surely deserves most of the credit for improvements at Eastern State during his 16 years there.

During the early 1940s, the American College of Surgeons (predecessor of the Joint Commission) made an inspection of Eastern State and reported that there was no hope that the century and a half old institution would ever be accredited.

Kentucky Commissioner of Mental Health, Dale H. Farabee, is right when he suggested that the "hospital staff, assisted by the chiefs of service, have worked with tireless dedication to pass a rigid inspection by the Joint Commission to win the accreditation."

Eastern now becomes the second of Kentucky's four psychiatric hospitals to be given the accreditation rating. Central State in Louisville was accredited in 1967.

The people of Eastern and Central Kentucky should be pleased with the progress which has been made at Eastern State, for in the final analysis, the new accreditation rating means that the hundreds of patients who annually use Eastern State's facilities will now have better care.

On April 30, 1969, Dr. Gragg had submitted his resignation as superintendent of Eastern State Hospital; he had been told by the current Commissioner of Mental Health that he could not continue in his current position, so he chose to resign. The commissioner had created a new policy in the State Department of Mental Health requiring every psychiatric hospital superintendent to have completed three years of psychiatric residency. Dr. Gragg's residency was in internal medicine, but he had passed an examination by the American Psychiatric Association that qualified him as a mental hospital administrator. That was not adequate for the new commissioner. It was also a foreshadowing of future ways when older employees were eliminated as newer employees were hired in mental institutions.

While Dr. Gragg was offered other positions in Kentucky state government, he refused them all. He did not want to work anywhere else. There were many published articles reacting against his resignation. The *Lexington Herald* criticized the Kentucky Department of Mental Health for forcing him out. That article stated, "In view of Dr. Gragg's record at Eastern State Hospital, we believe he should remain there. ... We do not want to see Dr. Gragg leave until we know how his departure will help Eastern State and its patients."

Two other milestones that Dr. Gragg achieved while at Eastern State Hospital need mentioning; first, he established a Bureau of Vocational Training where patients were taught work habits in a trade school. Patients were encouraged to follow the training opportunities for outside employment. Another program Dr. Gragg created was to educate workers in other fields, such as nursing, psychology, social work, seminary, or medicine, giving them practical experience at the hospital and opportunities for working with the mentally ill.

On April 25, 1969, Dr. Gragg's replacement was announced, while he accepted a position at the local Veterans Administration hospital. For years, employees continued to talk about how poorly Dr. Gragg had been treated, while many expressed anger over losing a friend and colleague.

As one interested in the hospital's history, I was fortunate to talk to Dr. Gragg about his experiences years later. He was not bitter but rather thankful for the experiences that he had had at Eastern State Hospital. He was a one-of-a-kind person who only thought of ways to improve patient care, always had their best interests in mind, and cared about his employees.

Sources for Chapter 8

Abrams, R. "The treatment that will not die: Electroconvulsive therapy." *Psychiatric Clinics of North America* 17 (1994): 525–530.

American Phrenological Journal. "A Life Illustrated." June 1861.

Armstrong, David, and E. Armstrong. *Phrenology: Bonehead Medicine, Great American Medicine Show*, 71–79. New York: Prentice Hall, 1991

Bolin, James. *Bossism and Reform in a Southern City: Lexington, Kentucky, 1880-1940.* Lexington, Kentucky: University of Kentucky Press, 2000.

Bridges, Dr. Drew. "Phrenology." *Hospital and Community Psychiatry Journal* (October 1994).

Courier-Journal. "Overcrowding Reducing Recovery Rate at Eastern State Hospital for Insane." April 1931.

Courier-Journal. "State Should Take Advantage of Developments." April 20, 1937.

Courier-Journal. "Treatment of Mentally Ill Is Advised." April 28, 1937.

Courier-Journal. "Why Did Dr. Gaines Resign?" November 25, 1956.

Cunningham, H. *Doctors in Gray: The Confederate Medical Service.* Louisiana State University Press, 1958.

Deese, W. "The Evolution of Psychology in the Early State Mental Hospitals." Presented at Centennial Annual Convention of the American Psychological Association, Washington DC. 1991.

Deese, W. Interview with Dr. Edgar Moles 1979. Discussion about his experiences at Eastern State Hospital in 1951.

Deese, W. Several interviews with Dr. Gragg about his recollections of the history of Eastern State Hospital.

Deese, W. "In Memory of Jessie Irvine." *The Kentucky Psychologist* 21, no. 7 (September–November 1987): 6–7.

Deese, W. "Phrenology on Old Postcards." *Postcard Collector,* 1997.

Deese, W. "Dr. Thomas S. Kirkbride." *Encyclopedia of Psychology.* The American Psychological Association, 1999.

Escape from the Cage. A videotaped interview of Dr. Gragg at Eastern State Hospital by Stephen Palmer in cooperation of the American Psychiatric Association on National Educational Television. 1957. Original copy was at ESH and copy was given to the author.

Fowler, O. S. "On Matrimony: or Phrenology and Physiology Applied to the Selection of Companions for Life." *Practical Phrenology.* New York: Fowler & Wells, 1890.

Gamble, Lucy. An interview taped upon her retirement from Eastern State Hospital, conducted by Dr. Gragg. June 12, 1968.

Gragg, Dr. Logan. Handwritten notes of treatment programs at ESH 1954. Found in history of ESH and confirmed later by Dr. Gragg.

Gragg, Dr. Logan. Handwritten notes of patients treated with Chlorpromazine. July 1956. Records of Dr. Gragg and given to author.

Gragg, Dr. Logan. Pictures and articles collected by Dr. Gragg. 1957–1969. Given to author in 1994.

Herald Leader. "Asylum Changes." June 1, 1900.

Herald Leader. "Asylum Employees." February 15, 1902.

Herald Leader. "Asylum Report: Seventy-Fifth Annual Report of the Eastern Kentucky Asylum for the Insane." January 4, 1900.

Herald Leader. "Fourth at the asylum." July 5, 1900.

Herald Leader. "Semi-Annual Inspection of the Eastern Kentucky Lunatic Asylum by the Board of Commissioners." May 17, 1901.

Johnson, Governor Keen. Official Kentucky Road Map, Issued by the State Highway Department 1939–1943.

Kerr, Judge Charles, ed. "Henry T. Duncan and James H. Reed." In *History of Kentucky*, Vol. IV. Chicago: The American Historical Society, 1922.

Lexington Herald. "Captain Charlton H. Morgan, Brother of General, Is Dead." October 11, 1912.

Lexington Herald. "Colonel John R. Allen." March 22, 1937.

Lexington Herald. "Dr. Robert L. Willis Made New Superintendent of EKLA, J. H. Reed Again Chosen Steward." June 15, 1908.

Lexington Herald. "800 Attend Open House at ESH. New Building at Hospital to be Named for Allen." May 18, 1958.

Lexington Herald. "Grand Jury Returns Indictment for Murder against 4 Attendants at EKLA." October 17, 1906.

Lexington Herald. "Irregularities, Including Murder, at EKLA Ordered Investigated by Grand Jury." October 2, 1906.

Lexington Herald. "J. H. Brand was Member of Notable Family." November 13, 1934.

Lexington Herald. "Ketterer Estates Suit with Dr. J. S. Redwine, Superintendent of EKLA Begun before Civil Court Judge Parker." February 26, 1907.

Lexington Herald. "Miss Lilly Duncan: A Memorial." April 12, 1931.

Lexington Leader. "New 100-Bed Building at Eastern State Expected Ready for Use Soon." July 12, 1957.

Lexington Herald. "Records & Equipment Displayed at Eastern State." September 27, 1957.

Mayo, W., ed. *Medicine in the Athens of the West, 1799–1950: The History and Influence of the Lexington-Fayette County Medical Society,* 1999.

Mental Hospital Committee. *Survey of the State Hospitals of Kentucky and New York.* Kentucky Archives, Lexington, Kentucky 1938.

Oliver, B. M. "Laundry Evolves into a Therapy Center." Abstract. *Mental Hospitals* (August 1961): 34–35.

Rogers, Anna. Recorded interview upon retirement of her years at Eastern State Hospital, conducted by Dr. Gragg. June 12, 1968.

Stout, G. F. *A Manual of Psychology.* New York: Hinds and Noble, 1899.

Wells, Samuel R. *New Physiognomy or Signs of Character.* New York: Fowler & Wells, 1894.

Chapter Nine

1990–1994

Since the time between the last chapter and this one at Eastern State Hospital, over twenty years has passed and a short explanation is needed. There were three major changes that had happened prior to the beginning of this chapter. First, the patient population had dropped from 999 in 1967 to under 300; most patients were being discharged due to increased medication usage and treatment programs. Second, the number of employees was being reduced as the patients decreased; they reached a maximum of 510 in 1967. This created stressful working conditions from threats or actual involuntary terminations of employees. Increasing educational requirements were added as the older or less educated employees were phased out. The state merit system was expected to protect those who did their jobs adequately; however, that interpretation was always disputed.

Dr. Gragg was at the beginning of that process when requirements for his position increased, and he was no longer qualified after fifteen years on the job. Another example happened with the social worker positions, which required a BA degree in 1960, but by 1990, the positions required a master's degree in social work. The current social workers either went back to school for that master's degree or they were fired.

Third, the older buildings were renovated as changing treatment methods required different spaces. The original building of 1824 was renovated for the second time with air-conditioning being was added. It was named for Dr. Logan Gragg on June 1, 1985; he and his wife were there to accept the honor. The commissioner who fired him had long gone, but Dr. Gragg was still remembered for his contributions to the facility.

In this chapter, the author goes back to that time to share her own experiences that were written down then. Anyone who might disagree with these interpretations is welcome to write his or her own understanding of that history.

The people involved include Winnie (the author), a master's-degreed psychologist at Eastern State Hospital since 1967, and Jean Newman, a new employee who worked in the Recreation Department. She and Winnie became close friends and shared events as they witnessed them.

The superintendent position historically required an MD; in 1990, the position was changed to director, and a PhD psychologist was required.

The psychology supervisor previously requiring an MA in psychology, now requiring a PhD, was Winnie's supervisor.

Dr. David Atcher, MD, was the medical director of the Geriatric Wards.

Other employees who helped with the History Celebration are identified later in the chapter.

*　　*　　*

Winnie entered the Allen Building, the very building where Jessie Irvine, as director of psychology, had hired her twenty-three years earlier. The Allen Building was opened in 1957 as a short-term intensive care facility and named for the first superintendent, Dr. John R. Allen. Although the Allen Building had changed in the last years, the other hospital buildings that were part of Eastern State Hospital had seen even more changes, which had started as the Kentucky Lunatic Asylum in 1824. That history had often been ignored except during the time when Dr. Logan Gragg was superintendent and Jessie Irvine was director of psychology. Now, they were gone, and geriatric patients occupied the Allen Building.

Winnie entered her psychology office to lock up her purse and check her schedule. She proceeded across the hall to the recreation room, where Jean Newman was busy hanging up decorations for Easter. The room was always cheerfully decorated and a source of enjoyment for patients and employees. Jean was always a ray of sunlight as she anticipated each holiday and planned for patient participation. After raising five children, she went back to school for a college degree and was hired in the Recreation Department at Eastern State Hospital. She had always enjoyed doing crafts, and now she encouraged patients to make crafts to hang throughout the recreation room. Patients loved her interest in activities and were eager to participate with her.

"Hello, Jean!" Winnie said as she took a chair next to her. "I cannot stay long since I hear we have a new patient on Allen II."

"Well, do you have time to drink a cup?" Jean asked, continuing to hang some crafts made by patients. "Coffee is ready, and oh, by the way, good-morning."

They both laughed at their own rudeness.

"No, I must see that new patient. I understand there is some controversy over her," Winnie said as she pushed up to get out of the chair.

"We have new patients all the time, why is this one different?" asked Jean, stopping to sit down in the next chair.

"Well, you know how the administration is around here; there is a lot of concern about this one, and I need to see what is going on. I saw our nurse in the parking lot as I was coming in and she said the hospital director and the psychology supervisor were looking at the new admission's chart. That is all I know, but I need to see for myself why they are so concerned," stated Winnie as she moved toward the door.

"I still don't know why they would care since they usually ignore the geriatric wards," stated Jean, picking up another decoration to hang.

"I don't know but I will find out." Winnie started toward the door.

"Oh, don't forget, you have the group discussion this afternoon; do you know what your topic will be? We can write it on the board for patients to read and discuss when they come to the morning activities."

"Yes, I found a newspaper article about Florida making their train tracks into walking trails. The article will encourage everybody to talk about the old railroad trains, so that will be our subject for group discussion this afternoon. You can start everybody talking about old trains and get them interested. I will be ready this afternoon for the group discussion." Winnie left the recreation room and went toward the wards where patients were housed.

She entered the nurses' station on Allen II and picked up the chart of Anna Rogers. She flipped through the chart and found no current information about the patient or even why she had been admitted here. Having given up on getting any useful information, Winnie went into the patient's room. The room was clean with new paint, and she noticed someone sitting next to one of two beds.

"Are you Mrs. Rogers?" she asked.

"Yes, I am," answered the tense female sitting in the chair by her bed. She had white hair, but it was well kempt and neat.

"Hello, I am Winnie, an employee here. May I talk to you?" She sat down in a nearby chair.

"Why, yes, but I don't understand why I'm here. I need a place to live, but I don't know why they sent me here. Who did you say you were?" Mrs. Rogers frowned with uncertainty.

"I'm Winnie, a psychologist here. I'm here to help all of us to understand why you are here."

"Oh, no one here can help me; I sold my farm and need a place to live. I didn't know why they would send me here."

"How old are you, Mrs. Rogers?"

"I'm eighty-eight, and I was doing all right until I had to sell the farm after Herman's death. I need a place to live, and someone sent me here."

"And what is today's date?" Winnie asked, trying to assess the patient's cognition.

"Oh, it is March 28, 1990," Mrs. Rogers responded quickly.

"That is correct; do you know where you are?" asked Winnie.

"Yes, of course! I'm at Eastern State Hospital in the Allen Building. I used to work here when Dr. Gragg was the superintendent; that was many years ago."

"Well, most people don't want to admit working here," responded Winnie in humor.

Ignoring the humor, Mrs. Rogers responded seriously, "It is true, I retired from here, but you young people have no idea how hard we worked against all odds here. Most of the buildings were not as nice as this one." She looked around at the newly painted walls and modern furniture.

"Yes, Mrs. Rogers, this building has recently been remodeled. But tell me, what did you do here?"

"I worked in Occupational Therapy. We made mops, brooms, draperies, and had a sewing room. I can remember all my past but I have trouble with today."

"But, Mrs. Rogers, you knew today's date. That is a good sign," replied Winnie. She started moving her chair closer to Mrs. Rogers so that they were not so far apart.

"I cheated," said Mrs. Rogers. "I saw the calendar in the next room."

"That is why the calendar is there," Winnie responded quickly. "You were looking for the date but there are people here who never bother to pay attention to any dates."

"Yes, I know, I used to work with those people, and I often posted calendars like you have done to help them," replied Mrs. Rogers.

"What has changed since you retired?"

"After many years, my husband, Herman, died and I just cannot manage the farm, so I sold it. Now I need a place to live until I can join Herman too."

"Do you have any children, Mrs. Rogers?"

"No, it was just Herman and me," she responded sadly.

"I'm so sorry about Herman," Winnie said. Their eyes met in a shared exchange.

"There is just no one left." Her eyes wandered away sadly.

"I am so sorry; have you talked to Cleo Coleman, your social worker?"

"I haven't talked to anyone but you. I certainly do not want to stay here."

"Since you worked here so long, I would think that you would feel comfortable being here; do you?" Winnie asked, hoping to tap into good memories of the place if she had really been a previous employee. Winnie was still unsure if Mrs. Rogers did work here in the past.

"Oh, no, in my day, all the elderly came here to die. I don't want that. I have a retirement from the state. Of course, not much now but I don't want to die here as I saw them do in the past. Certainly, there is a better place for me."

"Yes," replied Winnie, "I'm sure there is but since you devoted so much time here in the past, why not stay until things can be worked out for you? As you know, the state moves slowly."

"But the other employees I worked with are not here, those people I miss. It is not the same place to me. Mrs. Lucy Gamble and I were best friends, and she has been long gone. Mr. Reed and Dr. Gragg are all gone, even Jessie Irvine is gone, so it is not the same place."

"Oh, you knew those people?" Winnie remembered their names from the hospital's history. Now, she was convinced that Mrs. Rogers was not delusional because she gave real names of people in the history of the hospital.

"Oh, yes, we were all dear friends and we enjoyed working together," responded Mrs. Rogers.

"Well, Mrs. Rogers, I will talk to your social worker and see how soon we can find another place for you." Winnie stood up from the chair to excuse herself.

Mrs. Rogers quickly rose and said, "Thank you for talking to me; will you come back, please?"

"Yes, I will. I will read your chart and try to get you out of here." As Winnie started to leave, she reached for Mrs. Rogers to hug her and felt an instant bond. Mrs. Rogers quickly responded to the friendly hug. Winnie had learned from experience that elderly people responded well to such hugs while other professionals still criticized the practice. Mrs. Rogers showed personal warmth but was genuinely concerned over her situation. *She does not show any delusions,* Winnie thought to herself.

Winnie went to the nurses' station, hoping that new information had been added to Mrs. Rogers's medical chart; but as she reached for the chart, Dr. David Atcher grabbed it and said, with a silly smile on his face, "Nothing in there!"

"Oh, so you are also waiting," replied Winnie as she sat down next to Dr. Atcher. They had often complained together about how, even with all the well-educated employees, when it came to basics such as a current medical chart with all necessary information, data was often missing. They just looked at each other as Winnie shook her head. "Oh, this place stinks." They understood each other. The nurses' station was empty except for them so they often expressed their disgust when no one was around.

"Well, Winnie, did you see our new delusional patient? At least that was what the admission physician said," stated Dr. Atcher.

"Yes, I saw her but she is not delusional. She named people who worked here in the past. She might have other problems that I don't know about since there is nothing in the chart, but delusional? No," replied Winnie.

"Well, she claims to have worked here; isn't that delusional?"

"I have researched the history of this institution. She named several people who worked here in the past. I will check with the Personnel Department to see what they have on her, since we have no social history. Personnel should have something since she worked here." Winnie continued to ignore Dr. Atcher's disparaging comments about not finding any information.

"Now, Winnie," Dr. Atcher continued with his joking, "who in their right mind would want to admit to having worked here? Now, let's be real, she can't be in her right mind." He laughed. Winnie knew that he wasn't joking about the patient, but the stupidity of a system that was so dysfunctional that someone like Mrs. Rogers could not be properly placed except in a mental hospital.

"Oh, Dr. Atcher, you and your opinions are based on today's problems. There were earlier employees who really enjoyed working here, and that is part of our history that many current employees do not understand." Winnie realized that Dr. Atcher was teasing her when she was most serious. She sat back to relax.

"If I ever admit to being a part of this place, I will be delusional," stated Dr. Atcher as he returned to his charting. "Anyway, Winnie, at eighty-eight years old, what can you expect from her? She is actually in good physical condition."

At this point, Winnie was having difficulty accepting the casual way that Dr. Atcher was responding to this situation. She continued, "Can you see how this poor woman has been harmed? I believe that she may have been a pioneer here at this facility, and how does the facility react? I'll tell you how, she is called delusional! Instead, we need to be praising her. She is a hero here. This facility is so callous that we can't even recognize the giants in our history!" Winnie sat back in her chair, knowing that she was wasting her time complaining.

Dr. Atcher reached over and patted Winnie on the shoulder, "Now, Winnie, we all know how this place is; if you expect to see any important information in Mrs. Rogers's chart, forget that."

"Well, if there is nothing significant in the chart, how can we make any significant assessments? Where is all the professionalism that we have here? We need some outside collaboration to confirm what we are seeing," stated Winnie.

"Yes, I agree, but the wheels around here grind slowly," replied Dr. Atcher.

"I know. Cleo Coleman is her social worker, and she is usually on top of things, but she is so excited about her upcoming retirement that her work is not getting done. Who will do her work when she retires? Shouldn't someone be covering for her?"

"Well, Winnie, how should I know?"

"Isn't the second social worker helping out? Isn't that his job to cover?"

"He refuses to do the extra work, and his boss is over in the main office, so he gets by with anything."

Winnie looked disgusted at Dr. Atcher and said, "And you are medical director here. How can I do a psychological assessment without any history? I believe that Mrs. Rogers worked here but I have no information on how long ago or if she was really a good employee or some goof-off like our other social worker." Winnie was irritated but also realized that she was just wasting her time.

Dr. Atcher looked at Winnie and responded in his usual humor, "I just work here; you know the answer to that question since you have worked here longer than I." He was good at soothing and listening to employees. He was also good at using humor to defuse situations. Winnie decided to lighten up to his humor.

"Yeah, so don't rub it in," replied Winnie, laughing. "But you are younger than I and you have other job opportunities."

"Maybe I don't have any other opportunities," joked Dr. Atcher, "but don't tell anyone." He continued in his humorous way so that Winnie knew his intentions were to be a friend to a colleague.

"So, you are like me, lost in the state system, waiting for retirement time?"

"Yes, Winnie," Dr. Atcher said, becoming serious, "things could be worse here."

"Yes, and believe it or not, I actually enjoyed my job here. That was before my supervisor became boss and supervisor of psychology. I have never had one bad supervisor in all my twenty-three years of working here except for the current one. I still enjoy my friends and fellow employees here, though."

"Well, don't count me as one," Dr. Atcher retorted jokingly.

"No, not you," Winnie laughed at his humor. "But I still expect results after all these years, while you have already given up on anything getting done around here."

"Yes, I have," Dr. Atcher said as he returned to his serious side.

"Actually, I have to fight the system to keep myself from getting bored and depressed around here. I cannot accept the current administration but I love my job with the patients and some employees," added Winnie. "I just hate certain parts of it that are crazy."

"Well, I'm certainly not going to respond to that," smiled Dr. Atcher. Then, he leaned back into his chair and looked around the nurses' station to make sure no one was around. His expression grew serious as he lowered his voice so others could not hear him saying, "I did see your 'favorite supervisor' this morning looking around here for your mistakes."

"So, are you telling me this to make me more nervous or to keep me informed? I have known for some time my supervisor had plans to eliminate me from the state payroll," she whispered in a lowered tone. Both knew that there were many unhappy employees who thrived on the disputes around the hospital; any overheard information was often source for gossip so they continued to whisper.

"Your supervisor kept asking me questions about your work and arguing with me that your work was inadequate, even when I kept telling him that I was satisfied. He was not listening to me even though I am the one who should know."

Smiling, Winnie stated, "I thought you were not one to take sides in these personnel issues, at least you told me that."

"I don't take sides," he grinned, "especially since you are not a friend of mine." He smiled and then changed tone, saying, "Seriously, I just think you should know this."

"Thank you, Dr. Atcher, I will try to watch things, but as you know, I'm not perfect. I do try hard to keep my work up as I think it should be. But when my supervisor digs for dirt to fire someone, we all know that he will do it; he has succeeded with other employees, and now he is trying it on me."

"Are you able to defend yourself?" asked Dr. Atcher seriously.

"Yes, I have hired an attorney, and I will not go down as easily as I have seen other employees do. I will fight my supervisor in the State Personnel Department in Frankfort. My lawyer feels that I have a better chance in Frankfort, where certain employee rules are followed. My supervisor cannot fire me unless he can prove that I am incompetent on the job. I just hate to spend so much time and money defending myself, but I must and I will. I'm fortunate that I have friends who will help to defend me. Several are speaking to the Personnel Department in my defense. Since you are the physician on the two wards that I work on, you know my work best, but my supervisor does not want your opinion. How stupid is that when they do not use your opinion? Fortunately for me, my supervisor has become very unpopular for many reasons beside me, so I'm not completely hopeless."

Just then, Jean Newman entered into the nurses' station and interrupted the serious conversation; she said, "Oh, here are my two favorite people!"

Dr. Atcher responded, "Where? I don't see them."

Jean responded, "Oh, you know I'm talking about you and Winnie."

Dr. Atcher responded, "I'm not sure about Winnie," and he smiled at both women.

A nurse entered and asked Jean if she was looking for patients to attend her morning activity group.

"Yes, I am. I want those who are willing to play some games. Many are in bed. Do you have anyone who is up and willing?"

"Yes," the nurse responded, "the new admission is up and she is very alert. Most of the other patients are still in bed."

"I have already talked to her, but she refuses," responded Jean. "She said that she has done all that many years ago, claiming to have worked in the Occupational Department before. Is that true?"

"We don't know yet," stated Winnie, "since we have no social history available. I am still working on that. From my knowledge of hospital history, I would say she is correct."

"Just leave her alone since she is alert enough to know what she wants," added Dr. Atcher.

Jean left the nurses' station to find some other patients for her morning activities.

The hospital census was constantly decreasing as the local Community Mental Health Center developed more resources, all part of the growing community care trends throughout the nation. By January 8, 1990, Eastern State Hospital's census had 267 patients with 300 employees, more employees than patients. Unique to the whole history of the hospital, Dr. Gragg's belief in the value of equal numbers of patients and employees had been achieved. Yet, pressure was always present to prove that the old institution could provide "quality" care with fewer employees and more training.

While patients were always revolving through the hospital, employees were expected to adjust to the ever-changing expectations for more therapeutic programs. As employees became more professionally trained, employee ideals and supervisor expectations often clashed. Many new employees left in disgust, while others followed a middle ground or were fortunate enough to have a good relationship with their supervisor who protected them. Often the long-term employees found a comfortable middle ground while others gained power, either through relationships with more powerful supervisors or more training that gave them power to do as they wished. Often the physicians had the most power because they were the most difficult to replace.

Winnie returned to her office, hoping to find Cleo Coleman or any information about Mrs. Anna Rogers. Then Winnie went over to an older building of the hospital to see if the Personnel Department had any records of past employees. The Administration Building had been built in the early 1900s, and two others had been built in the 1800s. The older buildings had long been overcrowded with patients, but they were now facing major changes as more space was available. The Administration Building remained the same, while the old ballroom on the top floor sat empty and idle.

Discouraged by the lack of results, Winnie returned to the Allen Building before lunch time. That afternoon, Winnie and Jean held their usual afternoon patient group discussion, with trains as the subject of the week selected from a local newspaper article about Florida converting their old train tracks into walking trails. Since most patients could identify with trains from their past experiences, they enjoyed hearing about the story and looked forward to similar stories during the week. Since many hours of documentation were required for each activity, both Jean and Winnie spent the rest of the afternoon completing their paperwork. As they continued with their work, Jean said, "I really like your idea of having a subject of the week that the patients focus on."

"Oh, yes, I'm in favor of anything that helps. While some very isolated patients do not appear to respond, they do. You know Don on Allen 1?" asked Winnie.

"Yes, isn't he the brain-injured one?" responded Jean. "He usually does not respond to anything."

"Well, he even asked me the other day what we will be talking about this week. I was so thrilled because I thought he never listened or even appeared to respond," stated Winnie as she continued to write. "He even knew that I had subjects that we talk about; I was surprised that he remembered that! I was so shocked over his statements that I documented them in his chart."

"Yes, there are many other patients who get excited about the weekly subject." Jean continued to write her notes.

"And Jean, can you believe that the Personnel Department had no records on Mrs. Rogers? They claim that the records of anyone retiring from here after five years are sent to Frankfort, so they knew nothing. I can't believe the lack of interest in someone whom I believe was a pioneer here," stated Winnie. "But I must be careful not to mix my history of this place with my duties as a psychologist; I have no proof of what this patient is saying except for the history that I have collected."

The next morning, Winnie traveled her usual route on Fourth Street across the railroad tracks and into the original hospital entrance. While the second entrance was closer to the Allen Building off of Newtown Road, it was less historic and unappealing. When she arrived each day, she enjoyed seeing the old iron fence and older buildings closer to Fourth Street. These were the grounds of a mental institution over a hundred years old, and she could feel that history as it permeated the grounds. While many employees did not share her historical interests, Winnie was always reinvigorated with the historical ambience. She also enjoyed her coffee with Jean before work in the mornings, a ritual that developed after Winnie was moved to the Allen Building.

They were having the usual morning coffee before work time when Jean asked Winnie about the new admission. "What is wrong with her?"

"Actually, I don't think she should be here. She just needs help in getting a place to live. Someone diagnosed her as delusional, but the only delusion that has been observed is that she talks about working here in the past."

"Well, is that true?"

"I haven't gotten hold of Cleo yet, so I don't know Mrs. Rogers's background; it should be simple to find out if she really worked here. At least one would think so, but do you know that the Personnel Department is unwilling to call our office in Frankfort to look for her in their records? They say it is too much trouble. Well, Mrs. Rogers named people whom I know worked here at this hospital from my knowledge of that history. At this point, I have no reason not to believe her."

"I didn't see anything unusual from her except that she is elderly and her husband of many years has died," stated Jean.

"I saw her again in the hallway; she really likes you, Jean. You made her feel better. Mrs. Rogers is so receptive to caring employees, she is not like any paranoid or psychotic person," added Winnie.

"Oh, but Winnie, she still will not play any table games with me," Jean said sadly.

"She is just unhappy at being here and, I might assume, embarrassed over being here. She is depressed over losing her husband, selling the farm, and having to make changes in her life. But those are regular problems of life. Dr. Atcher has given her an antidepressant to help her. Actually, she is a very nice lady. Jean, can you imagine someone working here thirty to forty-five years and no one here knowing about it?" asked Winnie.

"Oh, if she worked here that long, she is a hero. She could help you with the history of this place," responded Jean. "I know you are collecting that history."

"I would think she could help me, but no one cares. However, I will wait to see what Cleo finds out. I do not want to mix my duties and my desire to talk to her about history will wait until I know she has no psychiatric problems. If she was an employee here, imagine all the history that she knows."

"Oh, yes!" Jean said as she became excited over the potential. "What do you have to do today?"

"Besides my usual morning staff meeting on the ward, I have a Fire and Safety Committee meeting this morning. It is one of my committees that I am required to attend."

"Oh!" Jean responded with a frown as she was shifting through her own daily schedule. "Why is that?"

"The director of the hospital decided that all hospital committees should have what he called professional leadership; he's required all physicians and psychologists to be on some committee. So the Fire and Safety Committee is mine," responded Winnie.

"Well, that just gives some of those who work here and never do anything something to do," replied Jean. "The supervisors are always in meetings and we never see them working with patients."

"Oh, do you mean like the psychologist on Wendell III? He claims to be attending meetings, but the ward employees and patients never see him," laughed Winnie. "There is also talk that he sleeps in his office, but that's probably just a rumor. Actually to be fair to the hospital director, this is a requirement of the Joint Committee of American Hospitals, so the director has to follow them. This is a national trend among mental hospitals."

"Well, it just makes more busy work, and the patients are neglected," stated Jean, who had come from eastern Kentucky, where the work was hard. She was often critical of other employees who did not do what she considered their work. She was also very caring with the patients.

"My committee is really not bad, at least for me. I volunteered to take this one because they really do something, not like many other committees that never achieve anything. No one else wanted to take my place on this committee because there are specific jobs, so I have been able to stay on it."

"What do you do?" asked Jean.

"We have two fire drills a month, a monthly meeting, and a quarterly safety inspection. At least we are doing something concrete. I enjoy doing my part," said Winnie. "It also requires one fire drill at five o'clock in the morning every quarter, but I get overtime for that. It is hard but I have adjusted to it. Oh, I need to go soon; what are you doing today?"

"My Recreation Department will be conducting a special meeting," replied Jean. "It involves plans for what is now the old dining room after the new Megowan Dining Room and Gym is opened. That old dining room has been here a long time, but I am anxious to see what plans they have for it. I understand the new Megowan Dining Room will be for the whole hospital and the old one will be developed for a 'new, innovative program.' That will be interesting to see!"

"That sounds interesting. I'll see you later." Winnie left and later, walked over to the Administration Building where the Fire and Safety Committee meeting was being held. While the Administration Building was built in the early 1900s, it was attached to another building that opened in 1824, now called the Gragg Building. Another large three-story building was attached to the other side of the Administration Building built in 1866. All three of these older buildings had been updated over the years. There were other unknown parts of the old institution, such as the two small octagonal buildings in the back of the three-story building. No one knew why the two octagonal buildings were there, since they were too small for anything but storage.

Winnie saw Cleo Coleman, the social worker, coming out of one of the buildings. Cleo apologized for the delay in getting to Mrs. Rogers. Both agreed that she did not show any psychotic symptoms, but there was no personal history to confirm that observation. "I don't see why she is here," continued Winnie.

"Well, the referring agency claimed that she was delusional, and the admitting physician took their word for it. Then, she came in at night, when there were no social workers on duty," stated Cleo.

"She is claiming that she worked here," responded Winnie. "Is that delusional? The Personnel Department could not be bothered with past employees, so they were not helpful. Mrs. Rogers named several of the early employees that I know about from collecting the history of this facility, so she knows more than Personnel," laughed Winnie.

Cleo shared the laugh and continued, "Anybody knows more than the Personnel Department does around here. I cannot believe all the trouble I have had getting the Personnel Department to help me with my processing for retirement. It has been a circus, and usually nobody knows anything or they give me the wrong information. I have given up on them here; I only go by what the Personnel Department in Frankfort tells me. So I am so fed up with these people here in this Personnel Department!"

"I'm so sorry! We will miss you. You at least cared about your patients."

"Well, I will miss you all, but this mess with the administration is senseless. They demand that I take days off because I worked overtime when they needed me, and they will not pay me for the time. So now I must take the time off before I retire, but they have no one covering my ward, and people like Mrs. Rogers often get ignored. I will be glad to leave here," stated Cleo. "However, I will see what I can find out for Mrs. Rogers; she deserves our best efforts."

"I would like to interview her about what she still remembers about this hospital," stated Winnie, "but I need to verify that she does not have a major psychiatric illness. If she was really here in 1922, she could be a wonderful historical source."

"Well, I will do my best. I understand that there are no living relatives, so it might be difficult." Cleo went back to her office to call her sources.

Cleo Coleman was a respected black social worker who had started working at Eastern State Hospital after getting a college degree in the 1960s. Through the years, Cleo observed that opportunities for advancement were decreasing without a master's degree in social work. She earned that master's degree by returning to school when her children were small. She gained financial aid from the State of Kentucky and paid back the obligation by continuing to work at Eastern State Hospital. Some employees did not have that option, so Cleo considered herself fortunate. Now she was able to retire at the age of sixty-five, with over twenty-five years of employment.

Winnie left work that day concerned over her limited information about Mrs. Rogers. Since Mrs. Rogers was still a psychiatric patient with reports of delusions, she felt restricted from gaining any historical facts from her. With her past problems with her supervisor, if she crossed that line into historian rather than psychologist with Mrs. Rogers, she could be in an indefensible position with her job duties. Only after Mrs. Rogers was confirmed as having no psychiatric history would Winnie be free to interview her about her earlier duties and experiences.

Mrs. Rogers was discharged by the time Winnie got to work the next morning. The history of Eastern State Hospital had lost a good resource. Winnie was upset and looked to see if Jean was in the Recreation Department.

"Jean, Mrs. Rogers was discharged last night. At least, that was what she wanted."

"Oh, but why discharge her so quickly when for several days nothing was done?" asked Jean.

"Yes, it was an embarrassment that she was here when everyone could tell there was nothing wrong with her. It shows that our admission doctor did not know what he was doing. The fact that she could have added to our history is unimportant to the administrators. That was not their interest. Also, the Personnel Department claimed to be unable to obtain any records, so there was no proof of her really working here. Yes, we lost a good opportunity," replied Winnie.

As a social worker, Cleo had done her job. She got Mrs. Rogers out of the hospital. Cleo, like several other employees who worked in the Allen Building, found more opportunities for professional enjoyment in that building. There was more pleasure for employees working with the elderly patients centered in the recreation room than on other wards, where patients were out attending activities off the ward.

The Allen Building was built with four wards in the early 1950s for admissions; the need for larger admission wards grew and another building, the Wendell Building, was renovated into a larger admission facility around 1960. Then, the Allen Building was changed into two Medical Surgical and two Geriatric Wards. As more patients were discharged into nursing homes in the 1980s, the two medical wards were changed into what was called Community Placement Wards, and the local Community Mental Health Center had administrative control of those two wards in the Allen Building, while the two Geriatric Wards continued to be part of the hospital.

The next week, Jean and Winnie met while in the hallway. Winnie had just left a staff meeting, and Jean was returning patients to the wards. Jean ran up to Winnie, excited about their upcoming trip. "Where are we going?"

"We are going to Massachusetts with the International History of Behavioral Sciences. I have been a member of that organization for years but never attended a conference. A history student of mine who got his PhD from the University of Kentucky, Dr. Ron White, did a dissertation on Eastern State Hospital and got me involved in that organization. Now, I am on the program using old postcards of American lunatic asylums, which includes our Kentucky Lunatic Asylum. It is a major attempt to call attention to the history of these early asylums and in particular to the history of our Eastern State Hospital, which has had little recognition or notice."

"Well, it doesn't matter to me, Winnie, I just like to travel with you; we always have fun," replied Jean.

"Well, I'm glad to have you traveling with me. My husband is pleased to have someone with me so that he does not feel that he has to go. The fun that we always have traveling is just icing on the cake for me. Seriously, I want to show that the history of Eastern State Hospital and other state hospitals is worthy of protection and research. There are a lot of American state hospitals including ours, but there is little interest in their long histories. Now, a long history of a state hospital is considered a negative rather than a positive asset." Then Winnie added, "That is also true of long-term employees," as they hurried down the hall.

"Well, I don't agree," stated Jean. "Long-term employees know more and are more valuable around here."

"The administration here doesn't see it that way," replied Winnie as they continued to walk toward their offices.

"Yes, I see that, but why is it that way?"

"Well, Jean, as I see things," replied Winnie, "new employees have a six-month probation period; the administration can fire them for any reason, even if the supervisor does not like them. It does not have to be any objective reason. After six months, employees can only be fired for proven causes of poor work, meaning that the supervisor has less control."

"But still, the longer one is employed, the more he or she has to offer," replied Jean. "I'm still new but even I know that the long-term employees know more. I always go to older employees when I want to know something."

"Yes," added Winnie, "but since the administration has less control, it often leads to conflict between supervisor and employee. There have been times when the administrators are out of touch with what is actually happening on a ward such as what happened on Intensive Treatment 3, the ward that I worked on in the Wendell Building before I was shipped here to the Allen Building." They both entered the Recreation Department, and since no one was there, they settled into chairs.

"What do you mean about being shipped here? I thought you chose to work here."

"Oh, I never told you about how I ended up here in the Allen Building?" Winnie asked. "I don't usually tell other employees since there is so much unhappiness around here. I just don't want to add to the misery here."

"Oh, I'll never tell," replied Jean. "I already know there is a lot of unhappiness among the employees. I just don't know why."

"Well, all the professional employees assigned on IT3 signed a request for concern. Of course, I was the one who wrote it but the other professional employees, including the psychiatrist, signed it. Our concern was about having psychotic patients on the same ward with mentally retarded ones. We had a bad problem on IT3, where two mentally retarded patients were constantly being beaten up by the psychotic ones. The hospital director had previously ignored our concerns, so we sent our request to the higher-ups in Frankfort. After our concerns were heard in Frankfort, the two mentally retarded patients were quickly moved to the other mentally retarded facility. Our hospital director was criticized for not acting sooner. Obviously, the hospital director and administrators were upset with us, whereas we felt we were acting on behalf of our mentally retarded patients. All of the professional employees who signed that petition were separated throughout other parts of the hospital, typical of how the hospital administrators handle those who disagree with them. I still miss working with some of my other friends on that ward, but I am happy here. I had no choice but to work in the Allen Building or else be fired."

"Wow! That is awful," responded Jean as she shrugged her shoulders, "all because you wanted to keep the mentally retarded patients away from the more violent ones. I have seen the mentally retarded ones get beaten up by psychotic ones. They should never be together on the same ward." Winnie was looking to see if any other staff or patients were around to hear.

"Yes, Jean, we have seen it happen often here, whereas our administration has said that there was never a mixing of the psychotic and MR patients. Anyway, as you know, it turned out best for me because I met you and a lot of the other employees in the Allen Building who have been put here because they have fallen into disagreements with their supervisor or administrators in the hospital. I enjoy working here and have made several friends on these wards. The administration stated that we were moved because we were all 'too close.' Sure, we were close, we agreed that the mentally retarded should not be on a ward with psychotic patients, but the hospital administrators continue to deny that. However, those patients were sent to the mentally retarded wards. Anyway, I'm happy to be away from all that." She moved toward her office door. She checked into her office and took out her purse from a drawer. She locked the door and waited for Jean as part of their ritual of going home.

Jean returned after she went into the recreation room to grab her purse, locked her office, and returned to where Winnie was waiting. "Well, I'm happy you came to the Allen Building; you have helped with our programs. The patients are responding better when you do the subject of the week and group discussions."

"I believe in activities that bring patients out; by my being around, helping with group discussions, and encouraging their interest in a subject of the week, they know me and are more active. Instead of talking to patients in an isolated office, they are more receptive to talking to me on the ward, and they gain more through regular interactions," stated Winnie as they walked out of the Allen Building together. They both had busy schedules the next day, so they did not talk again until several days later.

The next week, Jean and Winnie were sipping morning coffee and tea as they watched the other employees arrive. Jean was her usual cheerful self while Winnie was having difficulty adjusting to Jean's enthusiasm at such an early hour. "Did I tell you about the old dining room program?" asked Jean as she straightened up the chairs in the recreation room.

"Well, you did tell me about the new dining room and the gymnasium; both have been recently opened. Now, the question is what will be done with the old dining room?" responded Winnie as she sat down in one of the chairs.

"The new building is called the Megowan Building, named after someone in the past here." Jean continued to rearrange chairs. She ignored Winnie's negativism and continued her positive anticipation for the day.

"Oh, Jean," Winnie said, showing irritation for her friend's ignorance of the history of the institution, "Megowan was a patient here in the 1830s, and the family bequeathed a sum of money to be used only for patient recreation. The money was somehow diverted into other purposes, not for the original purposes of recreation. The new dining room and gymnasium was built with money that the State of Kentucky returned to Eastern State Hospital for the original purposes of recreation, and the building was named for the Megowan family." Winnie calmed herself. She added that she wasn't mad at Jean, but the continued ignorance about the history of Eastern State Hospital that she saw around was an irritation to her.

"I didn't know all that; they never mention that much," responded Jean as she sat down in the nearest chair. She continued to sort through papers while talking. "I didn't mean to make you mad at me."

"I'm not mad at you. It is just one more example of the administrators of this facility ignoring the interesting history behind everything." Winnie got up to get some coffee and continued, "I did the research a few years back on Megowan and provided information that his family specified that their money would be used for entertainment for patients. The financial manager proved that the money was diverted by the State of Kentucky in later years and that a new dining room and gymnasium with the Megowan name would satisfy the obligation that Kentucky had to the Megowan family."

"Oh, Winnie, I didn't know you had anything to do with it." She stopped to get her tea and returned to her chair.

"I didn't have anything to do with the money part, Jean, but I did provide the history of when the Megowan money was given and the historical facts. That is all in the history of Eastern State Hospital."

"Well, they certainly should appreciate your help, Winnie."

"Oh, Jean, you know how they are. My part has been completely ignored, but I don't want anything. Actually, the director did ask me for the information, so he at least knew who to come to. But he never gives me any credit for the historical data. That is the way he is; he expects help but never gives me credit for anything.

"Oh, how horrible," claimed Jean. "I just can't understand those people."

"I'm used to that, I'm just glad that they used the history to the benefit of the hospital. Actually that same history is in my home now because my supervisor threatened to, as he said, 'destroy everything in my office that was not related to psychology.'" Winnie reached for a refill of coffee.

"Do you mean that your supervisor threatened to destroy the history of Eastern State Hospital?" Jean asked as she stopped all activity.

"Oh yes, before I moved over here. Now, he denies it since I obtained a lawyer. But before, he stated that history had no place in a psychology office and since he was my supervisor, he had a key to my office and could destroy everything in my office that was not related to psychology. I didn't trust him and moved all the history boxes to my home. Now, my supervisor cannot get to them."

"Oh, when was that?" Jean's mouth was agape as she sat down with her partially filled tea cup. Surprised over the story, she became more attentive and sat down.

"Oh, I guess about a year and a half ago. I was working on IT3 in the Wendell Building. Some employees believe that my supervisor was just blowing threats since they say that they had seen him do that to others. They say he often makes threats and then denies it when officials ask. I believed his threats and hired a lawyer that my husband had recommended. Then, my supervisor tried to make it sound like I had a problem and denied his way out. My lawyer did determine that my supervisor had a legal right to ask me to move the history out of my psychology office, but he had no right to destroy it. Anyway, I moved all the history to my home where no one can touch it."

"Oh, that man is awful," replied Jean. "I did not know such educated people could be so cruel."

"You are not telling me anything!" Winnie replied quickly. "I just did not trust him enough to see if he was just bluffing, because once the history is destroyed, it is gone. Actually, I really believe that my supervisor is just too lazy to do much damage, but I still did not trust him."

"Why would he want to destroy the history of Eastern State Hospital?" asked Jean as she became engrossed in the conversation.

"Well, my lawyer did say that my supervisor was partly correct, that institutional history should not be in a psychology office. I disagree, because social histories of patients are now recognized as important to psychiatric care, and we hire social workers for that purpose. So, why not the history of this place?" asked Winnie as she stopped to sip some coffee. "I think we need to learn from our past, but I did as my lawyer suggested and moved the history of ESH to my home."

"Well, that makes sense." Jean sipped her cup of tea and said, "Why did you keep the history of Eastern State Hospital in your office?"

"I kept the original documents here in my office because many students and professionals who visited the hospital would ask about it, and I was always happy to show them the history. It started with Ron White, who came here as a PhD student. He did a lot of historical research and gave me copies of his results because I had given him copies of the original documents. Other students were always interested in the history, so I had it available. Since no one had made any threats to destroy it, I kept it in my office until my supervisor made his. Now, it is just my word against his, but the history is safe in my home. I'm not taking any chances."

"Well, that is awful. I knew that he didn't like you, but I didn't know why," stated a more subdued Jean. "I knew I didn't like him and now I know why; he doesn't like you, Winnie, and I don't like anyone who doesn't like you, my friend." She patted Winnie on the back.

"In spite of my interest in the history of psychology and this institution, my supervisor has not been able to prove that my work as a psychologist has in any way suffered! That I am proud of," stated Winnie. "If he could prove that my work has suffered, then he could fire me. That is the protection that we have as Kentucky state employees."

"Well, I know you spend more time with patients than I have ever seen any other psychologist do," stated Jean.

"Oh, thank you, Jean, but I know you are my friend, so I might expect you to say so. I appreciate your comments."

"No, Winnie, I mean it, I'm not just saying that because we are friends. You actually do more," stated Jean.

"Well, the PhD who previously had my job on the Geriatric Wards was also good," stated Winnie.

"Yes, he was good but he was always gone. He never helped with activities or attended activities to encourage the patients," replied Jean.

"Some psychologists feel that activities are not 'psychological enough,'" continued Winnie. "Whereas for our geriatric population, that is the best that we have from research that I done. It gives me a chance to observe the patients and lets them get to know me in a less fearful environment than an office. Your activities help to bring out their real potential rather than just observing them on the ward. Actually, I do both because I often need to evaluate their potential for training and/or nursing homes."

"So is that why the PhD did not bother with activities on this ward—they were not 'psychological' enough?" asked Jean.

"I don't know his reasons. Remember, psychology PhDs are trying to establish their credibility here at this facility, and they believe they cannot do the same activities that the less trained employees do. But since I don't worry about establishing my value as a master's psychologist, I still see activities such as you do, being very helpful for me in learning about my patients rather that talking to them in my office," responded Winnie. "However, the previous PhD is finishing his dissertation, so he might be too busy to work on the ward."

"I'm so excited about the Recreation Department getting the space of the old dining room. Things will be changing here." Jean looked at the clock on the wall.

"Oh, Jean, it is past time for us to leave. Grab your purse and I will get mine out of my office, then we can walk out together." They both scrambled to their offices.

Jean met Winnie on the way out of the building.

Winnie continued the conversation, saying, "Things will be changing but they have always been changing around here. In the twenty-three years I have been here, this institution has always been changing. It all depends on the people who work here, who has the power, the demands of the politicians, and social pressure. The question I ask, have the changes been beneficial or are they a repeat of the past? Until we know what that past was, that question can't be answered. Many current professionals choose to believe that everything that they do is beneficial. They do not want to be bothered with any other considerations," said Winnie as she looked for her car keys. Both Winnie and Jean said good-bye and agreed to see each other the following week.

Driving home, Winnie thought about their earlier discussions and pondered if she should have told Jean so much. Although they were good friends, the internal strife within the institution was difficult for new employees to understand, and Winnie did not wish to shatter Jean's innocence about the institution. While Winnie was not interested in getting employees to take sides or in spreading gossip around, she had discovered that the employees who knew what was going on were often best able to defend themselves when were they under fire by the administration. Many employees had suffered the loss of their jobs because they did not know how to defend themselves, whereas others had survived by keeping abreast of things. Jean was too honest and innocent to survive the current cut-throat world of Eastern State Hospital without someone preparing her.

The next week, Jean called Winnie aside and said, "I would like to talk to you later if you have time."

"Sure," Winnie said; "call me in my office when you are free."

Jean waited until the other recreation leader left to ask Winnie into her empty recreation room. She waited until Winnie arrived and then said, "I was really upset over what you told me the other day, and I didn't want my colleague to hear us talking. I did not realize that things were so bad around here at Eastern State Hospital. I know that there are many unhappy employees, but after hearing what you have gone through, I understand that other employees have similar difficulties. I understand better what is happening around me. I know that we are all here to help patients, but there are employees who use their power for other purposes. How can those people live with themselves?"

"I don't know, but I am amazed at how they justify what they do. But when you consider that there is no published history or standard whereby they can be judged, then these things happen. I did worry about telling you too much, but I feel you are better prepared to know if it should happen to you," stated Winnie. "All I know is what happened to me, but other employees can tell you other horror stories."

"I can't believe that the director and your supervisor are not happy over the history that you have collected; everyone should be proud of you," stated Jean. "I like history so much and can't understand them."

"Well, Jean, I am used to that. Can you believe that in 1970, the new employees of Eastern State Hospital were throwing away that history that Dr. Gragg had preserved in a closet? If I had not agreed to take it into my office, the information, which dated back to the 1800s, would have been thrown away. It was done through ignorance but there have been many other times when the history was thrown away due to the uncaring administration," stated Winnie. "There was one state employee who bragged about burning the old straitjackets, to hide the fact that straitjackets were used. They were used everywhere but to burn them is to destroy history of this old state hospital. How stupid are some people?"

"How can they be so uncaring about the history?" asked Jean.

"I don't see it as a matter of caring but rather ignorance; they do not understand psychiatric history. Every new professional assumes that what he or she is doing here is groundbreaking, when actually, much of it is a repetition of the past," stated Winnie as she looked at her watch. "Oh, I must go, I have a staff meeting in ten minutes. We have our trip to Westfield College in Massachusetts to look forward to next week, but I'll see you later, Jean, to talk more about our trip."

"Oh, yes, I'm so excited," stated Jean. "I can't wait."

The next week, in June 1990, Jean and Winnie went to Westfield, Massachusetts, for a conference by the International History of the Behavioral Sciences. Winnie was scheduled to present pictures of the early lunatic asylums in the United States, including Eastern State Hospital of Lexington, the second state hospital built in the United States. The meeting was attended by around two hundred participants. The organization consisted of psychologists who taught the history of psychology, historians, and sociologists.

They flew into Hartford, Connecticut, and rented a car to drive on to Westfield, Massachusetts. Winnie wanted to visit the Institute of Living, a private facility in Hartford that was opened in 1824, the same year as Eastern State Hospital. Winnie had already talked to the administrators and they were given a tour. Winnie was thrilled to compare the state and private facilities. Winnie concluded that the state facilities always had the more difficult patients, whereas the private facilities were able to eliminate patients if they did not have a family or resources to pay for their care. The private facilities were always seeking private contributors, whereas the state facilities were limited to what the state could pay. The private facilities could apply the newest methods, whereas the state facilities were often slower due to proving the value of each method. Winnie agreed to keep in contact with an employee of the Hartford facility. Jean was amazed and joked with Winnie about visiting another lunatic asylum.

Winnie responded by saying, "Now, you finally know me and my secrets!"

They arrived at Westfield College that afternoon and settled into the dormitory and met other participants. While Jean was not a psychologist, she had enough experience within Eastern State Hospital and had a friendly personality that won the attention of many participants. She fit in well with the professional atmosphere.

"Well, Jean," Winnie said, looking at her, "we will be meeting some interesting people. Since my presentation is tomorrow, I will pick out my best outfit to wear, tomorrow." They both giggled like schoolgirls since they both enjoyed nice clothes and often laughed over their own peculiarities.

"Good idea; so will they let me attend the meetings?" asked Jean.

"Yes, this is a small organization, and you will fit in well. If you remember, the New York meeting last year was restricted only to participants; it is different here."

"Yes, this is a friendlier conference," responded Jean.

"Well, Jean, the people in New York considered their organization too important for outsiders. This organization is more willing to tolerate others."

"Which one do you like best?" Jean asked.

"Actually, I like psychology best because I am one; however, I had the opportunity to talk about the history of Eastern State Hospital last year in New York City, so I took it. Remember, psychoanalysts make more money than psychologists, so they can afford to be less friendly," Winnie laughed. "That was also New York but we did have fun."

"We always have fun together," stated Jean. "We have already had a full day today."

"Well, we saw another lunatic asylum today," Winnie said, chuckling to herself while fixing her single bed. The beds were very comfortable.

"Yes, we saw some of Hartford, such as the old cemetery. I really like history," added Jean as she turned off the light.

The next day was exciting. "Oh, your presentation was so good," claimed Jean as they decided to take a break away from the other presentations.

"Oh, thank you. I knew you would like it; you're becoming a lunatic nut like me, but I was sure worried about the others," claimed Winnie as she walked outside.

"Well, you found out there are people here who agree with you that the history of old state hospitals is worth saving." Jean followed Winnie outside.

"Yes, and many of the people are psychologists who are members of the American Psychological Association. I was even asked to come with a presentation for the APA's convention next year." Winnie was looking around to see where they were walking. She had been told to follow a sidewalk.

"Oh, Winnie, how nice this area is," Jean said.

"Some of the people here are program chairmen at the APA, and they are encouraging presenters here to consider doing a presentation at APA," stated Winnie as she continued to walk for the exercise. Jean followed. They were both looking around while following a sidewalk.

Then they came upon a wall of trees, all contained in a large circle. They continued to follow a path when a beautiful garden of flowers inside the trees emerged. Both were surprised that they had not spotted the garden previously.

"Oh, it is so beautiful." Jean sat on a bench among the trees and flowers. The garden was away from the sound of the street and cut deep into a cave secluded among trees.

"I would not have seen this garden if someone had not told me to look for it," stated Winnie. "It is so nice."

"Can you believe that we are here in Massachusetts?" asked Jean.

"No, not really, it has been so exciting for me," claimed Winnie.

"I would never have believed that I could travel as much as I have with you. We were in Hartford yesterday, and last year we were in New York," stated Jean. "Where is the APA's convention?"

"It is in Washington," replied Winnie as she continued to look around.

"Oh really?" asked Jean. "I have always wanted to visit Washington DC; I would love to go!"

"Well, we will see. That is a year away, yet. I need to get a presentation together and then get it accepted, first. There is a lot to do yet!" responded Winnie. "While there were professionals who liked my presentation here, the growing trend in mental health is away from state mental hospitals into community care. There are those who agree that my research into the state mental hospital history is worthy of more research and presentations, while others do not like to talk about the old lunatic asylums."

"Well, they are just stupid," replied Jean.

"Especially that hospital director," added Winnie. Then she stopped and added, "Well, to be fair, the hospital director has not made any criticisms of my research as far as I know. He even got the Mental Health Department to accept my historical research. He was more accepting of historical research when Ron White was working on his dissertation with me several years ago. Now, Ron has finished his PhD in history and has gone. If I had not saved and preserved the history of Eastern State Hospital, Ron would not been able to get his PhD. At least, that was what he told me. So the director has tolerated my preservation of the history, but he has difficulty accepting me as a psychologist."

"Well, you certainly know what you are doing," added Jean.

"But they want me to have a PhD, whereas I only have a master's degree. When I started working there twenty-three years ago, few PhDs wanted to work there. Even with higher pay, many PhDs do not stay."

"But you do more than the other PhDs," stated Jean.

"Well, they assume that only a PhD can do my job, which I have done for twenty-three years; I got outstanding raises in earlier years. Now, they have decided that the job requires a PhD, not just a master's degree. This conflict is actually bigger than us. The director and my supervisor are trying to prove to the administrative powers that be in Frankfort that a PhD is required to do my job. They want to justify hiring only PhDs with higher salaries."

"But the PhDs do not do much. They just sit in meetings," stated Jean.

"Well, Jean," replied Winnie, "we know that, but the supervisors in Frankfort, whom the director answers to, do not know that. They only know what the director tells them. This gives the director more power to hire new PhD psychologists, and he is praised by the Kentucky Psychology Association.

"I know of a PhD over on the admission ward. I never saw him do anything, and others say that they never see him on the ward. There is a lot of talk about him sleeping in his office," added Jean.

"Yes, I have heard that too; I know who you are talking about. He had such a negative reputation on his previous job, and I begged my old supervisor, not the one I have now, not to hire him, but the director insisted. That PhD's wife is on the Board of Psychology and continues to be influential. At least, that is what I have heard, and we have all observed that any PhD at Eastern State Hospital is allowed to do as he or she wishes, while others are fired for less. The unfairness is known by everyone."

"Oh, I never realized there were such bad employees at the hospital," stated Jean. "I just assume people are good and that they do things for the good of patients. Now, I see that many employees are only out for themselves."

"Yes, you only see the good in people, which I admire about you," responded Winnie, "but in places like where we work, there is no fairness, and to assume so is naïve. But Jean, this conference has given me more confidence in what I am doing with the history of Eastern State Hospital."

They returned home and went back to their jobs as usual. Rumors continued to circulate that changes were coming to the hospital and that certain employees would lose their jobs. Jean and Winnie continued to discuss changes.

The following spring of 1991, Winnie and her lawyer were given notice of a hearing with the Kentucky Department of Personnel in Frankfort, Kentucky. They were appealing how her supervisor previously reduced her job duties and reassigned her to work in the Allen Building, which occurred in the spring of 1989.

The morning before the hearing date, Winnie decided to tell Jean about the hearing. Winnie came to work early, knowing that Jean would be in the recreation room. Winnie sat nervously in a chair while Jean got ready for the day. "Jean, I am appealing my supervisor's reduction of my work tomorrow. For twelve years, I ran a weekly outpatient therapy group at the local Community Mental Health Center. I had patients who were here on my ward attending my inpatient group therapy sessions, and when they were discharged, they would attend the outpatient group sessions because they benefitted from my previous groups. Usually, the Community Care Center has difficulty with our patients following up with their outpatient services, but that was not true of my patients. My patients attended the outpatient groups because they benefited from the support in my groups. But my supervisor did away with my group therapy, and I plan to show how that has been detrimental to patients and care that was not provided."

"Why did he stop them?" replied Jean as she stopped her busy work and sat down with her tea and poured coffee for Winnie.

"I believe in the value of group therapy, and many patients were helped by that follow-up from the institution to community care. No one in those groups had to be readmitted to the institution in twelve years," added Winnie. "No PhD can claim that much stability or success."

"But why are you protesting his doing away with the group therapy sessions? It is really less work; don't you want less work?" asked Jean.

"No, I believed in what I was doing. Often our patients do not want to attend the Community Care Centers because they do not know the employees or have no trust in them. My group knew me as their therapist in the hospital, and my involvement in the outpatient group made them more willing to get started at the Community Care Center. Those patients even took up a petition against my supervisor ending the group, but no one even responded to them."

"That all sounds good," Jean added skeptically. She still wondered why Winnie was protesting against less work. She had never known of any employee disagreeing with less work.

Winnie, feeling more relaxed, continued on, knowing that Jean had some real skepticism. "I believe that the group that my supervisor took away was therapeutically effective. I had many ex-patients who saw the group as essential to their succeeding outside of the hospital. That was all my idea; it was beneficial and provided stability for mental patients for twelve years."

"Oh, I can believe you did that," said Jean.

"Secondly, I do not believe that my supervisor is doing me any favors by taking away half of my work. I suspect he wants to force me into less work so he can later claim that I am not doing enough work. I have known of examples where my supervisor fired another employee because that employee was doing less work. My supervisor had relieved the employee of the work that he had felt good about. Then, my supervisor later fired him for doing less work."

"Those administrators are dirty and rotten."

"Also, I have always gotten positive praise about my groups, and my supervisor does not want me praised for my work. So, he took away one of my successful programs that I developed; he doesn't care about the patients who depended upon me."

"Oh, he is horrible," responded Jean.

"Since I had been doing an effective job by many people's standards, my supervisor eliminated all my therapeutic programs so that I would be seen as ineffective, giving him a cause to fire me."

"I've been told by others that you were showing up the other PhD psychologists who were not doing half the amount of work that you were doing," Jean said, as she seemed to understand better.

"Well, that might be another reason, but that is not completely true of all PhDs here; I know of several who are good. But I feel that my supervisor is just not fair to me, and I need to show that to the Personnel Department in Frankfort," she said. Winnie finally felt that Jean understood.

"But what will a hearing with the Personnel Board do?" asked Jean.

"Doesn't your supervisor have the power to do as he wishes with his employees?"

"Well, yes, as my supervisor, he has those rights. However, by having a hearing, I am making the Personnel Board aware of what has happened and have on record that it was against my will. Therefore, if my supervisor tries to fire me for doing less work, I am showing that he created the less work, not me. I am also showing that my supervisor eliminated some very effective treatment programs, which can only make him look bad."

"Ohhhh, Winnie, you sure are smart to figure all that out," Jean said, laughing. "I could not have figured it out like that. Why not just go to our Personnel Department here at the hospital?"

Winnie explained that the general belief among older employees was that the Administrative and Personnel Departments at the hospital never looked out for employee interests, but new employees such as Jean had not observed that. Winnie's lawyer had advised her to go higher up to the Personnel Department in Frankfort to be heard. Otherwise, the hospital offices would just hide things from those in Frankfort. The Personnel Department in Frankfort had the final say.

"So, you are going tomorrow?" asked Jean.

"Yes, I have taken a vacation day, so the administration cannot claim I was doing it on work time. My lawyer will be there to present my case of how my supervisor has continued to discriminate against me. I am asking for financial reimbursement."

"Do you expect any money from it?" asked Jean.

"Oh, no, but the Personnel Department will not hear my concerns unless I am requesting money. They will consider themselves winning if they don't have to pay me any money, and I will consider winning if they get my supervisor off of my back," laughed Winnie.

"Do you really want your old job back instead of staying here in the Allen Building?" asked a fearful Jean. "I would miss you if you returned to the other building."

"Actually, I like being in the Allen Building, but I'm not telling anyone but you. I wanted to expose my supervisor for the way he moved me without any justification and for his own personal reasons.

Just because I have developed good friends such as you is no reason to exonerate him."

"So aren't you nervous about tomorrow, facing all those people?" Jean shivered in her chair.

"Sure, I'm nervous, but I'm also angry and excited to be able to tell my side. However, my lawyer will do the talking, so I do not mess up. I will just follow his directions as he has told me. My lawyer has handled a lot of these personnel actions so he knows what to do. But guess what I will be wearing?" Winnie smiled, knowing that clothes were always a happy subject between them.

"Oh, what?" asked Jean quickly, jumping up out of her chair.

"I will wear my most expensive outfit! I want to look my best."

"Oh, yeah!" she yelled, laughing, "you can show them!"

"Yes, I have seen other employees go to these personnel hearings, all upset, crying, and begging. Not me! I will wear all my gold jewelry and my most expensive clothes. I'll not beg like they want me to," laughed Winnie.

"Oh, they are so ugly," stated Jean. "I used to think people here were so nice, but these are such ugly people." Jean added coffee to Winnie's cup.

"Well, Jean, I really don't think they started out being ugly, but they get caught in their own schemes and power trips. Everyone develops an ugly side when they are questioned. The State Personnel Department is a much more powerful group than the hospital director or my supervisor. While our Kentucky Department of Personnel is supposed to be neutral, if I can prove that what they did here was prejudiced toward me and nontherapeutic for patient care, then the director and my supervisor will look bad. At least I'll get them off my back!" Winnie relaxed and sipped some coffee.

"Well, I sure hope you win tomorrow." Jean shuffled some papers on her desk while checking the schedules for the day.

Winnie realized that Jean had difficulty with conflict and often did anything to avoid it, but she wanted her to understand. She asked Jean to stop shuffling papers and listen about some previous outstanding employees.

Winnie decided to tell her about Dr. Bob Deburger, a friend of hers who had died. "He was a PhD and a good one, who was working here when I was hired," Winnie said. "I really liked him. He was director of research here in 1967 and continued until 1970. The Department of Mental Health demanded that he move to Frankfort and work there rather than be based here at Eastern State Hospital.

"Dr. Deburger was not one to fit into Frankfort or office politics," she continued, "because he was a warm and caring person. He knew individual patients here and liked being part of their care. He did not want to go to Frankfort but they insisted anyway."

"Caring is unusual for a PhD," Jean said after returning to her chair.

"No, Jean, there are many caring PhDs, and Dr. Deburger was one. I saw him often for the next ten years, and I always knew I had a friend in the Frankfort office. However, he was unhappy with the cut-throat politics of Frankfort, and he died in 1980 from cancer. I blame the Department of Mental Health for his illness. He was so unhappy there."

"Why didn't he leave and work somewhere else?"

"He had so many years in the Kentucky retirement system that he could not quit his job. He had to do as the Department of Mental Health wanted. They gave him hell in Frankfort, and I still remember that. He was a real friend to me and often told me about the people in Frankfort. While I don't expect any understanding of my situation from the department in Frankfort, I want my proof of prejudice and reduced patient care by my supervisor to be of record. This is the only way to do it. I don't expect the people in Frankfort to be any nicer, but they have specific personnel rules to follow. A fair hearing is all I ask," Winnie said. "My lawyer thinks I have a good case." Winnie felt good that her friend, Jean, understood.

"Can I call you at home tomorrow night to see how things went?" Jean was aware that the time was approaching when other employees would be coming to work. Soon her fellow workers would be coming into the recreation room, and they would have to stop their conversation.

"Yes, you can. I don't expect an answer tomorrow, but I will let you know how things went." Winnie excused herself to return to her office.

The next night, Jean called Winnie, who was exhausted; it had been an emotionally draining day, but she was pleased with how things went.

Winnie was told by the Department of Personnel to expect a decision within a week.

The week came and went. There was no response. Winnie called her lawyer, who called the Department of Personnel lawyer. Two weeks later, she was notified that the Department of Personnel had ruled that the supervisor had a right to decide her work assignments but he should have considered her professional opinions and therapeutic programs. Her supervisor was told to leave Winnie alone, since she had a lawyer who could cause problems for them. Winnie felt like she had won!

While she knew it was a small victory, she still had shown that she was willing to fight for what she believed. She felt good.

For the first time in the five years that her supervisor had been her supervisor, Winnie had won a major battle against him. While she knew the Department of Personnel would favor him in her work assignments, her supervisor was recognized as the one who had eliminated effective therapeutic programs. This was a real professional blow to him. Since Winnie had never had such a difficult supervisor, others tended not to get involved. Except for personal friends who served to let Winnie ventilate her frustrations, there was not any support for her in a facility that claimed to provide mental health services, except for Jean. Also, Dr. Atcher had supported her in his own way.

Winnie had been contacted by peers in the American Psychology Association to conduct research into when the application of psychology became established in the early state mental hospitals. Psychiatry as a profession grew with the development of the early mental institutions, but not psychology. There were times when psychologists were hired in individual institutions, but it was not known when psychology became established in the early American mental institutions. Winnie agreed to do this project.

The research required a trip to the Archives of American Psychology at the University of Akron in Ohio. Winnie and Jean took vacation time in the summer of 1991 and visited the archives. Winnie determined what year psychologists appeared in each state's mental hospitals, and Jean helped her. She presented a paper at the American Psychological Association the following year.

That summer, Eastern State Hospital employees in the Allen Building had settled into a comfortable program of providing care for those who needed it. Many employees shared their talents with patients in various social events that the Recreation Department provided. Dr. Atcher enjoyed playing the fiddle, Jean had a good singing voice, and Winnie played the piano. The patients enjoyed the music, and other employees helped. They all viewed their responsibilities as including encouragement of the isolated patients to become more involved with any social interaction between patients and staff.

One day, Winnie and a new occupational therapist decided that patients could benefit from having a pet. Often employees would bring their pets for a temporary visit to the wards, and the patients were delighted. The occupational therapist suggested they designate a room where the local animal shelter could provide pets for a day. Dr. Atcher had agreed to the arrangement. But they were forced to discontinue the program because the therapist's supervisor had not been consulted first. The occupational therapist was moved to another part of the hospital.

Winnie and Jean were talking about it the next day. "Can you believe, our new O.T. worker was moved. Our patients had just gotten to know her and liked her."

"Yes, that is a shame," Jean replied. "I think the O.T. employee was also beginning to enjoy working with geriatric patients."

"Yes, it is a shame, but she was under her six months' probation, so she has to do what the supervisor tells her. I'm sorry for her, but she will survive. I'm sorry that the Allen Building patients will not be able to have pets now," added Winnie.

"Why not use the recreation room here? I am in charge of getting patients to come to the recreation room and animals in here would help. We can bring in some cats from the greenhouse and let the patients play with them in here," replied Jean.

"Oh, Jean, that's a good idea," Winnie replied, pleased.

"My supervisor doesn't care what we do as long as there are activities for patients, and I'm sure my coworker will agree to it. Anyway, we should have no problems," Jean said.

The next week, the recreation supervisor refused to allow a cat in the recreation room because she considered it to be "unhealthy." Jean just saw it as a way of the supervisors stopping a good idea; she said, "Those supervisors don't understand how much our patients love animals."

There have been several research studies showing that animals benefit their patients, especially geriatric ones. Winnie found some of those research studies and showed them to the supervisors, but they would not change their minds.

Jean later said that her recreation supervisor stated that if Dr. Atcher approved the cat, then the Recreation Department would certainly follow his decision. Jean believed that was just their way of getting around the issue, by shoving it off on somebody else.

"Well, Jean, that is our answer," said Winnie. "Let's take it up with Dr. Atcher. He knows these games that our supervisors play, and he might just help us to outwit them."

"Oh, yes!" shouted an excited Jean.

"Well, we can only try," responded Winnie. She went to find Dr. Atcher.

By the next day, Dr. Atcher had agreed to consider having a cat if Winnie and Jean would bring the animals in for his inspection. Several cats lived at the greenhouse to keep out the mice. They had been vaccinated and had been given regular shots, so they were the perfect solution.

Winnie talked to the supervisor at the greenhouse, and they agreed to provide two of their best cats for the Allen Building patients. Since the cats were around patients in the greenhouse, there was growing anticipation that these were two cats that the Allen Building patients could enjoy.

"Remember, Dr. Atcher must first interview the cats, according to our supervisor's requirements," Jean laughed. They carried the two cats to his office. Dr. Atcher was waiting and participated in the humor of the situation.

"I wonder if these cats will talk back to you, Dr. Atcher," Winnie said as they entered his office, laughing.

He responded, "Well, I hope not; if they do, they will have to be secluded." Dr. Atcher knew that the supervisor requirements were serious, and he followed the rules so that the hospital administration would be satisfied, but he always had fun with it.

Dr. Atcher interviewed the cats privately in his office and stated on a psychiatric interview form, "The cats are acceptable for staying in the Allen Building." Being the jokester that he was, Dr. Atcher made copies of what he called a *"psychiatric exam"* of the cats, stating that "they were not talking and self-isolating"; he recommended "that they needed to have more socialization." He sent copies to the necessary supervisors while patients and employees in the Allen Building anticipated the arrival of the two cats.

However, the weekly visits of the cats did not last long because the supervisor of the greenhouse was changed, and the new supervisor resisted the program. The Allen Building employees continued to resist pressures to do away with the cat program, as they witnessed the joy that patients gained from the cats. The real demise of the program came several weeks later, when one of the cats was killed by a car on Newtown Pike. However, the Allen Building employees had succeeded for a short time, showing that patient care was more important than whatever obstacles the administration provided. The camaraderie among employees improved. The Allen Building had become a fun place to work, and patients enjoyed the interaction and recreation with staff.

* * *

Several weeks later, the hospital director called Winnie on the phone. She was surprised since the director usually only communicated through the PhD psychologist program directors.

"Where is Dr. Atcher?" the director asked, without identifying who he was or even saying hello. "He is not returning my calls!"

"Well, sir, I have no way of knowing. He doesn't answer to me," Winnie replied in a somewhat baffled state.

"He needs to turn in an annual report as program director, and I have not gotten that report from the Allen Building," the director said.

"Well," she said, gaining courage, "don't bother me with that; you are his supervisor, and not I."

"I know that he is avoiding me by not returning my calls," the director said angrily.

"Well, I have no responsibility for him," replied Winnie.

"You are his assistant and are responsible for things when he does not do them," responded the director.

"No, sir, I am not his assistant," Winnie said as she was aware of becoming angry. She continued, "All other psychologists in this hospital are program directors, but you refuse to make me one; instead Dr. Atcher is the program director here. He wanted me to have that position but you insist that all psychology program directors be PhDs, which I am not. Although I have proven in the past that I can do the job, you have refused to give me the title. Now, you want me to take the responsibility because Dr. Atcher is not willing to do the job. I'm sorry but that is your problem and not mine." With that, she hung up on him.

Winnie left her office and saw that Dr. Atcher was sitting in his office. She entered and stated, "I guess you know that your boss is looking for you."

"Oh, yes, I know," said the smiling Dr. Atcher as he looked at Winnie.

"He called me and told me that I was your assistant, which is the first time I have heard of that," stated Winnie.

"Well, let's just ignore him," Dr. Atcher said, continuing to smile at her.

"Yes, I will be happy to," Winnie said as she left Dr. Atcher's office. She realized that Dr. Atcher was well aware of the games within the administration. As a physician, he had the power to do as he wished because no one would fire him. If other employees did what he did, they would have been fired.

Winnie and Jean were talking the next morning during a break. "Did you know that the director was looking for Dr. Atcher yesterday?" asked Jean. "I heard that from the nurses on the ward; evidently the director called for him on both of his wards, but he would not respond."

"Yes, and the director called his office, but he did not answer his phone. I understand that the director was demanding a yearly report from Dr. Atcher, who is refusing to do it. Dr. Atcher was avoiding him as usual," Winnie said as they both shared a laugh. Winnie had brought in her cup to see if any coffee was ready.

"Well, Dr. Atcher is not much of a paper person," responded Jean. She pointed out the coffee pot that was fresh and full. She looked for her cup.

"But, Jean, this is a bigger issue than just paperwork; the paperwork is a yearly requirement of the program directors. Since the director refuses to appoint me to that duty, he has shoved it off onto Dr. Atcher. Dr. Atcher feels that I should have the duty and resents the additional work. He enjoys playing games with the administration over that and other issues that he believes in." Winnie sat down sheepishly after pouring her coffee.

"Oh, but you can do the job," replied Jean.

"Yes, but if I did the job with only a master's degree, then there would be no justification for more PhDs and their higher salaries, would there?" Winnie shook her head.

"So, then it is just a game of the administration?"

"Yes, Jean! You see the veiled threats around here. Dr. Atcher does not like how they treat me, and he is irritated that he is stuck with the additional duties. It is a game played around here in many different ways."

"Oh, my," laughed Jean. "That is so funny."

"Yes, it is funny," Winnie said, but then she turned serious, adding, "often the patients are the ones who lose in these games. Dr. Atcher is fair with patients and makes sure that no patient is hurt in these games, whereas other employees are not so fair."

"Oh, I have seen that often, but it is funny to see someone winning such as Dr. Atcher!" Still laughing, Jean realized that she needed to return to work. "I have a meeting in a few minutes, so I need to go."

"Actually, the employees are funnier that the patients," said Winnie as she left the room with Jean. Both continued on to their work assignments.

*   *   *

In August of 1991, Winnie presented her paper on the evolution of psychology in the state hospitals to the American Psychological Association. The presentation showed that psychology was established as a department by the early 1950s in the first sixteen state mental hospitals. Most psychologists started with a master's degree, while other psychologists continued on to get their PhD. By 1955, psychologists were becoming more frequent; national requirements specified at least three psychologists in each state mental hospital. The lower salaries in the state mental hospitals contributed to many of the psychologist positions being left unfilled.

When Winnie returned from presenting her paper, there were rumors that the Allen Building patients would be moved to another part of the facility. The Allen Building, as a separate building, had become desirable to the local Community Care Center, which wanted to use it as a treatment center for alcoholics. While the local Community Care Center was established to provide psychiatric care in the community, they were requesting more institutional buildings for their programs; they now requested the newest building, the Allen Building, for their community program.

The old original buildings had been renovated with air-conditioning, creating more usable space for the remaining patients. Plans were being developed to move the geriatric patients from the Allen Building into the renovated original building, called the Gragg Building for Dr. Logan Gragg. For Winnie, it was a return to previous wards that she had worked on before but with modern changes.

However, the plans were still several months away, and employees were anxious about their jobs. While programs or patients were rearranged, older employees were often pushed aside as newer or more highly trained employees were promoted. These were common occurrences observed by the employees.

Jean and Winnie were talking one morning. Winnie was very excited and said, "Can you believe a friend of mine is coming to work here?"

"Oh, who?" asked Jean.

"Dr. Anne Shurling; we have been friends for years."

"Oh, that is nice," Jean responded, but with a negative tone at hearing that the friend was a PhD psychologist.

"Now, Jean, Anne is not your typical PhD. She is competent and caring, an unusual combination around here."

"Well, any friend of yours is mine, but why is she coming here?"

"She has been teaching at Transylvania and wants a change. Also, the hospital administrator is a friend of hers."

"Oh, no!" responded Jean, "not another you-know-what kisser!"

"No, she is much more diplomatic than I. She can stay friends with people without taking sides on issues. She knows how I feel about the director, but we stay friends anyway," added Winnie.

"How long have you known her?"

"I don't know exactly, but when she was a professor at Transylvania University, Dr. Shurling was bringing her psychology class here for me to talk about the history of this institution. She has really been the most encouraging of psychologists with my interest in history. I am so pleased that she is coming to join the Psychology Department of Eastern State Hospital," replied Winnie.

The year of 1992 brought a slowness that the employees of the Allen Building had not expected. Employees knew there were going to be changes, but those changes did not come, and the staff waited. Although daily supplies were needed for the wards, supplies were often not sent because they were expected to move. Employees were not allowed vacation time because they were expected to be available to help move. However, they did not move. It was frustrating to everyone. More patients were placed in nursing homes while the employees stayed. The employees continued to worry about their future employment, while others were frustrated over the lack of clarity.

$$* \quad * \quad *$$

Dr. Shurling and Winnie were eating lunch together one day. They went to a restaurant away from the hospital where they could talk. Anne was describing her duties in the Wendell Building as the program director; she said, "I really enjoy singing with my patients. We sing together and talk on the ward so I can know them and they know me. The other time is spent doing psychological tests, but mostly, I spend time with them on the ward."

"That is mostly what I do; it helps them to see me on the wards," replied Winnie. "That is the nicest part of our job. You are now on Intensive Treatment 2; do you know what psychologist was on that ward before you?"

Anne replied, "I do not think they had any psychologist on that ward."

"Anne, someone had to be on that ward; starting in the late seventies, each ward had a psychologist," added Winnie.

"Oh, I didn't know that there were that many psychologists here," said Anne.

"Oh, yes, there were up to ten here then, but when I came in 1967, there were only three psychologists for over one thousand patients. Now, there are at least ten with less than three hundred patients," responded Winnie.

"Well, I guess that is success: fewer patients," Anne said, jokingly.

"Oh, now I remember who was working on your ward before; it was Dr. VN. Oh, he was a real disaster!" Winnie laughed as she remembered.

"Oh no, not him!" exclaimed Anne as she put her head down on the table. "Now, I understand why other professionals are distant toward me. I never wanted to hear his name again." She looked up and shook her head.

Winnie responded by patting Anne on the head and saying, "I didn't know that you knew him."

"Yes, Winnie, I knew him but I wish I had never heard of him. He was my psychology supervisor when I took my practicum here several years ago. Oh, he was sicker than many of our patients. He had unrealistic ideas, and I had to seek the director's help from his excessive demands. Dr. VN had extreme delusions of grandeur." Anne relaxed back into her usual self.

"Oh, that is interesting. I had forgotten that you were a psychology student here. That was probably when we first met," stated Winnie.

"I have tried to forget that experience with Dr. VN. I would have never considered working here again if he was still here. When I was a student, he had control over my future as a psychologist. I had to keep the Psychology Department supervisor and director both informed, but fortunately, they knew of his problems. Whew! If he decided that I was not competent, it could have destroyed my career."

"Well, I am thankful that he was not my supervisor," responded Winnie, "although my current supervisor is not much better. While Dr.

VN was recognized as a troubled individual, my current supervisor is not, at least I'm not told. Dr. VN was one of several new PhDs who was going to 'improve' things around here; he left instead."

"Dr. VN was one of the worst I have known," Anne stated sadly. "I still shudder when I think about him. I'm sorry to know there are others, similar. Many employees question me." Anne smiled sarcastically.

"And you should consider that a compliment, because they are testing you, to see if you will be like the bad PhDs who have worked here," Winnie said. "Once they see how competent you are and that you can be questioned, then their respect will grow for you, Anne. I have no doubts about you! You just need to remember that there have been several incompetent psychologists who have abused their power here. That is why some employees are so distant until they get to know you; just hang in there." Winnie tried to make her feel welcomed.

Then, unexpectedly, Anne looked at Winnie and said in an unusually strong tone, "I could not believe that such bad psychologist had worked here until I remembered that Dr. VN was here; now, I can understand. Yes, I can see how individuals have misused their PhD status here."

"It really wasn't that way when I came in 1967. Dr. Boling was the only PhD here, and he had been moved to Eastern State Hospital from the Louisville State Hospital because of some trouble he had gotten into with the State Bureau of Health Services. I had observed that Dr. Boling was a homosexual but he kept his life very private, and I never saw any misuse of patients. While he was odd, he really did no harm," concluded Winnie. "Now, new psychologists have come, some have abused their positions, but no one has been able to criticize them because they are favored by the director."

"Also as the number of patients decrease, jobs have been eliminated and employees have lost their jobs. I know of several sad situations," added Anne. "But the Psychology Department stays the same, regardless of who leaves."

"I am now the only master's-degreed psychologist in a department of nine PhDs; no other department has that many PhDs," added Winnie.

"Well, we all know that the director has protected the Psychology

Department from job cuts when others were cut," replied Anne. She revealed a sarcasm that Winnie was unsure about. Was it anger at Winnie or her other friend, the hospital director? Winnie just kept quiet, knowing that Anne had to figure things out for herself. Their friendship was too deep for superficial problems.

"Of course there is resentment but it is also the unfairness that adds to the resentment. Do you know the PhD on Wendell III?" asked Winnie.

"Yes, I know of his wife, she is a psychologist on the Kentucky Board of Psychology. She is a very powerful person in psychology and misuses it."

"Her husband, a PhD, has been protected here; some employees on his ward do not know what he does while other employees get fired for doing more than he does. While there is a lot of resentment about him, the director continues to look the other way. The director's lack of fairness only adds to the resentments," concluded Winnie as they were finishing their lunch.

Winnie decided to drop the issue and focus on the fun things that she and Anne shared. They often visited antique shops; Anne had an interest in collecting a specific type of glass that her grandmother had used. Winnie had helped Anne collect it by visiting shops together.

Dr. Anne Shurling stayed at Eastern State Hospital for one year and moved on into private practice. She did stay neutral when others criticized psychology or the director at the hospital. When she was elected by fellow psychologists to the Board of Psychology, she told Winnie that she hoped to improve psychology as a profession and enforce stricter rules of professionalism. She was successful and well respected as a fair person; Winnie was proud of Anne's stand for ethical standards in the practice of psychology within the state of Kentucky.

In late spring of 1993, the Allen Building employees and patients were moved to the renovated Gragg Building. Winnie's new office was in two previous seclusion rooms. An elevator that had been requested since 1900 was placed next to the adjacent seclusion rooms. The whole building was air-conditioned, and all the wards were roomier since the census was down.

Jean visited Winnie in her new office for the first time. Looking around, she recognized it as two old seclusion rooms, long and narrow with windows at the end. Jean reacted negatively by asking, "Do you really like this office?" She shrugged her shoulders as if Winnie was hopeless.

"Oh, yes, I do. I know some others got better offices. You know the PhD on Wendell III? Well, he got an office with a beautiful front view, but he usually gets the best of everything, anyway. The talk is that since he sleeps in his office during the day, he now has the best office for sleeping," laughed Winnie.

"Oh, I still hear bad things about him not working," stated Jean.

"Well, I don't care what he has; I like my office best because I was here years ago. This is like memory lane for me, except it is cleaner."

"Oh, really?" asked Jean.

"I was working on what was called the Geographic Unit System with the Northern Kentucky Unit, around the 1980s. Then the whole hospital was organized into geographical units."

"Did you have this extra room too?" Jean looked into the adjoining second room and reacted as if something bad was in the room.

"Yes, I did, but where the elevator is, was a staff bathroom. I understand that the bathroom was added in an earlier renovation in 1944, but these were originally two long seclusion rooms, and the combination of two rooms gives me plenty of space; two windows for sunlight, next to my ward, so what else can I ask for?" Winnie asked, looking at Jean.

"It isn't as prestigious as the PhD's office," smirked Jean.

"I don't care. They hold no example for me," responded Winnie. "Anyway, Dr. Atcher got a nice office. It was offered to me but I told Dr. Atcher about it, knowing he would like it better. I did not want to be next to a lazy PhD. Anyway, everybody is happy, including me." They both parted to do their work. Winnie didn't care what others thought about her offices. She was back in the original building and feeling a renewed interest in the history. They settled into a routine.

During that summer, the director of Eastern State Hospital announced his retirement. Many were on vacation but Jean and Winnie rejoiced over the news. They could not believe it. There had been no gossip or even speculation that this could happen, and employees returning from vacations were overjoyed. Winnie was even glad to contribute to his retirement fund, not out of respect but for the joy of seeing him leave.

Jean's office in the Gragg Building was on the top floor; it was often full of recreation employees. So she and Winnie often met before work for coffee and tea in Winnie's office. Jean had learned to accept her office since it was quieter than others. They both were anticipating more changes; most employees believed that the hospital would improve. There were "friends" of the director who everyone knew would be leaving, since they no longer had his protection.

Then, around Thanksgiving, the supervisor of the Psychology Department resigned, giving Winnie more reasons for being ecstatic. The gossip had stated that the supervisor had applied for the director's position and was not accepted. Instead, the supervisor took another position outside of Eastern State Hospital, and Winnie could not have been happier. Jean celebrated with Winnie and her husband at their home.

One morning, Jean and Winnie were talking about some of the friends of the director who were leaving. Jean asked, "Why were there so many bad people here?" She was getting the coffee and tea ready.

"Jean, you need to remember that I am prejudiced against them." Winnie was feeling guilty over having talked too much about her problems with Jean. "Please don't let me harm you with all these 'games of power.' While I do think my supervisor was never fair to me, partly due to his own problems of a divorce and a rebellious daughter who became pregnant out of wedlock, it was his job to be fair to all employees under him. I would assume that he really believed in how he did things, but I believe he misused it against me. So, we were at odds all the time."

"That is what I mean; he is a psychologist. He is supposed to put aside all his personal problems and be fair," added Jean. She appeared to be depressed over the open criticism of the previous leaders. Jean still believed in the goodness of people, and while Winnie liked that about Jean, she did not want her depressed too much.

"That is the problem with some psychologists; they feel that they are scientifically trained, objective in all their decisions. Instead, they are blind to their own personal power plays," stated Winnie. "But again, that is my opinion." She was trying to soothe Jean's disappointments with all the criticisms of the past leaders.

"You would think that psychologists would know how power changes them," stated Jean.

"Yes, you would think so. Like the director, who was trained to be objective, but he would not tolerate anyone who disagreed with him. While I thought it was just me who did not like him, after he left, others who I thought liked him are now saying bad things about him, especially in the Personnel Department." Winnie took time to pour the coffee and tea. "I was really shocked to hear how they are talking against him," replied Winnie. "While it is human nature that they are jumping on the bandwagon of criticizing him, there was also fear by some who were afraid of losing their jobs if they said anything against him; everyone is talking." They both stopped to sip.

"I always believed that people were basically nice until I came to work here. I have really been disappointed at how some of the most educated can be so mean. I have never seen that before," responded Jean. She drank more of her tea.

"Jean, this is your first job in mental health, I have seen all these power plays in other facilities, but it has been worse here because jobs were decreasing. As the patients were being relocated out of the hospital, the census was dropping, money was being cut, and jobs were being lost. But people like the director, who favored PhD psychologists over others when they were losing their jobs, added to the resentment among the employees," replied Winnie as she stopped to drink some coffee. "Also, while there have always been power players in different mental health systems, they don't usually last as long as these did here."

"How awful," added Jean. Winnie realized that Jean was revealing her basic belief in the fairness of people, and she continued to admire her for that.

Trying to cheer her up, Winnie asked her, "Did you know the first PhD Psychology Department supervisor here?"

"No, I never knew him," responded Jean.

"He was a good PhD psychologist. He told me that there were several things that the director wanted him to do that he could not do, so he resigned. He implied that the director wanted him to fire me. He went into private practice instead."

"Good for him," cheered Jean. "He had principles that I like."

"Yes, we have had good employees here but many of them have left. My past supervisor was the only bad supervisor I have ever had, but he was willing to do whatever the director wanted him to do, including attempting to fire me. That was the problem with the director: employees had to do as he said or they had to leave. Many good employees did leave," replied Winnie. "It was the Kentucky Merit System that protected me. Employees cannot be fired unless their work is proven to be inadequate. He tried to find things wrong with my work but did not succeed, and I am still here, Jean. The system worked for me."

"I am so glad that you survived, but you have suffered," replied Jean.

"Yes, I have, but I had good friends like you who supported me."

"While I'm so glad the director and supervisor are gone, we have another PhD director taking his place," replied Jean.

"Yes, I have heard that, and we will give him our support. The new director has worked here several years, so he knows some of the problems."

They started putting away the cups, realizing that time was fleeting. Jean started getting ready to leave. Winnie stood up and drew her attention.

"Jean, think about it, we survived while many suffered in silence. I believe that we survived better because we supported each other. While some employees did not develop their own support friends, you and I did. Can you believe we used 'good psychology' on ourselves?" said Winnie laughing as they left, feeling better.

Several weeks later, Winnie told Jean of a plan that she was considering. "I would have never considered this if the previous director and my supervisor were still here," she said. Her excitement showed as she was beaming.

"Well, what is it, Winnie?" asked Jean.

"In May of next year, 1994, this hospital will be seventy years old. I want to plan a birthday celebration on May 2; the first of May is on

Sunday, so most employees will not be here, but they will be here on Monday. I think a celebration is needed."

"Oh, Winnie, that would be wonderful. How will you do it?" asked Jean.

"I plan to send a memo to the new director and ask him to establish a Birthday Celebration Committee to plan for the hospital's anniversary."

"Do you think he will agree to that plan?" asked Jean.

"Oh, I don't know, but if the past director was still here, the plan would have had a snowball's chance in hell," laughed Winnie. "But the new director is trying to be different, so we might have a chance. Anyway, he can always do like the other director and say no. As you know, I will try anything that I believe in."

"Let me know what happens," replied Jean. "I need to go upstairs now."

"Oh, I will as soon as I know anything." Winnie was excited over the possibility.

Several days later, Winnie asked Jean to come to her office after her work was finished. Jean could tell that Winnie was excited but waited until they were in the privacy of Winnie's office. Jean kept wondering if Winnie's idea would even be considered. Jean had difficulty waiting until after work. She kept wondering if the birthday celebration had really been approved. It had to be something good since Winnie was so excited.

When Jean entered Winnie's office, she excitedly waved a piece of paper and exclaimed, "The new director has agreed that I can appoint a Birthday Celebration Committee to celebrate the hospital's anniversary. Oh, Jean, I have dreamed of doing this for years. We now have support of the administration to do this." They hugged, laughed, and danced around the office. Finally the whole hospital will be able to celebrate its history!

"Oh, Winnie I'm so pleased."

"Well, I need to appoint a committee. Think about who you know that works here and is interested in the history of Eastern State Hospital," stated Winnie.

"Oh, I will; maybe we can get together next week. I know several people who I *don't* want on the committee," laughed Jean.

"Yes, me too," Winnie also laughed, "but we want people who are interested in its history, who can get along with each other on the committee, and who will add their special abilities toward developing a good program for the celebration. Of course, Jean, I expect you to help me with making history posters that will be hung on the walls. There will be displays of the history all around the walls for showing the hospital's history. You will represent the Recreation Department; we need to think of other departments that can help us," stated Winnie. "Oh, Jean, the director has agreed that all employees will be expected to do their usual work but can get overtime by working on the Birthday Celebration Committee."

They had several days to come up with a committee. Jean and Winnie met earlier than their usual worktime to discuss who would fit on the committee.

"Oh, I am so excited," stated Jean.

"Yes, so am I, Jean, but today I need to leave at the regular time. Can we meet earlier in the morning before work?"

"Yes, I am always at work by seven o'clock, so call me when you get here and I will come down to your office, Winnie." They both left.

The following morning, Jean and Winnie were drinking their tea and coffee and discussing their plans. The first person that Winnie suggested was Louise Thomas, director of supplies; she had shown an interest in the history of the facility by always collecting and preserving any historical items that she found. She often discussed her finds with Winnie. She was the only one in the Administration Department who had shown any interest in the history, and she could obtain supplies that might be needed.

"I don't know her very well," responded Jean.

"She is a long-term employee who was the administrator at the old Danville State Hospital. When the Department of Mental Health closed Danville in the 1980s, she was transferred here but her job education requirements had been increased and she was given a position as director of supplies instead."

"Well, as I said, I don't really know her. I just assumed that she was a flunky for the administration here."

"I can understand your assumptions, but she is different from the other 'ass-kissing' administrators here—please excuse my French," Winnie said as they both laughed. "That is one of several reasons why I think she will be good."

"Should we consider anyone else from the Recreation Department?" asked Jean.

"Do you know anyone who is interested in the hospital's history in your department?" asked Winnie.

"No," stated Jean, "no one in my department is interested in any history."

"Do you know of anyone in that department who can add to our program for that day or is willing to compile the history on posters?" Jean was the only one she wanted from Recreation.

"No, I just feel that I needed to ask. I know that some people in my department will become jealous of me for you picking me," stated Jean.

"Let them! This is a history thing, and employees who have never shown any interest in the history here will not have anything to add. Also, it will be a lot of work for anybody else, but we both like history, so it will be fun for us. But why would they be jealous?" asked Winnie.

"Oh, you know my Recreation Department. Everyone is competing and jealous of each other."

"Yes, I do," Winnie said reassuringly, "but you fit the requirements best. You are interested in the history of Eastern State Hospital, we work together well, and you are willing to help me make the history posters. The posters will require many hours of extra work. I will need help, and I know of no one else in your department who will be as good as you. The fact that we are close friends is not the reason you are on this committee."

"Oh, thank you, Winnie; I do enjoy working with you and learning more about the history here. I will enjoy this and have fun doing it."

"Yes, and we always have fun, but there are people who will always criticize us, especially when we do something worth doing like this. Just expect it. We have the support of the hospital administration, for once, so why should we care what some idiots think?" laughed Winnie.

Others considered for the committee included Dr. Mike Nichols, who was a good speaker and would be a good master of ceremonies for the afternoon program. He had encouraged Winnie with writing her first article in the *Kentucky Psychological Newsletter* when he was working at the University of Kentucky. Since the article was about the history of Eastern State Hospital, most psychologists had no interest, but he read the article and showed an interest that continued for many years.

"Oh, I never knew that," responded Jean.

"While Dr. Nichols is not known for excessive work production since his employment here, I have never observed him to be cruel or malicious to either patients or employees. He is actually well liked on his ward. He would be an asset to the committee."

"Well, see if he would consider doing it; I don't think he will if there is any real work involved," stated Jean.

"Now, Jean," Winnie said as she moved to the other chair, "Dr. Nichols will not do the work that we do, but he is good at public relations, which I'm not good at. Remember, he is also a psychologist. That is his excuse for being here, but I think we need him."

"Okay, if he will work on the committee. But I don't think he will; he is such a charmer and not a worker," Jean said negatively.

"You really don't know him like I do, but I will talk to Louise Thomas and Dr. Nichols today. I'm supposed to talk to everyone about being on the committee privately, and then the director will announce their names. Of course you, Jean, have agreed to be on the committee?" Winnie asked, smiling.

"Of course, Winnie, you know I wouldn't want to miss this," said Jean. "Oh, I need to go; it is time to start my regular work." She started to run out of the office.

"By tomorrow morning, maybe I'll know more," Winnie yelled as Jean left.

The next morning, Jean came to Winnie's office for tea and coffee. Winnie was moving her office furniture around.

"Why are you moving things around? You just got into this office several months ago," Jean said.

"We will need room for making the history posters. I need to keep my psychology work separated into one office and history in the other room." Winnie pointed from room to room. "The posters and supplies will be there."

"That will give us more room," stated Jean as she looked around.

"Oh, Jean, I talked to Louise Thomas," Winnie very excitedly stated. "She is very pleased to be on the committee. She had some good ideas also."

"Oh, like what?" asked Jean.

"She suggested that we have a secretary to do typing for us, which she can arrange. Then she suggested employees in the Maintenance Department will help with hanging posters and bringing in artifacts from the Kentucky State Archives. She said that a lot of old furniture from Eastern State Hospital is stored in the archives, and she can arrange to have the items loaned to us for a week."

"I never knew that," responded Jean, clapping her hands.

"I knew it but never knew how to borrow items from the State Archives. Louise knows how, and I like her ideas. She has suggested Connie Hopper for the secretary since she is one of Louise's secretaries. She suggested Gene Long and Orlie Wright to help from the Maintenance Department since they have had a long interest in the history here; both men know about the old buildings."

"Well, I never thought about using someone in the Maintenance Department, but that does make sense," stated Jean. "They will help with the heavy work of moving old furniture and displaying the posters on the wall."

"And they are good workers and interested in the history here."

"What about Dr. Nichols?"

"Well, he is thinking about it," responded Winnie. "But I think he will agree; he just never gives an immediate answer. He is actually an old friend, so I know he will. I will just give him more time."

"Don't we need someone for the food?" asked Jean.

"Yes, we do; I understand we only have two dieticians working here at the hospital. The main dietician is too busy, but Jackie Walters is new here and is interested. She wants to learn about the history of Eastern State Hospital and work with the committee."

Several days later, Winnie gave the names of employees for the committee to the new director. The Eastern State Hospital Birthday Committee consisted of Winnie as chairman, Jean Newman, Louise Thomas, Dr. Nichols, Connie Hopper, Jackie Walters, Gene Long, and Orlie Wright. Everyone had accepted and the committee started meeting before Christmas and continued on a weekly basis until May 1, 1994. The discussions included a sharing of historical information that each committee member had found, while Winnie and Jean showed copies from the original documents, starting with 1817, that were to be put on posters, and plans were made for the program to be presented on May 2.

Committee members agreed to take on specific responsibilities for the program. Dr. Nichols agreed to be the master of ceremonies and to seek professional support from local and state agencies, including the Department of Mental Health in Frankfort. Louise agreed to collect historical items from the Kentucky State Archives. Jean and Winnie continued to produce posters to be hung on the walls. Everyone on the committee agreed to work on the afternoon of Sunday, May 1, to stage the event.

The celebration was to be held in the Megowan Gymnasium, which had opened five years earlier. Since the Megowan Gymnasium was funded with money from the Megowan family, the committee decided it was more suitable for showing the history of Eastern State Hospital. Poster boards were to be hung on the walls prior to the celebration.

Winnie and Jean had agreed to compile the history of Eastern State Hospital on poster boards. Copies from the original data were put onto twenty-four-by-twenty-four-inch poster boards and covered with plastic. They worked many nights after work compiling the poster boards. They started with posters to represent each ten-year period and completed thirty-six posters.

Winnie discovered that specific themes, such as the sawdust beds and water closets, were not included in the ten-year periods. They made more poster boards for these themes, resulting in forty-eight more poster boards.

One night, as Winnie was copying newspaper pictures of previous employees to arrange on the poster boards, she recognized the name of Mrs. Anna Rogers, who had received a pin for forty-five years of employment in 1967. Another picture, from 1962, showed the same Anna Rogers with forty years of employment as director of the Occupational Therapy Department. Winnie was shocked to recognize the same person who was admitted in 1990 to the Allen Building.

Winnie was eager to share that information with Jean. Jean came ready to work, as they often did, until ten o'clock each night. When Winnie saw her, she said, "Jean, do you remember the eighty-eight-year-old woman who was admitted to the Allen Building in 1990?"

"No," Jean replied. She was looking for her unfinished poster from the night before and proceeded into the adjoining room.

"Sure you do!" Winnie followed Jean to the unfinished posters area. "She claimed to have worked here in the O.T. Department?" Winnie went back to her desk in the adjoining room, picked up the pictures, and returned to where Jean was. Winnie held up the picture as Jean looked up.

"Oh, now I remember her," Jean said. "Dr. Atcher considered her to be delusional. I never did know what to believe about her." She resumed her work.

"Actually, Dr. Atcher was not serious about the delusions but he was quoting what the admission doctor said. Since she showed no other signs of psychosis, she did not need to be here. I could find no history to prove that she worked here until now."

"Yes, I remember," Jean said as she was still fixing a poster.

"This is a picture of Mrs. Anna Rogers with forty-five years of service to this hospital; see, it is the same Mrs. Anna Rogers!" Winnie proudly held the picture up and Jean stopped working.

Jean took the picture and more carefully examined it. "Yes, that looks like her, even though she is twenty years younger here. Oh how sad; no one knew that she was correct when she said she worked here for forty-five years."

"That is sad. She should have been given a hero's welcome, instead the Department of Personnel knew nothing about her," Winnie said angrily. "That article shows a different time; when employees retired, they were featured in the newspaper. The employees were proud of their achievements here. Now, rarely do employees retire because they are fired or downsized. They were so proud of retiring from here that it was put in the newspaper!" Winnie exclaimed.

"It is a shame that no one knew about her years here," Jean replied.

"The only reason that I believed her was that she mentioned Dr. Gragg and Mrs. Lucy Gamble, whom I knew worked here. But when I told her that the Department of Personnel had nothing about her, her response was, "Well, the Department of Personnel is just made up of political stooges, so what can you expect from them?" So she still knew about the political control in Kentucky state government and Frankfort."

"Well, she was correct about the Department of Personnel." Jean laughed as she returned to the other room to make labels for the poster boards.

"I just wish I had been more forceful in getting some history from her. Imagine the wealth of information that we lost because we were so busy doing our own things. Now she is probably dead," Winnie replied as she continued to sort through old pictures. "She was director of the Occupational Therapy at one time."

"That is why we are doing this birthday celebration, to help employees and even Kentucky state government to realize that history has been here," replied Jean.

"Yes, you are correct, but we lost Mrs. Rogers's history," added Winnie. "A current problem with working in a state mental hospital is that the bosses and even some PhD psychologists see the work and history here as degrading or only for low-level employees. While it might be true for some employees, most were dedicated, and many came from very outstanding families in Lexington. Dr. John Allen was the first superintendent in 1844–1855, and his brother-in-law was Judge Buckner, a well-respected legal authority in their time. Dr. Chipley, the second superintendent, was considered, in his time, the best authority on insanity. Unfortunately," Winnie laughed to herself, "Dr. Chipley got on the wrong political side during the Civil War and was fired. But he was never fired for his knowledge or experience with the insane." Winnie continued to browse through old records.

"I'm sure no one knows about that," replied Jean as she finished another label.

"Then, more recently, James H. Reed came from two prominent Lexington families; his father was a Civil War hero. All these people were dedicated to the institution when it was not popular, nor did it pay well. That is why I wanted to do a poster on the past employees; the current employees have no appreciation for the dedication of past employees and their problems of working here," Winnie said as she continued placing data on poster boards.

They continued working at night on the poster boards. One night, Winnie asked Jean if she knew anything about her Recreation Department's history.

"Oh, no one knows anything. Of course, my department supervisor thinks that he created the department, but I know that is not correct because some of the older employees have talked about it."

"Well, I think we should ask all department chairmen to develop their own history. If they wish, we can take what we have and make it into a poster board to help them out. What do you think?" asked Winnie.

"Oh, that would be a good idea, but I suspect you will not get any cooperation."

"Well, if I bring it up in our next committee meeting and get their endorsement, then we would have the power to expect it from each department. We can work with them," added Winnie. "Oh, Jean, I forgot, there will be an article in the Lexington newspaper about the birthday celebration. They interviewed me yesterday. I am so excited, but you never know how it will come out."

"Oh, Winnie," Jean said, "this is so wonderful. This is your dream, and it is really working out."

That article was printed in the Community section of the *Lexington Herald* on January 12, 1994, and a second article was published in the same paper on April 27, 1994. In the first article, Winnie explained about her knowledge of the history of Eastern State Hospital. The second article interviewed previous employees whose names Winnie had given to the writer. They interviewed Bessie McCord and Edith Chumley, both with many years in nursing, and Dr. Logan Gragg, the former superintendent. All were retired but they all had their own stories.

The following week, Dr. Gragg visited Winnie in her office. They had developed a relationship in years past when he was working at the VA and she was collecting the history of Eastern State Hospital. He was retiring from the VA and now wanted to give her the prized possessions that he had retained from Eastern State Hospital. He was especially proud of the dinner bell that had been used to call patients to meals in the early days of the institution. There were many other items, including newspaper articles that he had preserved.

Jean was working on the posters in Winnie's office when Dr. Gragg arrived; she was very impressed since she had never met him. She observed him as a "very caring but humble person" and stated, "I can now understand why the older employees praised him so much."

One night, Winnie told Jean that Dr. Nichols had gotten the Cabinet for Human Resources involved. They would be sending out a press release. Winnie had also written an article about the celebration for the Kentucky Psychological Association's spring 1994 issue. The news was becoming known, and all members of the committee rejoiced. The committee had become a well-organized working group; each person had his or her own role and did it well. Everyone was happy to be involved.

One night as Jean and Winnie were working on the poster boards, Winnie brought up a subject with Jean, waiting to see how she would react. "Jean, I am going to suggest that the committee give our past director an award at the birthday celebration."

"Oh, no, not him, I can't stand him," Jean responded emphatically.

"Now, Jean, listen. After figuring out all the number of years of each superintendent or director that has worked here, the past director was here the longest: sixteen years."

"Well, he fired so many people, and I cannot stand him."

"Yes, I understand, but we cannot dispute the fact that he was here the longest," Winnie said.

"I had hoped that he would not even be there that day," replied Jean.

"But he did do the time," replied Winnie, "regardless of what we might think of him personally; you know how I feel about him! He was here the longest in that position."

"But why even suggest it?" asked Jean.

"Okay, Jean, as you know, I have a reason," Winnie continued. "Dr. Logan Gragg was here for thirteen years, and I want to give him an award for being the third-longest-serving superintendent. I cannot give that to Dr. Gragg without recognizing the previous one as being the longest."

"Now, I understand; you will need to convince the committee members. I have just read on this poster that Dr. Chipley served fifteen years," stated Jean. "He was the one who was here during the Civil War and was fired because he sided with the Union. It is interesting that the Southern sympathizers in Lexington had him fired because he required employees to swear an allegiance to the Union, when the asylum was supposed to be neutral during the war. How interesting," Jean continued to read.

"And Dr. Chipley served for fifteen years, while Dr. Gragg served thirteen as superintendent. We cannot recognize Dr. Gragg unless we recognize the previous director with sixteen years," stated Winnie.

"Well, anything for Dr. Gragg," responded Jean as she continued to make labels for the poster boards. "I really like that man."

"Well, if I can convince you," said Winnie, "I'm sure the committee will go along with it, especially when we include the honor to Dr. Gragg." They did.

All departments at Eastern State Hospital agreed to develop their own departmental history. Winnie had agreed to compile the history of the Psychology Department, since she had been the longest employed psychologist currently working there. She had already written a history of Eastern State Hospital and the Psychology Department in 1986 for the Kentucky Psychological Association, so she just had to bring that history up to 1994. The number of psychology positions had gone from three in 1975 to ten, including the director, by 1994.

Their work on the poster boards continued for three months, resulting in a total of ninety-nine posters, including ten-year time periods, special theme subjects, and the department histories. The Birthday Committee continued to meet on a regular basis; members were shown the posters as they were completed. When May 2 arrived, everything was ready.

Louise Thomas had succeeded in obtaining many old artifacts from the State Archives that had belonged to Eastern State Hospital. The ninety-nine posters had been hung on the walls of the MeGowan Gymnasium. Everyone was delighted.

Viewing time was permitted during the morning, and a four-hour program took place in the afternoon. While people viewed the exhibits, members of the committee were available to answer questions, since they all had gained knowledge about the history of Eastern State Hospital. Dr. Atcher had arranged for his band to play in the Allen Building while visitors looked at the exhibits. Jean sang as she often did with recreation activities. Visitors, former employees, patients, and official dignitaries from state government and mental health officials attended. They were surprised at the history of the facility and appeared to be pleased over the results. The committee was pleased.

After Dr. Atcher finished playing, Winnie asked him to look at one poster, the one with previous employees. He immediately recognized Mrs. Anna Rogers from the newspaper picture. He knew that it was the same Mrs. Rogers who had been admitted to the Allen Building in 1990 at the age of eighty-eight.

Winnie pointed to the picture and asked, "Now, do you still consider her to be delusional about working here? She retired in 1967 and started working here in 1922, according to the newspapers."

He responded in his characteristically joking way,· "Well, Winnie, I guess I was wrong, but let's not tell anyone. I don't want to ruin my reputation for being perfect, especially to the past director."

"Oh, I won't tell anyone; my past supervisor, who is also gone, can find out that Mrs. Rogers retired in 1967, the same year I came here, so I must have seen her, but I did not remember her. So don't tell my past supervisor that I could have made that mistake," laughing Winnie.

"Since both have been gone for at least eight months now, we are now safe." He smiled. Then he got serious, "Well, Winnie, you did win against your supervisor in spite of him claiming that he would fire you. He is gone and you are still here."

"Well, Dr. Atcher, as we both have observed many times, no one really wins in these situations. I'm just fortunate to still have my job." Winnie turned serious. "I was most fortunate to have friends who supported me during the process, and I thank you for being one."

"Well, I think you are a real winner, and I see it here with all this," he said, looking around. "I must say all this is so impressive, and it was all your idea. You must be pleased."

"Yes, this was a dream of mine, but I have had many others to add to all this. There is no way I could have done all this by myself." She waved her hands around the room and then looked seriously at him. "But, Dr. Atcher, I believe you are more serious than I have ever seen you. That is the nicest thing you have ever said to me."

"That was one of my temporary times of insanity." He smiled his usual silly grin that was so familiar to Winnie.

"Well, since we both have times of insanity, I liked your band, you sounded great, and I have heard good comments about the music," responded Winnie.

"Now, Winnie, since we both are having moments of insanity, I must go." Dr. Atcher wandered off into the crowd of people, standing around and looking at the posters.

Dr. Nichols was an excellent master of ceremonies for the program that afternoon with Dr. Ron White as one of the speakers. He had come from Cincinnati out of respect for having worked on his dissertation at Eastern State Hospital many years earlier. Dr. White was a real joy from the past for Winnie.

Dr. Gragg was another speaker. He was still loved by many past and present employees. He was well respected for his fairness to all and his interest in the history of Eastern State Hospital. He told many humorous stories about the institution. That day, he was exceptionally funny and clear in his memories of the facility even though he was showing his age.

Jean was very joyful that day, singing and greeting everyone. She helped to achieve a dream of Winnie's, which also became her dream: researching the previously unknown history of Eastern State Hospital.

As people continued looking at the exhibits and reading the poster boards into the afternoon, Dr. Nichols followed Winnie through some of them. Winnie had already complimented Dr. Nichols upon his performance during the program. He came up to Winnie and said, "I am so glad that you asked me to do this and be on the Birthday Committee. It has been a real experience, and I also appreciate your giving an award to our previous director."

"Well, Mike, as you know I am no fan of his, but he deserved the award. I feel we would have been incorrect if he was not recognized as the longest-serving director of this institution. It just would have been unfair to the history of this institution."

"He is really not as bad as you think," replied Dr. Nichols.

"Well, I guess not since he does have some good friends, such as you and Dr. Shurling. He must have some redeeming qualities," Winnie stated in a matter-of-fact way as they wandered around the hanging posters.

"I know you blame him for your supervisor's actions, but I don't think he was behind the attempts to fire you," responded Dr. Nichols.

"I'm sorry, Mike, but I still hold him responsible for many people being fired around here. Many of those employees were good at their jobs, but their supervisor found some cause to fire them. As director of the hospital, he had to know about it, and he did nothing to prevent them."

"But, Winnie, he was just doing his job, letting the supervisors do theirs."

"Yes, I have heard that explanation, but, Mike, I think he was just unfair. He favored some PhD psychologists who were known for not showing up at work or attending to responsibilities on their ward. Yet other nonpsychologists were fired for much less. As far as I know, he was not really unfair to me, but he was to others. Yet Dr. Gragg, who has been gone for many years, is still respected for his fairness to employees and patients. While the previous director can claim that he didn't know what was going on, we employees can observe who is fair and who is not."

"Well, Winnie," Dr. Nichols said, stopping to take a breath and hoping to change the subject, "you have survived, in spite of everything."

"Yes, Mike, I did. I am most proud that no cause to fire me was found and I am still employed. I also have many friends here, such as Jean and Dr. Atcher, who provided emotional support to me."

"And you were able to achieve all this," responded Dr. Nichols as he ignored Winnie's negative implications and continued to look at the displays.

"Yes, only after I was free to be creative and the hostile environment was gone," stated Winnie, knowing full well that her opinions were being ignored.

They walked toward the Psychology Department. Dr. Nichols read some of the history and commented, "Winnie, you have witnessed many changes here in psychology." He kept reading about the history of the Psychology Department.

While Dr. Nichols was still reading, Winnie pointed out another part she had written. In 1968, the hospital encouraged any type of intervention with patients that had the potential to be beneficial to them. There was a description of what she called "tunnel therapy." When a previously closed ward of isolated patients was opened, many patients were so uncomfortable that they disappeared.

Winnie explained, "My job was to find them and encourage some socialization or interaction. They were found in the old tunnels where most would not come out. So I started some simple group interaction techniques to help them to adjust to the outside world. That went on for several months until they were able to meet in a room. I always wore heels and dressed professionally, so I went into the dirty, unpaved tunnels with those clothes on." Both Winnie and Dr. Nichols laughed as they recalled the tunnels and her wearing heels in that dirty place.

"And the processes you observed have changed as more psychologists were added," added Dr. Nichols. The changing expectations of those psychologists grew into them being program developers with less of an emphasis on testing and therapy."

"Yes, as the Psychology Department expanded into ten people and earlier psychological tests were no longer used. The intelligence scales were discontinued, as emotionally disturbed people did poorly on them, and those scores often followed them even after they improved. The MMPI became recognized as culturally biased and not valid for employee selection. It was discontinued by the more recent Psychology Department," replied Winnie.

"Now, psychologists are more involved in the Court Commitment process of interviewing potentially dangerous patients. Since the Rorschach test is unacceptable in court now, personal interviews and ward observations are used instead," Dr. Nichols stated as he was still reading the Psychology Department history.

"Yes," responded Winnie, "testing has decreased as psychological examinations were based on interviews. Psychologists coordinated patient treatment programs on the wards or were in hospital committees, leaving them less visible to patients or to other employees. This left the impression to other employees, rightly or wrongly, that they were not working when their work had become more administrative than it was in the past. However, I still saw the importance of individual contact with the patients, while others saw committees as the way to work," stated Winnie.

"Yes, the image of psychology has changed here," responded Dr. Nichols as he continued. "My understanding of some PhDs was that they were on a committee that had special jobs for the director instead of putting them on a ward."

"Well, I've heard that explanation, but did you know that since the past director has left, two master's-degreed social workers have taken over empty PhD positions as program directors? I understand that they are getting praised for their work; that had never been done before. The past director was just blind to the problems of any PhD and critical to anyone else. Now, things have improved," stated Winnie.

"I can see where you are coming from," stated Dr. Nichols, "but, Winnie, you know I don't see the past director that way."

"Okay, Mike, I respect your position. There have been examples in this history, not only in psychology but in other institutions, where ideas were tried, lost, or maintained for various reasons. Even phrenology, which was taught here at the Transylvania Medical School, did not take hold. One main reason was the strong feelings against Dr. Caldwell, who was the father of American phrenology. Yet phrenology is now recognized as the forerunner of today's neuropsychiatry. How ideas were lost or maintained are part of the process of psychiatric care," said Winnie.

It was a great day and Winnie's dream had come true. The institution was able to celebrate over 170 years of history, as most state mental institutions were downsizing or even being closed in the current deinstitutionalization movement. Kentucky's first asylum did finally have its history told.

Chapter Ten

Two Sons of Henry Clay, Sr.

I n January 1988, Dr. Melba Hay, from the University of Kentucky, as
editor of the Henry Clay Family papers, contacted this author about
her historical knowledge of two sons of Henry Clay Sr. who had been
admitted to the Kentucky institution. Dr. Hay provided copies of family
letters and encouraged this author to write an article about the two sons.
This author did, and that article was accepted for presentation to the North
Central Sociological Association in April 15–18, 1993 in Toledo, Ohio. A
copy of that presentation follows.

Comparison of Treatment Outcome with Voluntary and Involuntary
Hospitalizations between Two Sons of Henry Clay

State legislatures in the 1960s required a strict proof of dangerousness to
involuntary commitment of a mentally disturbed person to a state mental
hospital (Stromberg, 1988). Historically, commitment to a state mental
hospital has served three social functions: (1) protection of society; (2)
treatment for the patient's own good; (3) mere custodial confinement
designed to care for the person's bodily needs. While custodial care which
includes #1 and #3 has been discredited in favor of #2 during the last
twenty years, dangerousness as criteria for commitment to a state mental

hospital is also being questioned. Teplin (1984) showed that the mentally disturbed were either too dangerous for treatment or not dangerous enough for commitment when the restrictions of dangerousness are too strict. Often the mentally ill do not qualify for treatment.

Since then, Mulvey et al. (1987) observed that state laws have shifted away from a strict concept of dangerousness toward more professional discretion. The shift to and from concepts of dangerousness have been based upon public pressure and not upon any longitudinal studies of voluntary or involuntary commitments within the state mental hospitals.

American psychiatric history of involuntary commitment has swung back and forth between legal proof of danger and professional discretion since the 1840s. Since the early methods of care are basic to our current therapeutic methods (Savino & Miles, 1976; Tourney, 1967; and Talbott, 1978), a study of early use of involuntary hospitalization can provide some necessary longitudinal data about court processes and psychiatric treatment outcomes.

Dangerousness as a criterion for admission is at least as old as the Kentucky Lunatic Asylum. It was opened for only "persons who are dangerous" and the "peaceable lunatics" were to be denied admission (Act, 1824). A specific example of involuntary hospitalizations can be found in the history of two of Henry Clay's sons. Theodore, who was involuntarily committed to the Kentucky Lunatic Asylum and stayed there for thirty-nine years until his death (Collins, 1924; *New York Times*, 1870), while John, who voluntarily went to the asylum for several short periods (*Lexington Transcript*, 1887), did not have extensive hospitalizations. Did Theodore have a less favorable outcome because he was court committed?

There are four confusing factors that must be analyzed before differences between treatment outcomes of the two sons can be clarified. Historical inconsistencies about Theodore's problem must be the first factor. There are at least three different statements about Theodore Clay suffering from a head injury at an early age. "The eldest son, Theodore Clay, in consequence of an injury, became insane, and remaining years of his life were spent in the asylum in Lexington" (Clay, 1910). A second family member, Mary R. Clay (1899), gave this account about Theodore:

"When a mere lad, a blow upon his head, which fractured his skull. It was trepanned [perforated] by Dr. Pindell, who expressed fear that, once reaching manhood, he would become insane but his boyhood gave exceeding promise for brilliant attainments." Then the third account was documented by Collins (1924) that "Theodore Wythe Clay, born 1802, lost his reason in his young manhood, from an accidental blow on the head with an ax in the hands of a slave and died in 1869, in the Insane Asylum at Lexington, of which he had been an inmate for forty years."

However, Theodore's behavior at his admission to the Kentucky asylum does not confirm the presence of any early life of brain damage. An analysis of the historical data about Theodore is needed to clarify confusion about his psychiatric problems and the need for involuntary admission.

The second confusing factor is that the Kentucky asylum had different time periods of treatment methods during its long history (Deese, 1983). The first two time periods, 1824–1843 and 1844–1870, comprise the times when Theodore and John, respectively, were admitted to the asylum. Since Theodore was admitted to the institution in 1831, he may have been the recipient of different treatment methods than John, who was admitted and discharged in 1845 when formalized moral therapy was established at the institution. Did the changes in treatment methods contribute to John's more favorable outcome? Did the lack of formalized moral therapy contribute to Theodore's longer hospital stay?

Thirdly, John Brand initiated the court commitment on Theodore Clay in 1831. He was also a member of the Board of Commissioners at the Kentucky Lunatic Asylum from 1824–1840 (Deese, 1985). As a member of the Board of Commissioners, John Brand helped to make all administrative decisions about the asylum, including who was admitted and discharged. Did John Brand misuse his authority? Did the Clay family disagree with what John Brand had done?

The fourth factor was the fact that Henry Clay Sr. was a candidate for president of the United States in 1832 and 1841. Many historians have researched the *Papers of Henry Clay* for their political value but few have considered the information of two sons admitted to the Kentucky Lunatic Asylum to be important or noteworthy. Since Theodore was committed to the Kentucky institution in 1831 and John was admitted in 1845, what influence did the presidential campaigns of Henry Clay Sr. have upon the emotional problems of his sons?

Method

Hospital information about the two sons admitted to the institution is still confidential. In reality, the old records at the Kentucky Lunatic Asylum were very inadequate and typical of that time. There is more information about Theodore and John being "deranged" in letters written by the Clay family from 1827 to 1851 and now published by Hopkins J.F. (1959–1984).

The first part of this study will reveal pertinent background information about the Clay family. The second part will isolate the problems of Theodore Clay, his court commitment procedures, hospitalization, family's response, and outcome with the problems of John Clay, his voluntary admissions, family's response, and outcome. Information about treatment methods in 1831 when Theodore was admitted and in 1845 when John was admitted to the Kentucky Lunatic Asylum will come from historical data found by this author (Deese, 1983). A final discussion of the four factors will help to summarize the different treatment outcomes for the two sons.

Results

The Henry Clay Family

As early as 1827, Henry Clay Sr. wrote letters stating that he did not have much hope for his two oldest sons (Theodore and Thomas) and "the hopes of all of us are upon Henry Jr." Thomas was an alcoholic at the age of twenty-five and Theodore claimed in a letter of February 25, 1828, that his health was good but not well enough to handle a "consistent task." Theodore admitted that he had over spent his allotment of money and felt that he would be happier if he was married. By April 1829, both Theodore and Thomas were living at home, unemployed, and Thomas was showing more physical signs of alcoholism. Henry Clay Sr. had offered Theodore the chance by June 1830 to be a farmer and cotton planter in St. Louis, but instead, by October 30, 1830, Theodore spent several months "consuming money and time uselessly." Theodore continued to "commit fresh indiscretions at home. On the subject of a certain young lady, he is, we all begin to fear, quite deranged. He seems to be doomed to misery and to render wretched all around him."

Henry Clay Sr. wrote that Thomas had spent time in jail in Philadelphia during the winter of 1828–1829 while his parents were in the social whirl of Washington DC. He was at home for about two weeks in October 1830 and in "two debauches, and the last threatened his life." He returned to Illinois and the family was "in constant dread of hearing other imprudences." Thomas was described as a "sot" in a letter of June 30, 1835, prone to "intemperate excesses and no fixed aim in life." Thomas settled in Lexington, Kentucky, with his father supporting him while one of Thomas's severe business failures resulted in Henry Sr. being on the verge of losing the family home in 1842.

Henry Jr., the third son, was first described in letters of 1835 as jealous and irritable in temper. He lost his wife in 1839 and the "tragedy was such a blow that he surrendered himself to melancholy, haunted by the idea of his wife and sister calling him to a place of more perfect rest." He continued to be depressed until he was killed in 1847 at the Battle of Buena Vista, ungallantly leading his troops of the 2nd Kentucky Regiment.

Henry Clay Sr. had only one of six daughters survive. She lived to marry but died in childbirth in 1835. She was "all that they could desire in a daughter."

The two youngest sons (James and John) were showing "no great promise of steadiness" by 1835. James Clay had a period of "indecision" which finally ended in his adoption of a legal career.

Henry Clay Sr. was a generous and kind father, but he interfered with the discipline of his sons. One example can be found in a letter of February 16, 1835, when John M. violated the rules of his school and was required to confess his error to the whole school. Henry Sr. claimed that it would cause permanent injury and withdrew John from the school.

When Henry Clay Sr. was severely criticized during his presidential campaigns for his gambling, dueling, and other wild behavior, information about Theodore and John was never part of public criticism (Hay, 1988). Henry Sr. had magnetism and charm that helped to hide the behaviors of his sons. While historians have emphasized the achievements of each son, those achievements were probably more a result of Henry Clay Sr.'s influence than the abilities of the sons. However, Theodore went beyond the usual family behavior.

Theodore Clay

Since Theodore was the first son of a famous statesman, everyone expected Theodore to follow in the family tradition. The fact that he disappointed everyone could have added to family claims of Theodore having brain damage. While it is impossible to currently disprove Theodore's brain damage, his achievements, while they were less than what the family wished, do not correspond with signs of brain damage at an early age. Such behavior as "Theodore's promise of eloquence and delivery of an oration in Lexington's fourth of July celebration in 1821 at the age of 19 years" (Van Deusen, 1979), does not confirm brain damage. Theodore was a messenger to Mexico in 1824 and conducted exploration expeditions in 1830. Then a final observation, Theodore's handwritten letters to his family were coherent and intelligently written. There was no sign of eye-hand distortions in the writings that are associated with various brain damages. While none of the sons achieved the same influence and status as Henry Clay Sr., Theodore was the first son to disappoint the family and they may have looked for any explanation.

Admission Procedure, Court Commitment

On October 3, 1831, the clerk of Fayette County ordered the sheriff to summons and impanel twelve good and lawful men, to enquire if Theodore Clay "is or is not a lunatic, and if so, when that infirmity commenced." This action come from a complaint filed on September 29, 1831, by John Brand and his son, William Brand, sworn that "they believe Theodore W. Clay insane, and of unsold mind, and they considered the lives of themselves and their family in danger from said Theodore W. Clay, provided he is not taken in custody and confined." The *New York Times* (1870) claimed that Theodore had used a pistol to demand the daughter of John Brand. The decision of the jury was that Theodore Clay was to be confined to the asylum (Commonwealth, 1831). The actual court record is now missing from the Fayette County Courthouse (White, 1984); only the family letters attest to that fact.

By January 8, 1832, Theodore was asking his father to get him out. Theodore kept requesting his "liberation," knowing that his father had "more weight than anyone to direct and superintend the institution." Theodore even promised to make his way to another city to earn his own living if his father would only help him to get out of the asylum. However, in another letter, Theodore agreed to live on his father's land in Illinois "with a small loan of $2,000 to make a retreat acceptable to me." In the same letter, Theodore expressed his "gratitude for all your kindness to me during the whole course of my life."

In a letter dated May 20, 1832, Theodore claimed to be "unpleasantly situated." He listed the names of the commissioners and he had "rewritten a respectful request, requesting his freedom." However, they had "given him no answer and had no reason to believe they would." Theodore demanded that "justice be done and hoped that it would be speedily." He never expressed any understanding of what he had done to get into the institution. He could not understand why he was "restrained" and said, "I will not if I can choose be a slave of any man." He did admit that "prejudice perhaps natural and right, exists in Lexington among many toward me, and for which also I can account, and which I confess myself both unable and unwilling to undertake to stem, if I have the option." There is no evidence that the involuntary commitment of Theodore Clay was for any specific time period but rather was dependent upon the family.

Treatment Methods at the Kentucky Lunatic Asylum: 1831

The first time period (1824–1843) was the beginning for the institution. At this time, only one other state-supported institution existed, in Virginia, and the field of psychiatry was just beginning. Physicians were part-time professors at the Transylvania Medical School and they handled the medical problems while the Board of Commissioners admitted patients, discharged them, and generally conducted the business of the institution. Moral therapy was not established until after 1844 when a full-time physician was hired and stability was established during the second and third time periods to 1870.

The method of treatment, called moral therapy, was based on teachings of Pinel, Turk, and Benjamin Rush. Four of Benjamin Rush's students were on the faculty of Transylvania Medical School, and they provided the leadership for the asylum. Moral therapy was closely allied to that of a well-regulated parental government. However, the "cold bath," leather shackles, tranquilizer chair, and straightjackets were used to restrain difficult patients.

Family's Response to Hospitalization

The Clay family members appeared to have some difficulty in accepting Theodore's commitment to the asylum. They provided him the use of a horse to ride about town, to visit home for days at a time and they provided him with his own library of political periodicals. By June 7, 1832, Henry Jr. wrote his father that he was convinced that Theodore was not restored. Henry Jr. further explained that he had planned to meet with the Board of Commissioners to request that Theodore be put in his care, but after discussing his request with Dr. Dudley, a prominent local physician, Henry Jr. decided that Theodore was best left at the asylum. Henry Jr. observed that Theodore's health was better and he appeared more content and happy than he had been for years.

Dr. Dudley was chairman of Surgery and Anatomy at Transylvania Medical School in Lexington. Dr. Dudley stated that Theodore was "deranged upon two subjects, love and ambition." Dr. Dudley felt that the love could be cured in time and that the ambition could only be cured by "humiliation." He recommended that Theodore be treated as an ordinary person, not be given so much liberty and the family should not send him any political periodicals. Dr. Dudley doubted if Theodore would ever become a useful member of society but felt that discharging him at that time would destroy any hopes of recovery.

Anne Clay Erwin, the sister, wrote a letter on December 1832, that Theodore was at home, "conducted himself quietly," and that "although Mama is now fully convinced that he [Theodore] is deranged, she is much happier than if he were anywhere else." Then on December 5, 1833, Henry Clay Sr. wrote to Henry Clay Jr. asking him to "ride over to Ashland occasionally and let me know how things go there. I fear from the tenor of the letters of Theodore that his mind is more unsettled than ever."

Henry Jr. responded to his father on December 14, 1833, and emphasized that the decision to recommit Theodore was mainly his sister Anne's since "he had become too dangerous to have in the house." His mind was filled with suspicions of plots and conspiracies. Henry Jr. emphasized that "when he [Theodore] was in the Hospital before, his health was reestablished and his mind certainly improved." Therefore, "let us curb our feelings. I have every hope that Theodore will be eventually cured if left in the Hospitals."

Theodore's obituary (*New York Times*, 1870) stated that in the early days following his admission to the Kentucky Lunatic Asylum he called it "a good boarding house but having some of the biggest fools he ever saw as boarders." In his years at the asylum, "he was considered one of the most noted members. He labored under the hallucinations that he was George Washington and was fond of assuming traditional attitudes of being the father of his country. At the weekly dances, he was always exquisitely dressed in the style of his day. Yet, during those years, he was reported to be restless, discontented and requiring close observation."

Theodore's condition became worse at the age of fifty-eight and he became "demented, in hopeless idiocy" until his death. Theodore's final behavior could be related to the onset of dementia, but his original and second hospital admissions were due to dangerousness in the community and at home.

John's Voluntary Admission

Henry Sr. first mentioned problems with John on March 17, 1845, when "John too has exhibited decided symptoms of mental aberration. Altho' now better, we have the greatest fears about him." On April 2, 1845, Henry Sr. stated that "I regret to inform you that John is becoming more and more deranged, and I fear there will be no alternative but the hospital." On April 5, 1845, Henry Sr. stated that "I lament to inform you that we have been compelled to place John in the Hospital. He was roaming about in the woods until two o'clock, although he offered violence to no one, he was wild, boisterous and incoherent. He threatened his own life and declared more than once that he intended to terminate it last night. His passion for Miss J— revived, he attempted to see her, but she, being advised of his situation, properly declined to receive him. He went in a carriage quietly to the Hospital. I was afraid of the effect of this last stroke upon your poor mother, but she was satisfied of the propriety of the measure."

Henry Sr. compared John's case to Theodore's in a letter of April 8, 1845, by saying, "I am afraid that John's case is hopeless. He exhibited a strong demonstration of derangement more decisively than his unfortunate brother when he was first put in the hospital. We shall make the best arrangements for the comfort of them. I have sent a servant to the hospital to attend on them." In a letter of April 27, 1845, Henry Sr. stated, "Poor John continues to be a source of great affliction to us. His case is that his reason is sufficient to enable him to comprehend his situation, to feel his confinement with the keenest pain, and yet is not enough make it to liberate him. If he were unconscious, we should be less affected. That is the condition of his unfortunate brother and I fear will ultimately become his own."

Treatment Methods at the Kentucky Lunatic Asylum: 1845

A second time period (1844–1870) has been called the golden age of the Kentucky asylum. By the beginning of this time period, there were many more state facilities and the medical knowledge had grown. This time period had two full-time superintendents giving a consistent period of care for the patients. The Board of Commissioners continued to handle the business affairs of the institution whereas the physicians admitted or discharged patients. The method of treatment was still moral therapy but it was implemented by a full-time physician. Restraints were minimized and rewards were used instead. Patients were classified according to their problems and behavioral expectations were established for each patient. Many activities were available to patient and work-training programs were established.

This second time period had the maximum ratio of employees to patients employed to carry out the methods (compared to other time periods until the middle 1900s). There was a general optimism and expectation of "curing" patients. This optimism continued until the institution became overcrowded after 1868. However, the physician's turnover rates of up to 1849 were still high compared to the following years of 1855 to 1870 or even current standards. Therefore, the time period of John's admission may have improved from the time of Theodore's admission, but the turnover rates of the physicians were still high for any stability by 1845. While the physician turnover rates stabilized later, they were not significantly different between the admission times of the two Clay sons.

Family's Response to Hospitalization

Henry Sr. did not mention any discussions with physicians as Henry Jr. had done with Theodore's release from the hospital. Henry Sr. stated that he was "inclined to make one more experiment with John home" on April 27, 1845, and would return him to the hospital if he exhibited "wildness of conduct as he did earlier." On May 6, 1845, Henry Sr. stated that he had again taken John out of the hospital and he "has been calm and rational. I pray to God that he may so continue." From the letters, one might be able to assume that Henry Sr. was around when John had his problems and was instrumental in helping at the time.

John was never hospitalized again. Henry Sr. wrote on November 14, 1846, "my son John is again restored to the use of his mind." However, on July 1, 1850, Henry Sr. received a letter from Thomas that "filled me with uneasiness about John." By February 11, 1851, Henry Sr. stated that from the last accounts of John, they "were good and I am all the time uneasy about him." Henry Clay Sr. died in Washington in 1852.

John continued to live at home with his mother, and he kept a diary from March 1864 to October 1866 that has been kept at Ashland, the family home in Lexington, Kentucky. This author has reviewed that diary, and the following significant information was picked from the written observations by John: His mother was 83 on March 19, 1864, and she died on April, 1864. John was forty-three that year and admitted to continuing to have difficulty with drinking too much. By December 28, 1865, he had decided to quit drinking but stated that he had made several attempts to stop drinking before. John started writing about seeing Mrs. Erwin (widow of Eugene Erwin, who was the son of James and Ann Brown Clay) about a year after his mother's death and they were married on July 1866. "On July 8th we rose. We formed some good resolutions about business and pleasure and put our trust in the powers above." They became known for breeding race horses.

John died in 1887 and Josephine managed the business after his death. Josephine Erwin Clay lived until 1920 and was known for her own accomplishments.

Discussion

This article started with the question, "Why did Theodore Clay have a less favorable treatment outcome than John Clay?" While both sons were reported to have been obsessed with a woman during their initial admission, what could have made the difference in their outcomes? There were four confusing factors that must be clarified before any causal conclusions can be made about the involuntary commitment of Theodore.

First, there were reports by family members that Theodore was brain-damaged as a child and that brain damage was the cause for his commitment. However, his behavior before admission to the Kentucky Lunatic Asylum and letters that he wrote to his father during his first admission do not confirm the presence of brain damage at that time. Instead, he was court committed because of dangerous or threatening behavior prior to both admissions to the Kentucky Lunatic Asylum. Data about his brain injury were written after his death and were never a part of the early Clay family letters.

The second factor is a consideration of differences at the Kentucky Lunatic Asylum between the time of Theodore's admission (1831) and John's admission (1845). Since the most therapeutic time period before 1900 has been identified to be from 1844 to 1869, was the treatment significantly better for John so that he had a better treatment outcome? While there were claims of improved treatment starting in 1844, the actual stability of employees and programs did not come until later. Any stability of employees did not come until after John had been discharged. Both sons were discharged after their first admission, Theodore after one year and John only a few days later, but the therapeutic effects of the hospital program do not appear to be significantly different for the two sons.

John Brand initiated the first petition against Theodore Clay. Did John Brand misuse his power as member of the Board of Commissioners to keep Theodore in the Kentucky Lunatic Asylum? While it is possible that John Brand could have misused his power, the Clay family letters did not criticize John Brand for his actions. The family was already aware of Theodore's behavior. Also, Mr. Brand was so concerned about his daughter's safety that she was sent out of town to stay with relatives. While Theodore's mother did not at first recognize that Theodore was "deranged," Henry Sr. was aware and did not use his power to remove Theodore early from the hospital.

The fourth factor related to Henry Clay Sr. running for president; how did that influence the outcome for Theodore and John? While there is little information about the effect upon the Clay family during the presidential campaigns, the fact that Henry Clay Sr. was the person most responsible for handling family problems, his absence from the home could have some influence upon the outcome of his sons. When Theodore was released from the hospital, Henry Sr. was away running for president of the United States. When John was hospitalized, Henry Sr. was at home and was willing to try John at home when his behavior was "calm." John succeeded on his second home visit and his outcome was more positive. It could have been due to the presence of his father or the father knowing better how to handle John; all these possibilities cannot be ruled out.

However, the major difference between Theodore and John was the fact that Theodore was determined by a court of law to be dangerous and was threatening or dangerous toward others. Even though John's initial symptoms were viewed as worse than Theodore's, he was only considered to be dangerous to himself. The family's fear of Theodore led to his second and final stay at the hospital.

There are two other factors that could have improved John's outcome. He went voluntarily to the hospital on each admission. John's acceptance of hospitalization indicates a different attitude than Theodore's. Secondly, the family recognized the symptoms earlier with John, and he was hospitalized before becoming dangerous.

Current involuntary commitment to a state mental hospital is an important social issue that needs longitudinal studies. Yet, the application of involuntary commitment in the early mental hospitals tends to get forgotten. This study attempted to show how historical data can be used for longitudinal information.

Sources for Chapter 10

Act to Carry into Operation the Kentucky Lunatic Asylum. *Senate Journal* (January 7, 1824): 137–138.

Clay, Mary Rogers. *Clay Family.* Louisville, Kentucky: John P. Morton, 1899.

Clay, Thomas H. *Henry Clay.* G. W. Jacobs & Son, 1910.

Deese, W. "The Keepers of the Kentucky Lunatic Asylum from 1824–1893." Unpublished manuscript, last modified 1985.

Deese, W. "Moral therapy at the Kentucky Lunatic of Asylum: Implications for psychology." *The Kentucky Psychologist,* Spring 1986.

Deese, W. "One Hundred and Fifty-Five Years of Mental Health Care" Unpublished manuscript, last modified 1983.

Hopkins, J.F. & Hargraves, M.: Vol. 1-6: Zeager, W. & Hay, M. Vol. 7 & 8: Hay, M. Vol. 9, *Papers of Henry Clay, Sr.,* Lexington, Kentucky: University of Kentucky Press, 1959-1984.

Hay, M. *Papers of Henry Clay.* Lexington, Kentucky: University of Kentucky, January 1988.

Lexington Transcript. "Obituary: John Clay." August 11, 1887.

Mulvey, E. P., J. L. Geller, and L. H. Roth. "The promise and peril of involuntary outpatient commitment." *American Psychologist* (June 1987): 571–582.

New York Times. "Obituary: The son of Henry Clay." May 19, 1870.

Savino, M. T. and A. B. Miles. "The rise and fall of moral treatment in California psychiatry, 1852–1870." *Journal of the History of Behavioral Science.* 1976.

Stromberg, Clifford. *The Psychologist's Legal Handbook*, Council for the National Register of Health Services, 1988, 551–553,

Talbott, John. *Death of the asylum.* New York: Grune & Stratton, 1978.

Teplin, L. "Criminalizing Mental Disorder." *American Psychologist* 39 (July 1984): 794–803.

Tourney, G. "History of therapeutic fashions in psychiatry, 1800–1966." *American Journal of Psychiatry* 124 (1967): 6.

Van Deusen, G. *The Life of Henry Clay.* Westport, Connecticut: Greenwood Press, 1979.

White, Dr. Ron. *A Dialogue on Madness: Eastern State Lunatic Asylum and Mental Health Policies in Kentucky 1824–1883.* Dissertation, University of Kentucky, 1984.